LATINA PSYCHOLOGISTS

In this book, twelve eminent Latina Psychologists illustrate how they practice gender- and culture-sensitive psychotherapy, counseling, research, pedagogy, social justice, and mentoring. They share how they create their own path in the midst of oppression – by becoming aware of the connection between their lives and their gendered, cultural, social, and political circumstances – and how they liberate themselves and those who seek their psychological services. Based on lived experiences, they reveal how they integrate a borderlands theory, a *testimonio* method, and an embodiment analysis into a Latina Feminist Psychology. More importantly, these Latina Psychologists offer easy-to-follow advice to help readers thrive while living in the cultural borderlands.

Lillian Comas-Díaz, PhD, is a clinical psychologist in private practice in Washington, DC, and a clinical professor at the George Washington University Department of Psychiatry and Behavioral Sciences. The author of over 150 publications, her scholarly work focuses on multiculturalism, women of color, ethnic minority mental health, psychotherapy process, social justice, and psychospirituality.

Carmen Inoa Vazquez, PhD, ABPP, is a practicing clinical psychologist in private practice in New York City and a visiting scholar/clinical psychology supervisor at Columbia University Teachers College. She has published several books, book chapters, and articles, and has made numerous presentations in the areas of gender, cross-cultural mental health, and training. She is a noted authority on Latin American mental health, particularly focusing on women and bicultural lifestyles.

"Many Latinas in the US feel overwhelmed and confused by constant questioning of our identity. For many of us, our bifurcated, walled up, and bordered selves are constantly fighting against our cultural roots as Latinas. It can be exhausting. In this book, Carmen and Lillian help us to understand the power we have within ourselves to navigate this internal struggle. They allow us to see that this conflict is not just in our minds and that there exists a transformative pedagogy through which we may find liberation."

– **Maria Hinojosa**, journalist, host of NPR's Latino USA, and president of Futuro Media Group

"*Latina Psychologists* examines how their lives connect with their scholarship and practice. A colleague once derisively called this connection 'me-search.' But, this book clearly shows how this connection gives their work strength, resonance, and vibrancy. It is a must read, not only for Latinas or others from 'minoritized' backgrounds, but also for those who have not had to confront how their history and identity affects their scholarship and practice."

– **Ana Mari Cauce**, Professor of Psychology and American Ethnic Studies, President, University of Washington

"Women's voices about their lived experiences are seldom documented. But, when they are, as in this book, they serve as a rich source of knowledge and have unique perspectives to bring us. This anthology is a special and important resource that brings new insights for those who want to be inclusive of all aspects of psychology and its ramifications."

– **Bonnie R. Strickland, PhD, ABPP**, Former President of the American Psychological Association

LATINA PSYCHOLOGISTS

Thriving in the Cultural Borderlands

Edited by Lillian Comas-Díaz and Carmen Inoa Vazquez

Routledge
Taylor & Francis Group
NEW YORK AND LONDON

First published 2018
by Routledge
711 Third Avenue, New York, NY 10017

and by Routledge
2 Park Square, Milton Park, Abingdon, Oxon OX14 4RN

Routledge is an imprint of the Taylor & Francis Group, an informa business

Library of Congress Cataloging in Publication Data
A catalog record for this title has been requested

ISBN: 978-1-138-03963-6 (hbk)
ISBN: 978-1-138-03964-3 (pbk)
ISBN: 978-1-315-17570-6 (ebk)

Typeset in Bembo
by Taylor & Francis Books

Lillian: To my female ancestors – a source of wisdom, guidance, and inspiration.

Carmen: To Victoria Vargas de Inoa – the best role model I could have had.

CONTENTS

ACKNOWLEDGMENTS

We would like to express our genuine gratitude to the contributors of this book for their significant and courageous contributions, diligence, and enthusiasm. Thanks also to Amanda Devine, Editor, and Nina Guttapalle, Senior Editorial Assistant, at Routledge/Taylor & Francis for their support and guidance and for believing in this work, and to Maggie Reid for copy-editing. We also thank two anonymous Latina Psychologist reviewers for their encouraging feedback.

Just as important, we would like to thank our life partners, who enthusiastically met with us on many occasions to offer their great ideas and tireless encouragement.

We also wish to thank our friends and families for their invaluable support throughout this project. Very specially and foremost, we want to express our deepest appreciation to David Comas-Díaz who so generously and expeditiously created the beautiful cover art for this book. He captured our sentiments to perfection.

CONTRIBUTORS

Margarita Alegría, PhD, is Professor of Psychology in the Department of Psychiatry at Harvard Medical School. She is also Director of the Center for Multicultural Mental Health Research, Cambridge Health Alliance, and Chief of the Disparities Research Unit, Department of Medicine, Massachusetts General Hospital.

Hortensia de los Angeles Amaro, PhD, during the writing of her chapter in this book, was Dean's Professor of Social Work and Preventive Medicine and Associate Vice Provost for Community Research Initiatives at the University of Southern California. Subsequently, she accepted the position of Distinguished Professor and Senior Scholar for Community Health at Florida International University in Miami to work on "big vision" projects with the university's leadership.

Patricia M. Arredondo, EdD, is former president of the Chicago Professional Psychology School, past president of the National Latina/o Psychological Association, and co-author of *Culturally Responsive Counseling with Latina/os* and *Becoming Culturally Oriented: Practical Advice for Psychologists and Educators.*

Carrie Castañeda-Sound, PhD, is an Associate Professor in the Psychology Department of Pepperdine University and faculty at Aliento, The Center for Latina/o Communities.

Lillian Comas-Díaz, PhD, is a practicing clinical psychologist in private practice in Washington, DC, and Clinical Professor at the George Washington University Department of Psychiatry and Behavioral Sciences.

Melanie M. Domenech Rodríguez, PhD, is a Professor of Psychology at Utah State University, TED Talk presenter of *No Way but Through*, and past President of the National Latina/o Psychological Association.

Oliva M. Espín, PhD, is Professor Emerita in the Department of Women's Studies, San Diego State University. She is co-editor of *Gendered Journeys: Women, Migration and Feminist Psychology* and *Feminist Therapy with Latina Women: Personal and Social Voices*, and author of *Women Crossing Boundaries*.

Pilar Hernandez-Wolfe, PhD, is an Associate Professor of Counseling Psychology, Lewis & Clark Graduate School of Education and Counseling. She is author of *A Borderlands View on Latinos, Latin Americans, and Decolonization: Rethinking Mental Health*.

Celia Jaes Falicov, PhD, is a Clinical Professor in the Department of Family Medicine and Public Health at the University of California, San Diego. She is author of *Latino Families in Therapy* and co-editor of *Multiculturalism and Diversity in Clinical Supervision*.

Ester R. Shapiro (Ester Rebeca Shapiro Rok), PhD, is an Associate Professor of Psychology at the University of Massachusetts, Boston, and a Research Associate at the Gaston Institute for Latino Research and Public Policy.

Melba J. T. Vasquez, PhD, is the First Latina President of the American Psychological Association (2011). She publishes extensively in the areas of professional ethics, ethnic minority psychology, psychology of women, and psychotherapy.

Carmen Inoa Vazquez, PhD, ABPP, is a practicing clinical psychologist in New York City and a visiting scholar/clinical psychology supervisor at Columbia University Teachers College.

PART I

Introduction

LATINA FEMINIST PSYCHOLOGY

Testimonio, Borderlands Theory, and Embodied Psychology

Lillian Comas-Díaz and Carmen Inoa Vazquez

> We as women should shine light on our accomplishments and not feel egotistical when we do. It's a way to let the world know that we as women can accomplish great things.
>
> *Dolores Huerta*

An Invitation

We hope that this anthology touches your heart. This collection of narratives may evoke both tears and smiles in your spirit. But more than anything, we hope that it inspires you. The rich tapestry of stories in this volume introduces us, a group of twelve Latina Psychologists representing psychotherapists, scholars, researchers, educators, mentors, leaders, and activists. We reflect on how our gendered ethnicity impacts our life and work. We share our ways of coping with intersectional oppression, adversity, and cultural conflicts. More importantly, we narrate how we became psychologists while struggling against sexism, racism, heterosexism, homophobia, xenophobia, and ethnocentrism. As a result of our lived experiences, we embark on a liberating journey to transform our work into a psychology that is relevant in gender and cultural terms.

Whether you are a Latina or not, a woman or not, a psychologist or not, we believe that you can potentially relate to the stories in this anthology. Maybe you will identify or empathize with, and/or connect to, some of our narratives. However, regardless of how these stories make you feel, we extend you an invitation: Allow yourself to develop a relationship with us, one that will encourage you to flourish.

As a group, we embody a variety of female experiences including identities reflective of the intersection of ethnicity, gender, culture, race, sexual orientation, socioeconomic class, age, (dis)ability, immigration status, nationality, language, religion/spirituality, place, and other diversity variables. Much like the Latinx community, we mirror the mosaic of our people. We use the term Latinx to designate the Latino/a community because this term is a gender-neutral concept that moves beyond binaries (McAlister, 2016). Moreover, the term Latinx includes lesbian, gay, bisexual, transgender, and queer (LGBTQ) (Sharrón-del Rio & Aja, 2015). In this volume we introduce a multiplicity of ancestry represented by women who are Mexican American, Puerto Rican, Cuban, Dominican, Colombian, Argentinian, and multiethnic. While several of us are immigrants and/or refugees, others are native-born and several are transnationals. Some of us are married, with or without children; while others are single, widowed, and/or divorced. Our sexual orientation includes heterosexual, lesbian, and queer. Since most Latinx people are of mixed race and heritage, we reflect a racial rainbow ranging from *mestizas*, creoles, indigenous, *LatiNegras* (AfroLatinas) to multiracial women.

Latinx spirituality functions independently from religion (Campesino & Swartz, 2006). As a consequence, numerous Latinas endorse spirituality as an important cultural value (Hunter-Hernandez, Costas-Muñiz, & Gany, 2015). Similarly, our spirituality and religions span from Christianity to Judaism to *spiritual mestizaje*. Originally coined by Gloria Anzaldúa (1987), the term *spiritual mestizaje* entails a transformative process of unearthing bodily memory to develop a continuous critical analysis of oppression and activism through a renewed relationship with the sacred (Delgadillo, 2011). As such, *spiritual mestizaje* is a method of transformation (Medina, 2014), one that involves an amalgamation of Western, indigenous, and African beliefs/rituals (Comas-Díaz, 2014).

The narrative tapestry in this volume illustrates how we, as a group of Latina Psychologists, *compose our lives* in the midst of oppression. Our approach is similar to autoethnography, a qualitative research method that goes beyond personal essays to connect lives with cultural, social, and political contexts (Chang, 2008, 2016). Here you will read about our challenges, disappointments, and failures as well as our strengths, passions, and successes. We describe what wounds us in addition to what motivates us. You will witness how each of us became empowered to alchemize pain into healing. Sharing our reflections from a Latina psychological point of view illustrates life lessons on coping with hardship, discrimination, cultural domination, and trauma. Out of our life stories you will witness how we develop and practice a feminist psychology in the cultural borderlands. More importantly, we hope that our *testimonios* offer you a roadmap to help you thrive.

Testimonio: In Our Own Voices

> It is the responsibility of those who survive the struggle for freedom to give testimony.
>
> *Julia Alvarez (2004)*

We use a testimonial voice to share our life reflections with you. A Spanish word meaning "witness account," *testimonio* entails a woman's description of her experiences with oppression, marginalization, victimization, and trauma (Aron, 1992). As a powerful healing tool used in psychotherapy with Latinx (Vazquez & Rosa, 2011), *testimonio* fosters empowerment, agency, and self-healing (Comas-Díaz, 2006). It reduces anxiety, depression, sleeplessness, and post-traumatic stress disorder (PTSD) (Agger, Igreja, Kiehle, & Polatin, 2012). Moreover, it facilitates the development of post-traumatic meaning-making (Akinyela, 2005). As a personal narrative, *testimonio* promotes strategies against patriarchy and oppression. Along these lines, it helps the development of an antiracist consciousness (Adleman & Enguidanos, 1995).

Born in a Latin American context, *testimonio* is a liberation method for the promotion of resistance, struggle, and social transformation (Cienfuegos & Monelli, 1983). As a form of life history, *testimonio* facilitates cultural survival, agency, and resilience (Smith, 2012). Just as important, *testimonio* is a gendered cultural script for understanding the relationship between self and other. As such, it allows the voices of the oppressed to move from the margins to the center (Brabeck, 2003). Therefore, when Latinas give *testimonio*, they reclaim their indigenous beliefs and practices, keeping alive their ancestral legacy. The structure of *testimonio* is consistent with the experiences of most people of color. Therefore, as a storytelling method, testimonio is congruent with the Latinx culture. For example, many Latinas use *testimonio* to offer powerful narratives and intersectional analyses of their struggle and resistance (Ortega, 2016). Likewise, as Latina Psychologists, we give *testimonio* to challenge oppression by rewriting gendered, ethnic, racial, sociopolitical, and psychological stories.

The definition of *testimonio* is fluid, including an individual strategy as well as a collective method. A single voice in *testimonio* goes beyond an individual occurrence, echoing the experience of many oppressed individuals. As an illustration, the sense of *I* explicitly stands for the sense of *We* of those who are oppressed (Brabeck, 2003). This way of sharing experiences informs individuals of their position within socially oppressive systems. As a result, *testimonio* generates knowledge based on individuals' lived experiences, rather than on the dominant culture's discourse. Since *testimonio* conveys the notion that truth is being revealed "under oath" (Smith, 2012), it grants cultural validity to the narrator, and encourages individuals to be experts of their communities (Ortega, 2016). At the same time *testimonio* also offers opportunities to individuals to critique their social contexts, fostering and thus empowering them to demand changes to transform the social structures that oppress them (Watkins & Shulman, 2008).

As a form of narrative inquiry, *testimonio* nurtures individuals' development of critical consciousness in order to acquire a thirst for justice and social equality. In this process, *testimonio* facilitates collective resistance and enhances the emergence of solidarity and coalition among the oppressed (Brabeck, 2003). It is important to note that *testimonio* differs from narrative research, where the psychologist shapes the unfolding of the narrator's story. Instead, *testimonio* presents an individual perspective, one that echoes a collective story that happened, and may continue to happen, in the Latinx community. Through this process, *testimonio* contributes to the growing scholarship on critical race methodologies, which aims to disrupt the apartheid of knowledge in academia (Pérez Huber, 2009). As such, *testimonio* advances the development of inquiry and research informed by gendered, racial, and social justice (Pérez Huber, 2009).

The practice of *testimonio* has been found to be empowering and emancipatory. Aside from revealing the effects of oppression on Latinas, *testimonio* elucidates women's strength to resist and overcome oppression. In this anthology, we share our experiences with cultural domination and describe how we challenged and transformed psychology. As women of color negotiating multiple cultures, we live at the edge of different and, at times, conflicting societies. Situated at such crossroads, we reconstruct our identity as we struggle against oppression to transform our lives and work. Most importantly, we document how we thrive while living in the cultural borderlands.

Surviving in the Borderlands

> To survive in the borderlands you must live sin fronteras, be a crossroads.
>
> *Gloria Anzaldúa (1987, pp. 194–195)*

A borderlands perspective is at the center of this anthology. Gloria Anzaldúa (1987) developed a borderlands theory to describe Chicanas' experiences living betwixt and between cultures. We have found that this theoretical perspective resonates with most Latinas regardless of national background. The concept of borderlands transcends geographical location to include cultural, conceptual, spiritual, and psychological spheres. Living and surviving in the cultural borderlands nurtures the emergence of a borderlands consciousness; in other words, the new *mestiza* (a mixed-race Latina) and the new mulatta (a multiracial Latina). While we celebrate the diversity among Latinas, we also identify Latinas' commonality of living in the borderlands. Therefore, we use the term *new Latina* to designate Anzaldúa's new *mestiza*. The new Latina's reconstructed identity affirms an intersectional self, one that embodies gender, ethnic, linguistic, psychological, spiritual, and geopolitical aspects of Latinas' realities.

Anzaldúa (1987) described the borderlands perspective as an interdisciplinary approach consisting of cultural studies, women's issues, indigenous mythology, spirituality, art, and Jungian psychology. Accordingly, Latinas become inner exiles as they straddle two or more cultures. In other words, Latinas are designated as the Other in the dominant culture. Notwithstanding these circumstances, surviving in the cultural borderlands generates *border thinking* (Anzaldúa, 1987). A fractured language born out of a subaltern perspective, border thinking is a reaction to the dominant cultural discourse (Mignolo, 2000). At the same time, border thinking empowers Latinas to transform obstacles into strengths or, in Anzaldúa's (1987, p. 247) words, "to dream the story into a virtual reality." Specifically, living at the cultural border imparts Latinas with a shift in perception, one that allows them to see accurately through people, events, systems, and dynamics. Instead of being divided by borders, Latinas are empowered by them, while they develop a specific way of perceiving power differences. This shift in perception is called *la facultad*, a keen spiritual intuition that emerges from the soul to deepen the way Latinas see themselves and the world (Anzaldúa, 2002).

Within the borderlands perspective, *nepantla* (a Nahuatl word for land in-between) is a liminal space of transforming possibilities. Latinas inhabiting *nepantla* feel the pain of oppression, an experience that fragments their sense of self. Paradoxically, this pain opens up multiple and alternative views of reality. That is, out of suffering emerges an awakening consciousness. The Aztec mythology serves as a vivid guide to understand inhabiting the borderlands. As an illustration, Anzaldúa (1987) reclaimed Meso-American goddesses as icons of feminist development and empowerment. She coined the term "Coatlicue state" to designate a female self-transformation process. An Aztec Earth goddess who embodies both creation and destruction, Coatlicue is a symbol of non-duality. In the borderlands context, the Coatlicue state refers to the negative feelings that Latinas experience as the Other in the dominant culture. To initiate the process of self-integration, Latinas can embrace the Coatlicue energy as a gestational state to give birth to themselves (Anzaldúa & Keating, 2002). During the Coatlicue state, Latinas descent to *el cenote* – a deep well where they come in contact with their cultural collective unconsciousness (Anzaldúa quoted in Román-Odio, 2013). Immersed in *el cenote*, Latinas use *la facultad* to access unconscious modes of knowledge in order to challenge the traditional ways of viewing the world. This new *conocimiento* (ancestral knowledge) emerges as an ancestral knowledge that is understood through a spiritual knowing-within.

The next Anzaldúan developmental step involves crossing over *nepantla*. To access this stage, Latinas can invoke the feminine energy of Coyolxauhqui, the Aztec moon goddess daughter of Coatlicue. According to Aztec mythology, Huitzilopochtli, Coyolxauhqui's brother, butchered her in an act of revenge. As a result, Coyolxauhqui became the Milky Way goddess. Out of Coyolxauhqui's dismembering, her head became the moon and the stars emerged out of her body. For this reason, Anzaldúa chose the Milky Way goddess to represent the integration of the fractured Latina, who gives birth to her-self. Like Coyolxauhqui, Latinas can pierce together their fragmented selves. To achieve this transformation, Latinas can use *testimonio*, memoir, and *autohistoria* (assemblages) as methods of self-integration (Anzaldúa quoted in Román-Odio, 2013). Interestingly, *autohistorias* are artistic modes of piercing fragmented parts of the oppressed self by embodying alternative visions of the person and the world (Anzaldúa, 2002). Due to this conceptualization, the borderlands theory is considered a theory of hope (Sandoval, 2005). We resonate with this description and believe that the borderlands theory offers a path for transformation and thriving for Latinas.

As Latina Psychologists, we reflect on our experiences of living in *nepantla*. Inhabiting *nepantla*, we share our descent into *el cenote* to initiate our identity self-integration. Out of this process, we initiate our decolonization. When we emerge from *el cenote*, we use our acquired *conocimiento* to embody a Latina Feminist Psychology.

An Embodied Psychology

Society exposes most women to negative cultural messages about their bodies, resulting in the embodiment of negative stereotypes. Originally developed to explain the effect of ageism on older individuals, we use Levy's (2009) *stereotype embodiment theory* to examine the process where the dominant culture assigns negative stereotypes to Latina bodies, leading them to internalize negative images. Unfortunately, Latinas' internalized negative body image affects their sense of self and agency (Delgado Bernal, Elenes, Godinez, & Villenas, 2006). For example, since microaggressions become an embodied oppression, most Latinas feel racism and sexism in their own flesh. As a result, Latinas inherit stories that are stored in their bodies (embodied). Sadly, this experience frequently results in the development of a negative embodied self.

Following the embodiment method, we borrow Cherie Moraga's (1981) *theory in the flesh* to describe how we, as Latina Psychologists, embody a Latina Feminist Psychology. Moraga advanced a theory where Latinas' bodies become an ideological site. Therefore, *theory in the flesh* is a feminist conceptualization that identifies how Latinas' physical realities, such as skin color, phenotype, hair texture, body type, place where they grew up, and sexual desire, all fuse to identify Latinas as the Other. Additionally, when Latinas speak English with a Spanish accent and/or use Spanglish, they are exposed to *linguistic* terrorism, an attack ranging from microaggressions to xenophobia (Anzaldúa, 1987). As a non-essentialist Latina feminist concept, *theory in the flesh* offers a method for examining the sociopolitical and psychological effects of living in a specific social space (Anzaldúa & Moraga, 1981). Moreover, it nurtures the emergence of *conocimiento* to foster survival and an urgent need for liberation. Through this process, *theory in the flesh* establishes new categories of analysis, including storytelling and spirituality, to subvert the dominant psychosocial discourses (Hurtado, 2003).

Like most Latinas, we live and work at the intersection of mind, spirit, and body. Therefore, we utilize embodiment as a method of analysis and inquiry (Perry & Medina, 2015). The development of our embodied feminist psychology can be understood as follows. First, we master the language of psychology. Then, we become painfully aware of how Eurocentric worldviews of individualism, meritocracy, and objectivity dominate mainstream psychology. As psychologists trained in mainstream psychological paradigms, we resist intellectual colonization.

We become aware that due to our combined legacies of *coloniality of power* and *coloniality of gender*, we can act as agents of an oppressive status quo. *Coloniality of power* refers to how the European colonial structures of power and privilege continue to affect Latin Americans, supporting a social system based on the intersection of race, politics, and class, and assigning privilege to Whites while disenfranchising people of color (Quijano, 2000). Even more, coloniality of power exposes individuals with a legacy of colonization to neocolonization (Comas-Díaz, 2016). Additionally, *coloniality of gender* ranks men as superior to women while oppressing both women and men of color, resulting in the interruption of solidarity (Lugones, 2008). Our awareness of these dynamics nurtures a psychological decolonization. Accordingly, we open up counter-spaces to challenge scholarly imperialism, thus resisting the hegemonic forms of psychological theory, research, and practice. In this process, we recover our discounted *sabiduría* (wisdom) and use this insight to create alternative ways of thinking. As *pensadoras* (creative thinkers), we inhabit a *thinking-space* (Mignolo, 2011) where we generate new psychological possibilities. In such a thinking-space, we employ our *facultad* to engage in transformation. Through this process, we reclaim our discounted *sabiduría* and create new *conocimiento* leading to a culture- and gender-appropriate psychology.

Finally, as we embody a Latina Feminist Psychology, we embark on a personal and collective liberation journey. We reconnect with our ancestral calling to heal, educate, empower, and liberate. Notably, we enact the contemporary roles of *curanderas* (healers), sages, warriors, and change agents. In this path, we commit to sharing our *conocimiento* and wisdom to benefit others. We advocate for the wellbeing of the Latinx community through a *servidora* (committed to serve) system. Moreover, as *promotoras*, we educate and promote health and wellbeing in our communities. In this process, we combine healing with science, scholarship with social justice, and solidarity with leadership.

Weaving a *Testimonial Arpillera*

Twelve Latina Psychologists share their life stories in this anthology. As psychologists, we understand that writing life narratives and reflecting upon them promotes personal healing as well as social transformation. Similarly, we chart a course for decolonization and liberation. We embark on this path to rescue repressed gendered cultural knowledge and to integrate it into a Latina Feminist Psychology.

As a whole, this anthology offers you a *testimonial arpillera*. *Arpilleras* are brightly colored tapestries woven by Latinas to protest oppression. *Arpilleras* emerged during Augusto Pinochet's dictatorship in Chile, when women created complex tapestries to preserve the memory of the disappeared and to protest against the suffering and hardship of living under systemic oppression. *Arpilleras* are forms of artivism, art to promote social justice (Sandoval & Latorre, 2008), that have become a symbol of resistance against oppression. Moreover, *arpilleras* have been embraced internationally, becoming an icon for indigenous empowerment against the state violence in Columbia, Perú, and other countries. You will read in this anthology how our *testimonios* create a healing and empowering tapestry.

To produce this anthology, we invited ten eminent Latina Psychologists to join us in sharing *testimonios*. We identified a series of areas to guide the writing. In essence, we asked our contributors to reflect on how their personal story influenced their life and how their lived experiences affected their decision to become a psychologist as well as the choices they made in their career. To facilitate this task, we developed the following testimonial questions and asked the participants to reflect on them.

Testimonial Questions

1. *How did gender, ethnicity, culture, socioeconomic status, sexual orientation, age, physical (dis)ability, religion/spirituality, nativeness, etc. and their intersectionality impact your role as a psychologist? Here it might help to indicate life experiences in the world of academia, professional psychology, etc. while training and in the development of your career.*
2. *What effect does intersectionality have in your life and in your work as a psychologist? Here again the idea is to contribute your specific experience including your struggles, coping style, and triumphs.*
3. *How do you conceptualize your identity? Ethnic identity? Latina identity? Latinx identity? National identity? Sexual orientation identity? Socioeconomic identity? Religious/spiritual identity?*
4. *Does your Latina identity have a role in your psychological work? If so, how?*
5. *Do you consider yourself to be mixed race (*mestizaje, mulataje, *LatiNegra, other) or mixed ethnicity (Anglo Saxon and Latina, Jewish and Latina, etc.)? If so, how does this identification influence your life and work? Here you may consider any impact on your clients/patients, supervisees, trainees, and colleagues and on any other aspects of your life that will help the reader.*
6. *How do immigration and/or refugee experiences (your's and/or your family's), acculturation, biculturalism, bilingualism, monolingualism, and accent influence you in your personal life as well as in your role as a psychologist?*
7. *Are you first generation, immigrant, several generations after ancestors' immigration, or native (ancestors always lived in the U.S.)?*
8. *If you are an immigrant, did you come to the U.S. as child, adolescent, or adult?*
9. *Where were you raised? How many countries have you lived in?*
10. *How do you describe yourself as a girl and/or teenager? Were you athletic, a tomboy, studious, popular, a nerd, a Goth, unpopular, and/or other?*
11. *What is your racial identification? Do you "look" (phenotype) or do you consider yourself White (Guera), Mestiza, Indian, Creole, Mulatta, and/or LatiNegra?*
12. *Is there any difference between how others label you ethnically and racially and how you see yourself ethnically and racially?*
13. *Have you experienced discrimination, prejudice, racism, sexism, heterosexism, xenophobia, trauma, ageism, and/or oppression? Do you have significant others who have*

experienced these types of discrimination? If so, do you feel comfortable sharing how these experiences shaped your life and work?

14. *Have you experienced post-traumatic growth? If so, please explain.*
15. *What are your areas of privilege? How have these influenced your life and your role as a psychologist?*
16. *Have you been (or are you) in an interracial/interethnic/interfaith romantic relationship? Can you share your experience? What about being in a same ethnic/racial/faith/nationality romantic relationship? Please share.*
17. *Do you have children and/or engage in mothering? Can you share your experiences of mothering?*
18. *If you have children, are they children of color, Latinx, White, AfroLatinx (Lati-Negro)? Within this context, do you socialize your children in ethnic, racial, and/or gender terms? If so, how?*
19. *If you do not have children, can you share how this experience has been for you? For instance, were you an early articulator, or did you decide later to be childless? Or perhaps you have stepchildren, or "culturally" adopted members of your family, or legally adopted children.*
20. *Can you describe your theoretical orientation as a psychologist, psychotherapist, researcher, and/or scholar? Can you narrate the reasons for making these choices? Also, have you been faced with a need to amend these theoretical orientations while learning, working, mentoring, teaching, or doing research with Latinas? If so, please share.*
21. *Are you monolingual, bilingual, multilingual? Which languages do you speak (please note that Spanglish is considered a language)? Do you engage in transnationalism, and if so, how does it affect your psychological work?*
22. *Can you provide an illustration of your psychological work (therapy, research, teaching, social justice work, etc.) with Latina/os or Latinx families and/or communities?*
23. *What are the stresses, gifts, burdens, and blessings of being a Latina Psychologist for you? Here you can focus on your own personal experience (i.e. seeing patients/clients/students/supervisees/mentees) in gatherings outside the consulting room, university, etc., or whether this gives you a special place/role in your family? Is there a clear difference in your experience with non-Latinx patients/clients, students, mentees?*
24. *Besides being a psychologist, do you have avocations or passions (art, sport, etc.), take part in community service, and/or have any other wellness activities?*
25. *Do you engage in self-care and wellness? If so, please share.*
26. *Do you practice faith, religion, and/or spirituality? Conversely, are you agnostic?*
27. *Can you relate in any manner to ageism? That is, ageism relating to yourself, your relatives and/or your patients/clients or students/supervisees, their relatives, or people they interact with? If you are a therapist/counselor, have some of your patients/clients considered you to be too young or too old? Have some of your patients/clients presented intergenerational problems where parents, grandparents, grandparents-in-law cannot understand certain values that differ from theirs? For example, have you worked with clients experiencing acculturation and other cultural conflicts?*

28. *Have you experienced grief? If so, how did you cope?*
29. *Is there anything about you that most people don't know and you would like to share with the reader?*
30. *Anything else you would like to share?*

We invite you to use, modify, add, and/or delete the above questions to examine your life and work in your *testimonio*. Please answer them as best as you can. Afterwards, you can reflect on what these questions bring up for you. When you contemplate your answers, we hope you will envision your journey of transformation.

Reading Ahead

This anthology is divided into six parts. In this Introduction, you have found a description of the Latina Psychologists, as well as a discussion of *testimonio* and the Latina feminist perspectives of the cultural borderlands and *theory in the flesh*. You also saw how these concepts relate to the development of a Latina Feminist Psychology. Part II presents how the lived experiences of three Latinas shape their psychological practice, focusing on a gendered and cultural adaptation of psychotherapy. Part III brings the life stories of three more Latina Psychologists who concentrate on research and scholarship. Additionally, in Part IV you find the *testimonios* of three Latinas who share how their lived experiences influence their social justice action. Likewise, Part V offers the reflection of three Latinas who are mentors and leaders in the field of psychology. Finally, in Part VI you encounter an analysis of all the *testimonios* as well as a section on ways to thrive.

Conclusion

> It's important to have strong images of women out there, women who aren't afraid of expressing themselves, women who aren't afraid of taking chances, women who aren't afraid of their own power.
>
> *Gina Torres*

Like other Latinas, we write to survive, resist, and overcome oppression. As a result, our life stories reveal enduring lessons in living, working, and thriving in the cultural borderlands.

Finally, we ask you to bear witness to our *testimonial arpillera*. We invite you to connect with our life stories, hoping that you become inspired and, thus, benefit from our collective wisdom. Our deepest wish, however, is that you thrive in your life.

References

Adleman, J., & Enguidanos, G. (Eds.). (1995). *Racism in the lives of women: Testimony, theory, and guides to anti-racist practice*. New York: Harrington Park Press.

Agger, I., Igreja, V., Kiehle, R., & Polatin, P. (2012). Testimony therapies in Asia: Integrating spirituality in testimonial therapy for torture survivors in India, Sri Lanka, Cambodia, and the Philippines. *Transcultural Psychiatry*, 49(3–4), 568–589.

Akinyela, M. K. (2005). Testimony of hope: African centered praxis for therapeutic ends. *Journal of Systemic Therapies*, 24(1), 5–18.

Alvarez, J. (2004). *Before we were free*. New York: Alfred A. Knopf.

Anzaldúa, G. (1987). *Borderlands/la frontera: The new mestiza*. San Francisco: Aunt Lute Publishers.

Anzaldúa, G. E. (2002). now let us shift … the path of conocimiento … inner work, public acts. In G. E. Anzaldúa, & A. L. Keating (Eds.), *This bridge we call home: Radical visions for transformation* (pp. 540–570). New York: Routledge.

Anzaldúa, G. E., & Moraga, C. (Eds.). (1981). *This bridge called my back: Writings by radical women of color*. Westertown, MA: Persephone Press.

Anzaldúa, G. E., & Keating, A. (2002). *This bridge we call home: Radical visions for transformations*. New York: Routledge.

Aron, A. (1992). *Testimonio*, a bridge between psychotherapy and sociotherapy. *Women & Therapy*, 13(3), 173–189.

Brabeck, K. (2003). *Testimonio*: A strategy for collective resistance, cultural survival, and building solidarity. *Feminism and Psychology*, 13(2), 252–258.

Campesino, M., & Swartz, G. E. (2006, January–March). Spirituality among Latinas/os: Implications of culture in conceptualization and measurement. *Advances in Nursing Science*, 29(1), 69–81.

Chang, H. (2008). *Autoethnography as method*. Walnut Creek, CA: Left Coast Press.

Chang, H. (2016). Autoethnography in health research: Growing pains? *Qualitative Health Research*, 28(4), 443–451.

Cienfuegos, A. J., & Monelli, C. (1983). The testimony of political repression as a therapeutic instrument. *American Journal of Orthopsychiatry*, 53(1), 43–51.

Comas-Díaz, L. (2006). Latino healing: The integration of ethnic psychology into psychotherapy. *Psychotherapy, Theory, Research, Practice & Training*, 43(4), 436–453.

Comas-Díaz, L. (2014). La Diosa: Syncretistic folk spirituality among Latinas. In T. Bryant-Davis, A. Austria, D. Kawahara, & D. Willis (Eds.), *Religion and spirituality for diverse women: Foundations of strength and resilience* (pp. 215–231). Santa Barbara, CA: Praeger/Greenwood.

Comas-Díaz, L. (2016). Racial trauma recovery: A race-informed therapeutic approach to racial wounds. In A. N. Alvarez, C. T. H. Liang, & H. A. Neville (Eds.), *The cost of racism for people of color: Contextualizing experiences of discrimination*(pp. 341–375). Washington, DC: American Psychological Association.

Delgadillo, T. (2011). *Spiritual mestizaje: Religion, gender, race, and nation in contemporary Chicana narrative*. Durham, NC: Duke University Press.

Delgado Bernal, D., Elenes, C. A., Godinez, F. E., & Villenas, S. (Eds.). (2006). *Chicana/Latina education in everyday life: Feminist perspectives on pedagogy and epistemology*. Albany: State University of New York.

Hunter-Hernandez, M., Costas-Muñiz, R., & Gany, F. (2015, December). Missed opportunity: Spirituality as a bridge to resilience in Latinos with cancer. *Journal of Religious Health*, 54(6), 2367–2375.

Hurtado, A. (2003). Theory in the flesh: Towards an endarkened epistemology. *International Journal of Qualitative Studies in Education*, 16(2), 215–225.

Levy, B. (2009). Stereotype embodiment: A psychosocial approach to aging. *Current Directions in Psychological Science*, 18(6), 332–336.

Lugones, M. (2008, Spring). The coloniality of gender. *Worlds & Knowledges Otherwise*. Retrieved from: https://globalstudies.trinity.duke.edu/wp-content/themes/cgsh/materials/WKO/v2d2_Lugones.pdf

McAlister, J. F. (2016). Making feminist, queer, Latinx, and #BlackVotesMatter. *Women's Studies in Communication*, 39(4), 353–356. doi: 10.1080/07491409.2016.1230988

Medina, L. (2014). Nepantla spirituality: My path to the source(s) of healing. In E. Facio & I. Lara (Eds.), *Fleshing the spirit: Spirituality and activism in Chicana, Latina, and Indigenous women's lives* (pp. 167–186). Tucson, AZ: University of Arizona Press.

Mignolo, W. (2000). *Global histories/global designs: Coloniality, subaltern knowledges, and border thinking*. Princeton, NJ: Princeton University Press.

Mignolo, W. (2011). *The darker side of Western modernity: Global futures, decolonial options*. Durham, NC: Duke Univeristy Press.

Moraga, C. (1981). Entering the lives of Others: Theory in the flesh. In G. E. Anzaldúa & C. Moraga (Eds.), *This bridge called my back: Writings by radical women of color* (pp. 85–90). Westertown, MA: Persephone Press.

Ortega, M. (2016). *In-between: Latina feminist phenomenology, multiplicity, and the self*. Albany, NY: State University of New York Press.

Pérez Huber, L. (2009, November–December). Disrupting apartheid of knowledge: Testimonio as methodology in Latina/o critical race research in education. *International Journal of Qualitative Studies in Education*, 22(6), 639–654.

Perry, M., & Medina, C. L. (2015). *Methodologies of embodiment: Inscribing bodies in qualitative research*. New York: Routledge.

Quijano, A. (2000). Coloniality of power, Eurocentrism and Latin America. *Nepantla: Views from South*, 1(3), 533–580. Retrieved on November 19, 2013, from: https://www.unc.edu/~aescobar/wan/wanquijano.pdf

Román-Odio, C. (2013). *Sacred iconographies in Chicana cultural productions*. New York: Palgrave Macmillan.

Sandoval, C. (2005). Unfinished words: The crossing of Gloria Anzaldúa. In A. Keating (Ed.). *Entre mundos/among worlds: New perspectives on Gloria Anzaldúa* (pp. xiii–xvi). New York: Palgrave MacMillan.

Sandoval, C., & Latorre, G. (2008). Chicana/o artivism: Judy Baca's digital work with youth of color. In A. Everett (Ed.), *Learning race and ethnicity: Youth and digital media* (pp. 81–108). The John D. & Catherine T. MacArthur Foundation Series on Digital Media and Learning. Cambridge, MA: MIT Press.

Sharrón-del Rio, M. R., & Aja, A. A. (2015, April 8). The case for "Latinx" – and why this term matters for intersectionality. Retrieved from: https://everydayfeminism.com/2016/04/why-use-latinx/

Smith, L. T. (2012). *Decolonizing methodologies: Research and indigenous people* (2nd ed.). London and New York: Zed Books.

Vazquez, C., & Rosa, D. (2011). *Grief therapy with Latinos: Integrating culture for clinicians*. New York: Springer Publishing Company.

Watkins, M., & Shulman, H. (2008). *Toward psychologies of liberation*. New York: Palgrave McMillan.

PART II
Psychotherapy

1

LIVING AND WORKING IN CULTURAL BORDERLANDS

Celia Jaes Falicov

> Today's links across national and cultural borders bring about the ambiguities of living with two hearts instead of the old living with a broken heart.
>
> *Falicov (2014a, p. 114)*

Our names can be a door to our personal culture and migration story. My complete name is Celia Haydee (Zisman) Jaes de Falicov, although I grew up as simply Celia Jaes. One may guess from this name that I am an Argentine Jew, Argentina being the country in Latin America with the largest number of people that have Spanish first names and Jewish last names. Both my life and work embrace cultural complexities and span several ecologies. These involve migrations and transnational journeys "in-between" countries, language and accent, social class and education, ethnicities and religion, generations and types of family organization. Living in cultural borderlands – i.e. zones of overlap and similarity between cultures and cultural borders or barriers, or zones of difference or exclusion from other cultures – has shaped my personal and professional life in inseparable ways.

Migrations and Cultural Borderlands in my Early Development

Both of my parents' families were painfully aware of the fact that sociopolitical and economic events shape crucial life decisions such as migrating to an unknown, very distant land. They knew from their experience that to understand family distress, one must always include events that are beyond the control and wishes of each family. My father's family moved to Argentina in about 1919 from either Lithuania or the Ukraine – it is unclear – escaping religious persecution and utter poverty. These paternal grandparents arrived in Argentina with seven of their eight children, one baby girl having died on the boat during transit. My mother's family was smaller; they came to Argentina from Rumania later, probably 1931 or 1932. They were escaping pogroms after my mother's grandfather was shot to death by Cossacks in the public square, a common anti-Semitic violence in those years in Eastern Europe. My maternal grandfather journeyed alone to find work and save enough to bring his nuclear family, consisting of his wife and four children. The oldest was my mother, who was 15 years old at that time. A testimony to my grandfather's grit and pluck, or perhaps despair, emerges in one of the stories I heard many times growing up. Apparently, he first went to Colombia to find work; on his boat journey back to fetch his family, somebody told him that the future looked better in Argentina, so he decided to bring them all to that unknown and remote country. My parents met as adults in Argentina, and I was the first one born in Latin America, followed by a sister and a brother.

As the first child in my family born in a foreign land, I witnessed the silent yearning for absent members, so often woven into the fabric of immigrant family life. In order to accompany her husband and four children to safety, my maternal grandmother, known as Rivska in Rumania but as Clara in Argentina, had left her own recently widowed mother behind. In Buenos Aires, my grandparents lived around the corner from my parents, and when I was born, my grandmother asked that her first grandchild be named in tribute to her mother, to whom I owe my Hebrew name: Ziporah. Throughout my childhood, my grandmother provided me with many ethnic foods, which she prepared with the most unconditional and secure loving attachment I have known. Today, more and more Latinx children are being raised by or live with grandmothers. Yet we know very little about how these family arrangements affect the lives of both. In my courses and writings, I encourage Latinx psychologists to develop frameworks capable of addressing collectivistic multigenerational families with attachment bonds that may differ from the Western Euro-American and middle-class mainstream mother-child models that still narrowly permeate much of the psychological normative literature.

Neither one of my parents or any of their siblings went to school, in contrast to the stereotype of educated Jews but not so unusual for the very poor of Eastern Europe. There, they were isolated in Jewish enclaves where they were not allowed to attend school. In Argentina, they had to work and schooling was not compulsory at that time. My father worked as a delivery boy for a noodle company, and his father was a pickle maker at the market. My grandfather on my mother's side learned to do picture framing of such things as family photographs, working in a small neighborhood shop.

I was the first in my nuclear and extended family to have Spanish as a native language and to have any schooling. Like many children of immigrants, I absorbed the new culture and language for many hours of the day while also living partially in the old culture of my family. The position of oldest daughter granted me the responsibility of "helper" to my parents and my siblings from an early age.

This situation prepared me to understand what I have called the "roots and/or wings" metaphor to describe the dilemmas of the second generation; i.e. the wish to always honor the original culture along with the wish to become accepted and integrated into the majority culture (Falicov, 2014a).

My roots were to be a dutiful daughter, a girl trained in "feminine" skills of cleaning, knitting, embroidering and obedience. My wings were aspiring to the many freedoms that an education would grant me, freedoms I never witnessed in the women, or even in the men, of my extended family. Everybody had jobs; nobody aspired to an education. A bookworm by nature, as a teenager I came across Simone de Beauvoir's *The Second Sex* (1949/1970). This book stirred me: a woman needed to fight for her rights to be respected and to be educated.

My best friend's mother, an Argentine neighbor, enrolled me in high school simply because she believed that I should study. Although high school was not compulsory at that time, my friend's mother thought her daughter should go on studying, and she worked hard to convince my parents to allow me to take the competitive entrance exams. My friend's mother, as well as the encouraging words of my fourth- and fifth-grade schoolteacher, taught me that small acts of caring are not trivial; they can change a person's life. I dedicated my first professional award to her.

The long subway ride to high school took me away from the neighborhood and opened up a wide new cultural world. But it also confronted me with being the "other" in at least two ways. While school was exhilarating, it also was a place to feel like a new immigrant in my own country, fearful of not knowing the ways, fearful of not belonging or being found out as ignorant. Children who are the first to enter school in their families may feel very anxious, even scared, with no role models and few or no supports at home for this journey. The second way of being "other" had to do with ethnicity and religion. Jews are a small minority in this very Catholic country, and in an all-girl class of 55, only 5 of us were Jews. Public education was not entirely secular and not co-ed in Argentina as Catholic religious instruction had been reinstituted between 1943 and 1955 for political reasons (Rein, 2005). The five Jewish girls were taken out of class every day at catechism time to attend Morality class. This practice was of course respectful of religious differences, but it singled us out. The Jewish girls were also discouraged from joining field trips on the basis that there would be prayers before meals and other religious rituals that would make us uncomfortable. All of this may have been well intentioned. Yet, as an adult, I have become aware many times, both in Argentina and in the U.S., of exclusions or disparaging comments, microaggressions about Jews or other minorities based on widespread and inaccurate stereotypes. Years later, my own therapist in the U.S. told me that she was incredulous that I had come from an uneducated family who lived in a small rented apartment in which three children slept in beds that got pushed against the wall to make room for a table and chairs where our family of five could eat our meals. She thought all Jews were rich and educated. Over the years, I have come to appreciate that even the most educated often uncritically fall prey to ethnic or racial stereotypes. One should not ignore the internalized racism that comes from these experiences. I cannot deny that getting off the subway two stops before the Jewish neighborhood was one of the attempts I made to hide where I came from. So were the vague answers I gave when people inquired about my family. Only many years later was I able to recognize that I was trying to "pass" for non-Jewish and perhaps for being from a higher social class. I reflect often on how easy and yet how painful it is for a person from a socially stigmatized group to feel ashamed or fearful of being seen with those negative attributes.

Getting an Education

Throughout my adulthood, I believed that my parents' reluctance to allow me to go beyond primary school was only another instance of sexism; as my father often warned me, "Nobody is going to want to get married to you if you know too much." Yet it did not occur to me until much later that the intersection between my gender, my education (and theirs) and my family's migration to an unknown land played a role. Many immigrant parents have a need to remain close to their children at all times, not only out of cultural collectivism or economic hardship, but also because their separation anxiety and protectiveness gets reactivated when entering yet another unknown context (Falicov, 2014a). Girls may even become more "*encerradas*" (Smith, 2006) or conflicted over separation in late adolescence (Zayas, 2011). These complex intersections that crystallize in gender-based controls became illuminated for me in the movie *Real Women have Curves*. Immigrant parents who have not gone to school may fear that education could take their children further away, propelled by ambition or assimilation towards what the parents fear will become "a different mentality."

So getting an education was an uphill battle. Once I finished high school, not only did my father not want me to continue studying but, in particular, when I entered the University of Buenos Aires, he did not want me to major in psychology. This was not such an unusual career objection in the late 1950s, but my father's vehemence on the subject was odd because he was mild-mannered, soft-spoken, not a domineering man. Men like him who undoubtedly have their measure of sexism but are not necessarily "*machista*" inspired me to write many years later about the complexity of Latino manhood (Falicov, 2010). What my father asked me at the time was: "What can you do by talking? Isn't talking what you do with your girlfriends all the time? What kind of work is that?" Even though I opposed his views, he taught me to question whether a profession based on listening and talking makes sense, and whether listening and talking is a universal need or a culturally and socially constructed enterprise.

My father's questioning began to take on a conceptual meaning many years later when I began to think about how to introduce cultural perspectives into clinical practice. For a man like my father, who was an immigrant, who labored from an early age and never went to grade school, who became literate on his own, how could he imagine talking as work? Or talking therapy as useful? It seems plausible that my father's plight became my inspiration when years later I began to question whether the "one size fits all" approach to therapy really works for everybody? What do we have to be willing to learn so that the contributions of psychology can apply to all sectors of society? Much of my work questions the uncritical application of theories, models, interventions and techniques based on one size fits all, and it supports collaborative approaches rather than top-down models and simple cultural adaptations of mainstream approaches (Falicov, 2009).

Growing up in Cultural Borderlands

Inhabiting cultural borderlands became part of my identity. I lived in a Jewish and in a Catholic world, in an educated and a non-educated one, in an immigrant and a national world, speaking in Spanish and broken Spanish with Yiddish words – the language that adults in the family used when they did not want children to understand – living in a very modest apartment and neighborhood and beginning to observe the more beautiful and affluent homes of my classmates in a different part of the city. All this was happening in the same day. Thus, multiple contexts and multiple identities describe my early experiences much more accurately than single monolithic labels, an issue that would mark all my written and applied work over time.

Migrating to the U.S. as a Young Married Woman

Getting married in Argentina at age 20 opened up a different cultural world and a new borderland. My husband was a newly graduated physician. His parents were an Argentine-born, middle-class, Jewish, cultured professional couple. They taught me how families function when they value reason over emotion, and education and assimilation over tradition and religion. These experiences got me closer to understanding the white, Euro-American values that later on I would find embedded in so many professions and institutions.

Neither family could help us economically to get settled after marriage, and Argentina was once more in economic and political turmoil, facing again the proverbial brain drain that was precipitated by having more educated people than the country could employ. So we went away, hoping that a U.S. postgraduate medical education could secure a future return to Argentina. The paradox of this decision for me was that getting an education had always been the dominant motif of my life, yet I left Buenos Aires after three hard-won years of university without graduating to get married and migrate to Chicago, Illinois, in order to support my husband's education and our livelihood. Perhaps this was excessive gender-based sacrifice, akin to the behavior of many immigrant women who follow their husbands to unknown futures. Nevertheless, I exercised one crucial assertive negotiation: I asked my husband to sign an informal written contract (we kept it inside a vase) stating that if within a year I could not resume my graduate studies in the U.S., we would both return together to Argentina. That year I worked full-time as a file clerk and "moonlighted" as a hospital technician. But I also started to take evening college courses so that I could take the GRE and apply to graduate school. Courses like American civics and American geography hit me in the face with the fact that I knew nothing about the American constitution or American rivers and mountains. It was like the icy weather waiting outside that I had never known before; and with barely knowing English, I really did not know where I was. Another disconcerting identity transformation came out of the fact that nobody could pronounce my first or last name. To this day, I am more often called, and even written, by others as Cecilia rather than Celia, even when people look at my name tag. Because my maiden name, Jaes, required constant spelling and explanation, I opted to use my husband's surname, Falicov, an expedient decision I have never lived comfortably with.

My Graduate Education and Political Engagement

One year after the migration, I obtained a part-time research assistantship that allowed me to enroll at Loyola University in Chicago, a Catholic University where I obtained a Master's in Psychology. This led to a clinical practice externship at the Neuropsychiatric Institute of the University of Illinois. At this institute one of my supervisors, a well-known researcher, coaxed me to apply for government tuition and a stipend to attend the University of Chicago full-time for a PhD. Once again in my life, I met a stranger, a mentor who, like my childhood neighbor, encouraged me to go on with my education. Research shows that the growth of children of unschooled immigrant parents often depends on the foresight and generosity of mentors or teachers who encourage them (Suárez-Orozco & Suárez-Orozco, 2008). Of course, the serendipity of the historical time helped too: those scholarships were much easier to get then than they are now, particularly for a foreigner. These opportunities granted to me have spurred me to give back by supporting and mentoring young people who are the first to be educated in their families. I was one of the first volunteers to the now very successful Barrio Logan College Institute in San Diego. I feel deep empathy for the fearfulness that accompanies a sense of not belonging, the threat of being thought to be an interloper or a fake, the test-taking anxiety or just simply the shyness that many young people from underserved populations feel when entering college.

A couple of years ago, I had the privilege of sitting on a public stage interviewing students from Mexico and Central America attending Freedom University, an underground university for undocumented students who are being taught at an undisclosed location by a socially conscious group of professors from the University of Georgia in Athens, Georgia. Hearing their harrowing stories made me appreciate not only the courage it takes to study without role models or parental assistance, but the determination to learn and grow while living in the dark and in fear.

Academic Exposures

Entering the University of Chicago was a profoundly transforming life experience, an exhilarating and demanding life of the mind that was taking place on a university campus, a completely new experience for me as I had not gone to college in the U.S. My psychology doctoral education was in the Committee on Human Development, an interdisciplinary field that studies and integrates borderlands among biology, sociology, psychology and anthropology. The mandate was clear: to understand each stage of human development, the biological, psychological, anthropological and sociological levels need to be included. I had inspiring, even electrifying, teachers; mostly white men, of course, each with a different angle but nonetheless having a broad view of what mattered in the human sciences: the anthropologist Robert Le Vine, the brilliant developmental psychologist Lawrence Kohlberg, the Rorschach expert Samuel Beck, the TAT expert William Henry, the scholar Bernice Neugarten who specialized in late adulthood and aging, the humanistic philosophers Eugene Gendlin and David Bakan, the groundbreaking psychologist Carl Rogers. They all taught us to adopt a questioning attitude towards all intellectual outputs, including theirs – an attitude that fit me well. Growing up during a dictatorship, I have never been able to follow a leader, and even less so a guru promoting a unitary way of thinking. The dean of our graduating class of psychologists told us that we had just entered a life of learning to live with and tolerate ambiguity. Although this was a disconcerting view at that time, I have come to agree with it totally.

The prevailing view in the Committee on Human Development was that to understand any complex phenomena, two, three or more disciplines are needed. This view makes studying the subject matter even more complex, but in the long run it clarifies connections that would otherwise remain obscured by the isolation between disciplines. These layered cultural borderlands between disciplines sparked my interest in how culture and context are embedded in the fabric of all of our lives and marked my way of thinking from then on. Today when I write, I am likely to integrate readings in the social sciences when they appear to illuminate psychological behavior.

Political Engagements

The time and place of my graduate school years were ones of profound ideological upheaval. For many students, these were very liberal times: the civil rights movement, the opposition to the Vietnam War or the protests at the democratic convention of 1968 in Chicago. Every Tuesday night I went to a consciousness-raising feminist group; every Monday night, I worked with a group of health service providers to create a free health clinic for poor people, primarily African Americans; many of us campaigned against nuclear arms by using the rise of psychological anxiety as our argument. With other graduate students, we created a local chapter of Psychologists for Social Action (which became a chapter of the national Psychologists for Social Responsibility) and edited the local newsletter of *The Radical Therapist.* Our motto was "Therapy is for Change not Adjustment"; i.e. therapy is for social change, not adjustment to social conditions. The inspiration came from an address delivered by Martin Luther King to the American Psychological Convention in the summer of 1967, a speech as just and as riveting today as it was then. He exhorted psychologists to examine the word "maladjusted" and recognize that we must never adjust to racism, religious bigotry or unjust economic conditions. King aptly called this opposition to injustice a necessary "creative maladjustment."

The community mental health movement flourished in the 1970s. We subscribed to the view that therapists should work in the community and help change the conditions that produce psychopathology. Matthew Dumont (1994), one of our heroes, argued that significant changes in individual mental health can only come through social change. Furthermore, he believed that mental health professionals have a particular expertise to bring to the enterprise of urban renewal, community development and social planning. I worked part-time at the Southeast Community Mental Health Center while studying for the PhD. Therapy was regarded as a legitimate and useful tool that should be as accessible to the poor as it is to the rich. Community members defined their needs and devised the strategies for change, while the mental health worker was a collaborative facilitator.

These were years of enormous consciousness-raising and radical thinking about race, class, gender, and ethnic and gender prejudice and discrimination. I was a committed student and a committed social activist. Students in Argentina had always been politically engaged, so I was already carrying that expectation within me. Undoubtedly, the political climate of the late 1960s and 1970s is a decisive background to my career-long commitment to cultural diversity and social justice. Nevertheless, there is also a deep emotional impetus in my personal story of how or why I become a family psychologist focused primarily on Latinx immigrants at a time when neither the profession nor the topic of Latinx mental health were central concerns for most. While I was fascinated by anthropology and sociology, my ultimate decision to become a psychologist was based on a drive to understand the intimate impact of larger societal forces and processes such as migration on individuals, families and communities. My focus on Latinx can be explained by my professional experiences as a bilingual, bicultural person.

Professional Experiences

I graduated with a PhD in 1971 and spent the next year as a postgraduate student at the Tavistock Clinic in London, U.K., an experience that marks my discovery of family therapy as a field of study and practice. As a foreigner with a Spanish accent, I felt more accepted in London, where I could open my mouth to say hello without people immediately questioning where was I from. I could relate to Salvador Minuchin with his strong Spanish accent when he arrived at the Tavistock Clinic to spend a sabbatical. He had already published *Families of the Slums* (Minuchin, Montalvo, Guerney, Rosman & Schumer, 1967), which documented his research and practice with Black and Puerto Rican families whose children were in a school for delinquent boys in New York. His way of thinking left me with the indelible notion that the whole family needs to be helped and that the context of poverty often devastates their lives. I began to see families as part of the solution, much more than as having the blame for their children's problems. I returned to Chicago determined to learn to work with families in therapy.

I went to work full-time at the Pilsen Little Village Community Mental Health Center, one of the first large Latino neighborhood outposts. It was my first full-time job as a clinician, one where being bilingual and bicultural was a rare and great asset. While working with the Latinx community, family therapy seemed to be just the right fit with the family and collectivist orientation of so many of my clients. So I went for training at the Family Systems Program of the Institute for Juvenile Research in the west side of Chicago. Staying there nearly a decade, I worked first as a family therapy trainer and eventually became the director of the program. Every day I was immersed in family work, videotaped my sessions and gave supervision with the one-way mirror. I came to value these technologies enormously as a means of learning with transparency and accountability. The Institute was funded by Chicago County Mental Health and served a large inner-city area. Clients were from the low socioeconomic level of all races and ethnicities. I worked primarily with Latinx and African Americans and also with some disadvantaged Whites. Taking summer practicums at other family therapy training centers in Philadelphia and in Palo Alto, I came to appreciate the value of a simpler technology: the audiotape. Perhaps because I grew up hearing many *radionovelas*, I knew what an incredible window to relationships it is to listen carefully to people talking to each other. The fact that I could do it in Spanish and then listen intently to the tapes to continue self-learning doubled my pleasure. I always tell stories to my students about how much they can teach themselves by listening critically to their clinical work.

Writing as Giving Voice

During those years, I started to write and publish, first in collaboration with colleagues at the Institute for Juvenile Research and then alone. We had a great deal of enthusiasm for a new multidisciplinary field, so the writings were about models for training in family therapy and shortly after about therapeutic strategies for working with Mexican Americans (Falicov & Karrer, 1984) and variations in the family life cycle of the same population compared to mainstream normative models (Falicov & Karrer, 1980).

Putting in writing my thoughts about family therapy theory while researching the many cases in my clinical practice became a passion, and it also kept me abreast of other people's work. My publications led to being on editorial review boards for domestic and international journals. They also led to involvement with AFTA, the American Family Therapy Academy, an organization of teachers of family therapy. Years later I served as their president. This network of colleagues became and still is a great source of intellectual nourishment through exposure to other people's thinking, invitations to present or contribute chapters or articles, and many other forms of professional support.

The sparkling doors and even the homes that writing opened for my professional life have motivated me to encourage students both in the U.S. and abroad to write about their work as much as possible. I stress to them that the desire and commitment to write about one's own work need not be driven by academic advancement at a university. Argentines have an intellectual tradition of writing outside academia, so perhaps that gave me some cultural impetus. I am convinced that culturally diverse groups in the U.S., such as Latinx, must share their work experiences, be it a case study or a theoretical or personal reflection. Sharing these writings can help discern the extent to which we can accept and apply findings or clinical interventions based on the mainstream Euro-American cultural models that have been advanced in the mainstream literature as universal truth, unwittingly marginalizing other cultural values, family forms or societal experiences. For example, I believe that there is enormous emphasis in the mental health field on parental responsibility for mental health outcomes and not enough on the positive or not so positive effects of sibling relationships – a topic that becomes evident when interviewing families, particularly those with large sibling groups. Writing is giving voice, and giving voice is a form of social action.

From the Midwest to Southern California: A Second Relocation, a Personal Loss and Professional Development

Another Migration

The rule of a brutally inhumane military dictatorship made a return to Argentina onerous and risky. Instead of going back, my husband and I decided to relocate with our two daughters from Chicago to Southern California in the fall of 1979. New jobs, new schools, new climate, new social relationships, new lifestyles, but the same language and more cultural know-how than the first migration. In addition, living in San Diego, a border city with Tijuana, Mexico, seemed to bring us a step closer to Latin America. In April and May, San Diego explodes with a purple passion of jacaranda trees that is so evocative of Buenos Aires' streets in bloom … it does bring me a little closer to home.

I worked at the San Ysidro Mental Health Center, a large county program for Latinx, very close to the Mexican border. A third daughter was born and I wanted to have an office nearby home, so I started a private practice where I rented two small contiguous rooms and installed a one-way mirror that I could use to train and supervise therapists interested in learning to work with families.

During these early years in San Diego, I edited a book titled *Cultural Perspectives in Family Therapy* (Falicov, 1983). Using a definition of culture much broader than just ethnicity, I invited chapters on race, class, gender, migration, international views – all geared to throw light on the question of what it takes to become a culturally attuned therapist. These perspectives were different than the prevailing approach to cultural competence as based on describing broad ethnic-specific values for Latinos, African Americans, Asians, etc. It contested the idea of set cultural themes for ethnic groups and instead offered therapy avenues for inquiring about culture with curiosity and respect.

Writing, teaching and supervision opened doors to academic affiliation. I became a non-salaried clinical professor in the Department of Psychiatry at the University of California San Diego (UCSD), supervising child psychiatrists who wanted to learn family therapy. My experiences in the psychiatry department were painful. I wanted to formalize the teaching of family therapy to child psychiatry residents. Later on, I explored getting a small space that would allow me to accept an offer to become editor of a premier family therapy journal. But it seemed that being a psychologist, a woman, a Latina, a family therapist and a mother of three perhaps represented too much diversity to a male-dominated, biology-oriented and psychoanalytic department.

A Family Turning Point

A few years after moving to California, my husband died, at a time when we had two young teenagers and a new second-grader. His untimely death made it patently clear that one person can embody and signify a country and a culture for another person. Although I had reflected before on family transitions during migration, becoming a widow at a relatively young age brought another dimension. To the ambiguous losses of migration, the non-ambiguous loss of the premature death of my sole immigration life companion caused me to reflect on the intersection of migration with unexpected and untimely losses (Falicov, 2016).

I had to face anew the issue of belongingness, the agony of whether to return with my American-born children to my native home or stay close to the new life in my adoptive country. Economic considerations had weight: both my mother and my younger sister were also widows, living together in one small apartment in Buenos Aires. They were dependent on my remittances, so in spite of my emotional distress, it was more feasible to survive with my children and continue to help my long-distance family if I remained working in the U.S. six days a week. My well-meaning American friends questioned my not stopping the remittances. I was asked once whether I had calculated how much more money I would have if I added what I gave to my mother and my sister, including the monthly interest it could have accrued. I struggled to understand what seemed to me to be foreign views about money, eventually putting in writing my thoughts on variations in the cultural meanings of money (Falicov, 2001).

The answer to the dilemma of staying or leaving after I became a single parent represented another cultural borderland: I belong here *and* there. I had to learn to live with two hearts instead of a broken heart – a metaphor that I began to utilize when talking about how many immigrants today differ from those of the past because they can remain connected at long distance through the new technologies of communication (Falicov, 2007, 2014a). The meaningful system in the case of immigrants comprises those who have migrated but also those who stay behind, perhaps never seeing each other again. Concerned about the consequences of the feminization of migration that separates mothers and children, I have elaborated on conceptual and technical ways to develop transnational elements in therapeutic practice. An example is what I call therapies of separation and therapies of reunification, which involve special interventions, such as catching-up life narratives, certificates of legitimization of parenthood or celebrations of reunification (Falicov, 2014a).

This transnational being in-between, although painful at times, has become second nature for me, and perhaps it is enriching in its own way. I am emotionally attuned to this cultural borderland in many of my immigrant clients who teeter between returning and staying as they see the pros and cons in both.

The Focus on Cultural Diversity and Sociopolitical Contexts in My Work

From the late 1980s to the mid 1990s I wrote a number of theoretical and applied articles on learning to think culturally, articles that became the basis for all my future work (Falicov, 1988, 1995b). I introduced an ecosystemic lens to the study of culture by proposing a multidimensional and multi-contextual view. I also proposed that the therapeutic encounter is not culturally neutral: practitioners bring their cultural ideas derived from psychological theory and their cultural personal upbringing or preferences.

Cultural Borderlands and Ecological Niches

Inspired by Latina writer Gloria Anzaldúa (1987) and by the anthropologist Renato Rosaldo (1989), I adopted the notion of cultural borderlands as it resonated so well with my personal and professional experience (Falicov, 1995b). I found the idea of an ecological niche, a concept from biogeography denoting the environment and the resources influencing an organism, useful in encompassing two ideas: the inhabiting of multiple contexts for each individual and the interactions with others that creates borderlands. So today I describe all clients, therapists and supervisors as belonging to ecological niches that encompass both multiple contexts and cultural or personal borderlands. These concepts prevent us from describing a client's culture in stereotyped ways.

I did not feel that culture should be the sole focus of an individual's description, but rather that we should always take into account four levels for each person: the universals that unite us, the particulars (or idiosyncratic and unique features) that distinguish us, the culture-specific aspects (such as predictable religious rituals) and each person's ecological niche; i.e. the cultural and sociopolitical contexts of insertion and exclusion that create bridges of human connectedness or separation from each other. Thus, a Latino client who is a scientist from humble origins, an agnostic, a democrat and a feminist who is helping raise adolescent girls may share significant cultural borderlands with a White Anglo scientist who is also an agnostic, a democrat and a feminist, who was raised with modest means and is also the father of adolescent girls. Of course, both men also have significant differences, like their race and color, experiences of discrimination, religious backgrounds, languages, food, music and family structures they were raised in. Acknowledging our multiple identities affords the possibility of appreciating both the cultural borderlands that we share and those that separate us.

MECA: A Multidimensional, Ecological, Comparative Approach

I proposed a framework that I called MECA (multidimensional, ecological, comparative approach) that could encompass four basic universal domains (migration, ecological context, family organization and family life cycle) in which cultural and sociopolitical variations manifest themselves. MECA allows for embracing and comparing the diversity among Latinos rather than lumping them in one monolithic category. Furthermore, the same basic parameters can be used by therapists to compare their own theories and personal values with those of the clients they are seeing and, thus, gain awareness of cultural borderlands with their clients. MECA became the framework I used to organize my first book about Latinos, *Latino Families in Therapy* published in 1998, which now has an updated second edition (Falicov, 2014a).

Continuing with MECA applications, I have recently unearthed old work of mine on intercultural couples (Falicov, 1995a) as the increase in these types of marriages is staggering and Latinx are part of these new relationships. MECA has been useful for premarital counseling and for couple therapy because it provides a method for understanding and hopefully bridging cultural and sociopolitical differences in these relationships.

Distinctions between Cultural Diversity and Social Justice

In the second edition of *Latino Families in Therapy*, I use the four domains of MECA to make clearer distinctions between cultural diversity and social justice approaches. These concepts are often conflated in the literature when, in reality, each requires different types of therapeutic practices.

Writing a book gave me the exciting opportunity to integrate a lot of current clinically relevant research literature and my own practice-based research as well as popular novels, poetry and films relevant to working with the diversity of Latinos. Further, in chapters of a book on diversity and supervision, I extended the use of MECA to the self-examination of the therapist and the supervisor's own ecological niche. This cultural self-examination insures a comprehensive cultural view of the therapeutic system while also gaining awareness of one's own overlaps or distances towards clients, unrecognized racism or ethnic prejudice, and the power differentials that may promote social injustice in treatment (Falicov, 2014b).

Cultural Humility versus Cultural Competence

Seeing therapy as a cultural encounter, I favor the notion of cultural humility over the construct of cultural competence (Falicov, 2009). Cultural humility originated in family medicine (Tervalon & Murray-Garcia, 1998) in an effort to have practitioners recognize their own cultural values and behaviors and engage in self-reflection about their own culture in order to avoid imposing it on their client. In fact, cultural humility stresses clear awareness of the hierarchical nature and power differentials in the relationship. Thus, cultural humility sees clients as the experts on their culture. Rather than practitioners becoming "competent" about the culture of patients, they need to inquire about this with curiosity and respect and not impose their own cultural values.

Migration-Specific Competencies

Cultural competence courses have been more concerned with values tied to ethnicity, religion or gendered behaviors and how these may change with acculturation. In contrast, I have always been deeply interested in including the emotional impact of migration at an interpersonal level. I focus on migration relational stresses, such as ambiguous losses and gains, separations and reunifications, couple polarizations, the trauma of coaxed or unprepared migrations and the transformation of all relationships between those who came and those who stayed over time. These migration relational stresses have fairly defined clinical presentations at various life cycle points and require targeted therapeutic practices that are seldom addressed in cultural competence courses (Falicov, 2012, 2014a, 2014b).

Weaving and Reweaving the Past in the Present

My Current Family Life

I am blessed with three wonderful daughters, all bilingual, bicultural academic or professional women, happily married to men who either speak Spanish or are very appreciative of Latin American countries and cultures. They all have children, which makes me *una abuela* of five grandchildren. I am delighted that each of my daughters is engaged in work that has involvements with Latinx, through various venues. One is a professor of film studies focused on Latin American and Latino film production; she conveys a vibrant panoply of Latino cultural products to her students. My second daughter is Development Director of Mujeres Unidas y Activas, a very large old organization in San Francisco, California. She truly believes that Latina immigrant women themselves are uniquely equipped to find individual and community solutions to the problems that affect their lives, such as immigration rights, domestic violence or work development. My youngest daughter is a labor lawyer working for the City of Buffalo, New York, with a commitment to better the working and living conditions of minorities in that area, particularly African American and Puerto Rican families, defending their rights to a lead-free home, the justice of a living wage or being trained in a trade.

After 28 years of widowhood, I am now in an intercultural marriage. I married last year to a wonderful man, a professor of political science and international relationships. He was born in the U.S. of Russian socialist refugee parents, so we share the experience of growing up in an immigrant household. He speaks adequate Spanish, loves Neruda's poems, admires Mercedes Sosa's voice, but favors mariachi music over tangos(!). He has two terrific sons, one a left-wing political philosophy professor and the other a democratic political consultant. My husband also has five grandchildren. So altogether we are a whopping 22 people; it looks like I may have finally reproduced the size of the extended family I grew up in.

My Current Professional Work

For the past nine years I have been involved with the UCSD Student-Run Free Clinic Project. I started as a volunteer in the medical clinic, which serves undocumented, uninsured and underserved adult Latinx immigrants. After three years of doing therapy and teaching the medical students, who were studying medicine for the underserved, it became clear that the clinic (which had operated for 12 years in three trailers in the parking lot of a public school) needed to develop a larger mental health component.

Faced with budget constraints and as a believer in volunteerism, I proposed organizing a group of Spanish-speaking, bicultural volunteers who were licensed, experienced professionals to serve as mental health workers. I am currently the director of these services. It has been an exciting and rewarding project, its success due to the fact that the volunteer professionals fall in love with a population of patients that is always giving back by loving in any way they can, from cooking tamales to knitting scarfs or just offering simple human warmth.

As part of this project, a support and empowerment group takes place every week; the facilitators are two community *promotoras*, and the group sometimes meets at a nearby park when there is no room at the clinic. I have learned a lot participating in this group, which is based on discussions of abstract topics such as compassion, forgiveness, fatigue or self-care. No one is forced to reveal anything personal, but the topics inevitably mobilize personal thinking if not disclosure. The attendees report tremendous changes in their outlook and behavior and describe how these changes also stimulate family change. Witnessing the strengths with which these immigrant clients face many adversities, I have developed tremendous respect for the healing and solace they find in religion.

This past year, I became a coördinator, along with seven other Latinx psychologists, of a group dedicated to creating a Latinx local mental health organization. Every three months we offer a free community event, which about 40–50 mental health workers attend. The last topic was titled *"Amor en tiempos de locura: what can mental health workers do about current immigration stressors?"* We invited the Mexican consul's office and distributed many resource materials to give to clients. There is always food, music, dancing and open community announcements at these network-building events.

When I reflect back on my own trajectory and that of the field of Latino psychology, perhaps my greatest regret is the relative lack of interest in family therapy that Latinx professionals have. The levels emphasized in theory, research and clinical practice are the individual and the sociocultural. The relational level, so intensely studied by family therapists, has not really made significant theoretical, research or practice inroads among Latinx. The absence of this level of thinking is difficult to understand when it comes to working with Latinos and particularly for the first- and second-generation immigrants, who are all purported to be family oriented. The reasons for this relative absence are complex and societal, such as the emphasis on individual pathology and diagnosis, research methodologies and the way the entire system of mental health reimbursement is constructed. I often feel I could have done more to legitimize and train Latinos or to transmit my passion for family systems thinking and therapy.

This regret notwithstanding, there are moments when I feel a strong mutual connection with the growing world of young Latinx working in mental health. Some time ago, the National Latino Social Work Association gave me an award. After my presentation, a long line of young second-generation Latinx waited to greet me, thank me, kiss me or take a photograph. One of them said to me: "Thank you so much for migrating all the way from the south to be with us; we really need you here because when we read you, we find ourselves in what you say. You speak for us." Her words were my biggest award and reward ever.

References

Anzaldúa, G. (1987). *Borderlands/La frontera: The New Mestiza*. San Francisco: Aunt Lute.

de Beauvoir, S. (1949/1970). *The Second Sex*. New York: Bantam Books.

Dumont, M. (1994). *Therapists in the Community: Changing the Conditions that Produce Psychopathology* (Master's thesis).

Falicov, C. J. (Ed.) (1983). *Cultural Perspectives in Family Therapy*. Rockville, MD: Aspen Systems Corp.

Falicov, C. J. (1988). Learning to think culturally in family therapy training. In H. Liddle, D. Breunlin & D. Schwartz (Eds.), *Handbook of Family Therapy Training and Supervision* (pp. 335–357). New York: Guilford Press.

Falicov, C. J. (1995a). Cross-cultural marriages. In N. Jacobson and A. Gurman (Eds.), *Handbook of Marriage and Marital Therapy* (2nd ed.) (pp. 231–246). New York: Guilford Press.

Falicov, C. J. (1995b). Training to think culturally: A multidimensional comparative framework. *Family Process*, 34(4), 373–388.

Falicov, C. J. (2001). The cultural meanings of money: The case of Latinos and Anglo-Americans. Special Issue: Ethnicity and the Meaning of Money and Property (ed. K. Doyle), *American Behavioral Scientist*, 45(2), 313–328.

Falicov, C. J. (2007). Working with transnational immigrants: Expanding meanings of family, community and culture. *Family Process*, 46(2), 157–172.

Falicov, C. J. (2009). On the wisdom and challenges of culturally attuned treatments for Latinos: A commentary of evidence-based practices. *Family Process*, 48(2), 295–312.

Falicov, C. J. (2010). Changing constructions of machismo for Latino men in therapy: "The Devil never sleeps". *Family Process*, 49(3), 309–329.

Falicov, C. J. (2012). Immigrant family processes: A multidimensional framework (MECA). In F. Walsh (Ed.), *Normal Family Processes* (4th ed.) (pp. 297–323). New York: Guilford.

Falicov, C. J. (2014a). *Latino Families in Therapy*. New York: Guilford Press.

Falicov, C. J. (2014b). Psychotherapy and supervision as cultural encounters: The MECA framework. In C. A. Falender, E. P. Shafranske & C. J. Falicov (Eds.), *Multiculturalism and Diversity in Clinical Supervision: A Competency-Based Approach* (pp. 29–58). Washington, DC: American Psychological Association.

Falicov, C. J. (2016). Migration and the family life cycle. In M. McGoldrick, N. Garcia Preto & B. Carter (Eds.), *The Expanding Family Life Cycle: Individual, Family and Social Perspectives* (5th ed.) (pp. 222–239). New York: Pearson.

Falicov, C. J. & Karrer, B. (1980). Cultural variations in the family life cycle: The Mexican American family. In E. Carter and M. McGoldrick (Eds.), *The Family Life Cycle: A Framework for Family Therapy* (pp. 383–425). New York: Gardner Press.

Falicov, C. J. & Karrer, B. (1984). Therapeutic Strategies for Mexican American Families. *International Journal of Family Therapy*, 6(1), 16–30.

Minuchin, S., Montalvo, B., Guerney, B., Rosman, B. & Schumer, F. (1967). *Families of the Slums: An Exploration of Their Structure and Treatment*. New York: Basic Books.

Rein, R. (2005). Nationalism, education and identity: Argentine Jews and Catholic religious instruction, 1943–1955. In Marjorie Agosin (Ed.), *Memory, Oblivion and Jewish Culture in Latin America* (pp. 163–176). Austin: University of Texas Press.

Rosaldo, R. (1989). *Culture and Truth: The Remaking of Social Analysis*. Boston: Beacon Press.

Smith, R. C. (2006). *Mexican New York: Transnational Lives of New Immigrants*. Berkeley: University of California Press.

Suárez-Orozco, C. & Suárez-Orozco, M. (2008). *Learning a New Land: Immigrant Students in American Society*. Cambridge, MA: Harvard University Press.
Tervalon, M. & Murray-Garcia, J. (1998). Cultural humility versus cultural competence: A critical distinction in defining physician training outcomes in multicultural education. *Journal of Health Care for the Poor and Underserved*, 9(2), 117–125.
Zayas, L. H. (2011). *Latinas Attempting Suicide: When Cultures, Families and Daughters Collide*. New York: Oxford University Press.

2

UPROOTED AND TRANSPLANTED

The Trajectory and Development of a Latina Psychologist

Carmen Inoa Vazquez

> I grew up in a dictatorship, where you couldn't talk about difficult situations – there was this culture of silence. We would run into a problem and have no one to talk to.
>
> *Julia Alvarez*[1]

I also grew up under the dictatorial ruling of Rafael Trujillo, an unfortunate occurrence that determined the fate of a nation for nearly three decades, applying torture and persecution to the citizens of my birthplace, the Dominican Republic, while simultaneously launching me on a life trajectory full of significant losses that gradually evolved into wonderful gains. Let's walk together through my life narrative, which illustrates the losses and gains I have experienced since being transplanted to the East Bronx in New York City at the age of sixteen. The loss of my voice was preceded by the loss of an intact family, a culture, and a support system. It has been clear to me that although this experience occurred so many decades ago, it continues to be relevant to many aspects of my personal life today, particularly in my relational roles as daughter, spouse, mother, friend, and psychologist. This experience has been the pillar of my definition as a Latina Psychologist, serving as a role model to other Latinas while also functioning as practitioner, supervisor, researcher, and author.

Development as a Latina Psychologist

There are many well-respected theoretical foundations that contribute to the training of a psychologist; mine was anchored in psychodynamics. I was trained by accomplished psychologists, among them Paul Wachtel, who provided me with theoretical teachings and direct supervision while at the City University of

New York (CUNY). Wachtel's psychodynamic thinking encapsulates a combination of "insight and action" (Ziv-Beiman et al., 2016; Wachtel, 1977, 2014). His model considers psychopathology as the result of a relationship involving unconscious intrapsychic processes and overt interpersonal behaviors (Wachtel, 1997). This training has been fundamental to my development as a clinical psychologist while simultaneously expanding the cultural specifics necessary to be of assistance to Latinas and others who have sought my psychological help. At the same time, I have been able to guide future psychologists, either through direct supervision or coordination of their training, to become culturally competent mental health providers to the Latinx population in the U.S.

How should a Latina Psychologist be defined? One way to respond to this question is through the narration of my own *testimonio*, a concept described in the Introduction of this book. My *testimonio* has become an important component in my professional development as a clinician, particularly in my practice helping Latinas and others from diverse backgrounds. At the same time, the application of intersectionality – another concept illustrated in the Introduction – during my clinical work has facilitated the therapeutic dialogue between patient and therapist, helping in obtaining an easier resolution and processing of unconscious conflicts brought to the treatment room by the patient. Intersectionality considers the relevance of different identities existing concurrently within a person, including attributed social positions such as race, gender, sexual identity, and class (Rosenthal, 2016). My viewpoint adopts the position that there is no need to deny an existing societal reality, whether exemplified in rejection through discriminatory practices and/or oppression due to gender-related issues. On the contrary, validation of the societal reality helps the Latina patient connect with her intersecting identities, whether related to aspects of the immigration history of self or family, socioeconomic hardships/privileges, language, skin color, age, sexual orientation, or familial/cultural values. Each of these components describing the Latinx experience can surface in the treatment room, and the inclusion and systematic consideration of such experience within the psychotherapy process with Latinas not only enhances important aspects of the patient/psychologist interactional stance, but also facilitates the therapeutic relationship while providing the patient with a sense of "feeling understood" through the therapist's self-disclosure.

The decision to self-disclose with patients or students requires continuous scrutiny by the therapist or the teacher, who must constantly consider the benefits to the patient or the student. While the application of therapist self-disclosure in psychotherapy has achieved prominence, particularly in Integrative Psychotherapy (Ziv-Beiman et al., 2016), addressing caution in its application is pivotal in order to avoid injurious side effects for patients (Berg, Antonsen, and Binder, 2016). Deliberations on the effects of self-disclosure are not new among psychotherapists, and many have written on the subject (Farber, 2006; Ziv-Beiman, 2013; Henretty and Levitt, 2010). My consideration to self-disclose, when appropriate, during my treatment of Latinas and my recommendations to selectively self-disclose during supervision of students who treat Latinx, regardless of their ethnicity, are based on the belief that knowledge can be transferred to those who may not have lived a similar experience in order for them to attain a level of empathy and understanding that can benefit the patient. I also believe that this is an effective way to operationalize useful information learned from the narratives of other Latinx, in addition to my own personal experience, including the portrayal of acculturation stress, a topic that has been amply covered by John Berry (1990, 2009), one of the most cited authors addressing acculturation and related stress. Acculturation stress is a salient topic for psychotherapy with Latinx, and it is a reason for seeking psychological help for themselves and/or their families. While it is recognized that not every member of the family experiences stressful acculturation uniformly, and that the process does not have to be stressful per se, there is empirical evidence and consensus that acculturative stress can result in higher levels of anxiety and depression for those exposed to it (Crocket et al., 2007; Vazquez and Rosa, 2011). The immigration experience is one important aspect of the intersectionality of Latinx that requires exploration in the treatment room, in particular when experienced during the formative years, especially when one takes the position that acculturation is not necessarily linear and can take variations across generations and gender. This aspect of the intersectionality of Latinas can affect different areas, such as parenting skills, grieving practices, familial interactions, level of assertiveness, and socialization. My work as a Latina Psychologist with patients from diverse backgrounds has been framed by the recognition and understanding of the dynamics surrounding the immigration experience of my patients. This frame of thinking has also helped me to recognize the complex structures presented by the many Latinx I help, which could simultaneously include the experience of oppression and discrimination based on gender, ethnicity, language, socialization in separate cultures, age, physical infirmity, and social orientation. These are circumstances that must be considered a possible explanation of the inner conflicts presented by Latinx seeking psychological help in the treatment room.

The Beginning Struggles of my Immigration Experience

The following statement uttered by my mother still echoes in my mind to this date: "Carmen, your father and I and the [extended] family have decided that the time has come for us to move to New York." My feelings must have been very transparent, and my mother's wisdom filled in the rest: "Don't you want to go to New York? You don't look excited?" And so began my uprooting from the Dominican Republic and transplantation to the Bronx at the age of sixteen. My mother's name was Victoria, and she liked to remind my brother and I, as well as others, that her name was associated with a queen. What she said was the law. In all fairness though, I must admit with great pride that she was the best role model I could have had.

I do not remember witnessing any sense of passivity or obsequiousness in her actions, even during very dangerous and difficult moments. She had to be strong because she feared, due to Rafael Trujillo's indomitable path of destruction intended to eliminate anyone who did not see the world as he did, that my brother would be killed and/or I would be tortured, violated, or killed. This was not a far-fetched fantasy as attested in Julia Alvarez' historical novel *In the Time of the Butterflies*, her account of the four sisters who publicly objected to the torture and killing practiced by Trujillo's regime, one of them also having resisted Trujillo's sexual advances. Three of them were eventually tortured, imprisoned, and killed when their vehicle was pushed off a cliff after returning from visiting their husbands (who had been imprisoned for opposition to the Trujillo regime) in jail (Alvarez, 1994). To this day, I have an unresolved fear of riding in automobiles. At the age of twelve, I could not understand my mother's intensity in admonishing me not to let Trujillo's brother touch my hair; years later I learned that he had a house near our town, in an area named Caracol, where he kept a harem-like group of young women who were his mistresses. Although it is said that some fathers obsequiously offered their daughters to him, he allegedly intimidated young women and, using his power and influence, persuaded them to become his concubines. My mother shared with me that she had returned several negligees sent to her younger sister by Petan, as he was called, with a note reminding him that her sister was a married woman. This was not a small task for a citizen living during Trujillo's dictatorship. My mother's assertiveness provided me with a survival mechanism; although this was somewhat lost initially upon my arrival to this country at the age of sixteen, it was later regained and put into good practice. Assertiveness can also be learned by identifying and becoming familiar with the many different role models available through literary works of gendered cultural resilience.

Although awareness of Trujillo's absolute power never deterred my mother from speaking her mind against what she deemed improper, it is important to be cognizant that dictatorships all over the world foster conformity and obedience through directly imposed guidelines, particularly during the socialization of young people, which is often achieved via propaganda using imagery of power (Moghaddam, 2013). Trujillo's power was feared by most people, and they refrained from offending him lest they lose their lives or have their relatives tortured; yet I don't recall my mother ever acting in a sycophantic manner with Trujillo. A vivid memory in my mind is witnessing her confrontation of one of Trujillo's *guardias* as he demanded the purchase and placement in my parents' store of a plaque depicting the inscription: "In this house Trujillo is the Boss." She bluntly told the guard, "No, we are not buying it. Trujillo is not the boss in this house." She handled this very dangerous and tense situation all by herself because my father was at his farm that day. Years later, I asked her how she had found the courage to confront this guard and whether she had been afraid of risking retribution from Trujillo, to which she replied, "Partly because of my youth; but also I had to do it." I think on this occasion she did not give herself the credit she deserved, because I witnessed so many other courageous behaviors on her part that showed what an accomplished feminist she was, though at the time I did not recognize the term as we know it today.

During my early years growing up in the Dominican Republic, I heard very frightening stories of killings, incarcerations, and disappearances of loved ones, including families and friends. There was no freedom of the press, no freedom of ideas, no freedom of speech, and citizens were not allowed to listen to certain foreign radio stations deemed enemies of Trujillo's regime. I have memories of my parents locking themselves behind closed doors in their bedroom to secretly listen to the "forbidden" news on foreign radio stations. Many of those who were found to have dared to violate or disobey these sanctions lost their lives.

My parents were very careful not to express their opinions in front of us, the children, yet I always managed hearing their personal views uttered behind the closed doors in hushed tones. I perceived their frustrations, helplessness, and fears. As a child, clearly I did not know how to resist or protest what I already perceived as "evil," but I remember feeling compelled to do something, probably in an attempt not to feel helpless; this prompted me on one occasion to "act out" by placing a piece of chewing gum on the forehead of one of Trujillo's busts displayed in the school. The panic that gripped me once I came home for the midday meal, realizing I had dared to protest against Trujillo, not only took my appetite away but also gave me the courage to run back to the school, while my family took their siesta, to remove the piece of chewing gum. My fear-induced fantasies were appalling to me. I remember feeling terrified, thinking that if anyone found out what I had done, my whole family could be executed. I am sure that many Dominicans who experienced those years can relate similar stories that include intense fears produced by such a cruel dictatorship.

At some level, I understood that my parents had no choice but to leave our country in order to escape the oppression we were suffering. Yet leaving my friends and sense of wellbeing was, and is to this day, a very painful and defining experience for me. I also understood that my mother left behind her husband, her son, and a zone of comfort where she had a loving supportive system that included her own language, culture, and an extended family and friends. My father and brother stayed behind, also deprived of having an intact family and a sense of safety, peace, and wellbeing. My father and brother were not allowed to leave for New York with us because during Trujillo's rule, both landowners and physicians were deemed essential to make the country prosper. My brother eventually obtained a visiting visa to the United States and was granted asylum for political reasons, but my father was never allowed to travel and join us while Trujillo was alive. To this day, I have unresolved separation anxiety despite years of therapeutic work on the subject. My memory of my father disappearing at the airport at the moment we were boarding the plane to come to New York City is embedded in my mind forever. I later realized that in his traditional thinking, he did not want me to see him cry – "men do not cry" was the gender-specific cultural motto – and he went to a private place to cry. I did not want to leave without hugging him and receiving that last-minute moment of comfort from my father, but he was nowhere to be found. I vividly remember hearing the last announcement for boarding and my mother literally pulling me to follow her onto the plane. As I turned my head while ascending the stairs to the plane, I saw my father's face, which exemplified the pain of separating from us. I saw his Adam's apple moving up and down his throat. He had big ears and, in my imagination, I saw his ears flapping. When I tell this story, many people laugh, but to me, even at the present time, it is not a laughing matter; it is a reminder of the experience of pain brought by separation from those we love, regardless of the reasons. To this day, and while writing these memories, I still feel the pain of that separation moment from my father and the rest of my family and friends. It is a dormant pain that reignites like fire with every visit I make to the treasure chest holding my memories – with every visit.

The Loss of Innocence – The Language/Education Issues – Losing the Voice

Upon arrival in the Bronx, my first impressions were confusing and alienating, even with the wonderful support of my aunt Josefa who was herself an immigrant undergoing her own acculturation struggles. The closed doors of a Bronx apartment were restrictive, foreign, and unpleasant to me given that in my home town the windows were only closed during the day when it rained and doors were rarely locked. I missed my father, my brother, my friends, my world; but there was no return and we had to "*adaptarse y punto*" (adapt to it, period). This was my immediate survival option in order not to feel so impotent while witnessing my mother's nightly cry.

I arrived in the Bronx during the month of July having completed the junior year of high school in an academic track. I had studied French and English but was still not fluent in either language. In September, on the first day of school at James Monroe HS in the Bronx, the "foreigners" were placed in a Tower of Babel where none of us spoke the same language; to add insult to my injury, I was set back a year, repeating the same grade through no fault of my own. Among the many memories etched in my mind was the frustration and humiliation I experienced in a history class when the teacher made a mistake and I corrected him, as best I could. I knew the subject well, having just studied the topic the previous year in Spanish, but I could not express myself in English with the needed eloquence to defend my point. I was ridiculed by the teacher and the entire class. From that moment on, I decided I was going to master English as fast as it was possible. I started by learning from the dictionary twenty new words daily, and I attended night school for adults with my aunt Josefa. Besides attending school during the day, I managed to convince my mother and aunt to allow me to work on a part-time basis, packing lace into boxes, in the factory where they were working. I cajoled them and was very explicit that I was not neglecting my studies, but I felt that this was the least I could do to help my mother. Once my English improved, I started working in a Woolworth store as a cashier, but I was quickly fired when I refused to press some handkerchiefs that had gotten wet in a flood in the store. My refusal to do the task was due to my awareness that I was the only person from the group of cashiers who had been asked to do what I considered at that age and time to be a menial job that was beneath me; I was still adjusting from a time back home when someone else pressed my clothes. It took me a while to face my reality at the time.

As my English improved, my role as the translator and facilitator for the family solidified. Later on when I became aware through the relevant literature of children's role reversals in Latino immigrant families, it felt like *déjà vu*. My familiarity with the experience of such a fast "growing up" and role reversal has been quite enlightening for my subsequent understanding of other Latinx who shared a similar plight, and to this day, this reality allows me to better understand similar experiences in others. Role reversal in children is not always the result of immigration, but regardless of the reasons, the end result of the experience can affect the ability to feel empathy toward oneself or others (Herer and Ofra, 2000). Luckily, my ability to feel empathy was not affected; on the contrary, my role reversal augmented my understanding of others. On the other hand, I have worked with Latinx whose self-esteem and self-worth has been significantly affected by these difficult experiences; even though they were too young to handle insurmountable problems facing the grown-ups, they still blame themselves for wrongly perceived failures.

In terms of linguistic skills, and having an accent, I have been amply exposed to microaggressions, a term coined by Chester M. Pierce in 1970 (DeAngelis, 2009) and broadly addressed by Derald Sue et al. (2007). I have also experienced many direct linguistic aggressions and have been the recipient of very offensive and difficult treatment. Let me explain: On one occasion while working in an office, I asked a supervisor for clarification in order to find some documents – it is important to note that at that time I was already attending college and my English was quite appropriate. However, I had an accent that brought out xenophobic reactions in this supervisor, and she responded by calling me a "helpless creature" who "can't even understand English well." A few words of clarification are important here: These blatantly painful experiences of rejection happened many decades ago, and I have mostly resolved the negative effects they have exerted on me. On a positive note, this experience has allowed me to help and understand others from an advantageous position of "having been there in my own flesh." On the other hand, the reality is that although the content, in terms of the words used, has changed, the context has not. Aggressions due to speaking another language are not only exemplified in my patient's experiences, but in my own present situation as well, where microaggressions are still firmly very well represented.

Even now, I am still ridiculed and/or laughed at because of my accent. Individuals who have limited experience speaking any language other than English, and might have unconscious but misplaced perceptions of people from other cultures who have learned English as a second language, have mocked my accent, finding it funny and uttering phrases such as: "I don't understand what you are talking about? Speak English." Others find my accent "sexy, like a hot Latina" or declare my utterances unacceptable even when I am correct. For example, if I say "jalapeño," I am told "No, it is jalapiiiiino." Also, the moment I utter any words, I am immediately asked "Where are you from?" Luckily, the many years undergoing my own personal psychotherapy and exploration of self have provided me with a balanced understanding so that I am not personally affected but, rather, can move on, seeing the reality as it is.

The Secretarial Years

It is relevant to share the secretarial years because they are an important part of my *testimonio* and have afforded me experience that clearly portrays other gender-specific components very informative to my development as the Latina Psychologist I am today. Two years after my arrival in the Bronx, a lack of understanding of the educational system and my limited mastering of English left me graduating from high school with a General Diploma, which excluded the required Regents Exams and precluded my continuing on to a college education. Victoria, my formidable role model, sent me to the Latin American Institute, a school for Señoritas (young ladies) on Fifth Avenue, where I became an executive bilingual secretary; this was a prevalent practice at that time for the education of young girls, particularly immigrants. I would be remiss if I did not emphasize the tremendous financial sacrifice my mother made to put me through that school. She was not able to get financial support from my father due to the political situation in the Dominican Republic. While at the Latin American Institute, I became aware that I was without question the "poorest" girl in the entire school. This is difficult for an eighteen-year-old to understand, particularly when my life in the country of my birth was completely different. Now I look back at those years with amusement because I held the illusion that I was Rich and White, but suddenly became poor, a woman of color, and a Latina. Now, this identity is my badge of honor. While at the Institute, I constantly received invitations to my friends' houses in Dobbs Ferry, Larchmont, Mineola, and Floral Park, and I understood I had to reciprocate. While in the Dominican Republic I would have had a similar position to my classmates, this was not my reality in the Bronx. My pain was intense when after inviting some school friends for a Thanksgiving dinner, my mother asked me to disinvite them, reminding me that we did not have the means for such a dinner and that although these friends were from a similar ethnic background to mine, they were not immigrants. They were attending the school to learn English as an enhancement to their careers of law and business. Their relatives' elegant houses, where they were living, were very different from our Bronx apartment. Needless to say I was furious with my mother, but I later understood her feelings of shame to be living where we lived. For her, working as a laborer in a factory, while back home she had lived in a totally different world, was too difficult to accept. I called this period "my growing up fast years."

On another occasion, I was invited by a friend and classmate to visit her father's restaurant to eat lunch. I was aware that this restaurant was very expensive, and I definitely did not have that kind of money; but I surmised that her father was treating us and took the risk of accepting the invitation, saying to myself, "If I am asked to pay, I will say I forgot my wallet, and my mother will have to give me the money the next day." Immigrants learn to survive very fast. Needless to say, just as I predicted, I was treated to lunch by my friend's father. I understood all of a sudden that I was "poor," "nonwhite," "the other." That sense of shame of being "poor" has been the narrative of many of my patients. Being "poor," in particular for adolescents, can produce very strong feelings of confusion, sadness, low self-esteem, and rage. I can only imagine what a difficult experience my mother faced when she had to remind me that we did not have the means to entertain my friends. I lost my innocence through an awareness of a loss of status and identity, albeit only for a while. The effects of economic hardship of immigrant children have been amply addressed in the literature with recognition of the high representation of Latino children living in poverty (Mendoza et al., 2017). An understanding of the dynamics of poverty is of benefit in walking the patient through the path of their story in their *testimonio* and in validating their experiences with the therapist's self-disclosure, when deemed applicable. In these cases, I have found that self-disclosure has been very helpful in my work with Latinx, particularly when my "poverty experience" was primarily associated to living in the United States and being an immigrant. It is representative of the millions of immigrants who face a similar fate but, at the same time, thrive through their adversity. As is evident by now, I feel strongly that the therapist's self-disclosure can occupy a place of prominence in the treatment of Latinx, similar to its application within relational therapy and also within Integrative Psychotherapy, where it has been deemed an integral intervention (Ziv-Beiman, 2013; Ziv-Beiman et al., 2016). This idea will be expanded on in the Conclusion of this book.

It is worth repeating at this juncture that the decision to disclose my personal narrative is based on significant deliberations in an attempt to determine the value of sharing my life experiences and the possible benefits or harms to others in doing so. I have spent a great deal of time pondering whether, as a psychologist, the sharing of my personal experiences with my patients and/or supervisees could be beneficial to them. I have reviewed the relevant literature on self-disclosure, consulted with trusted colleagues, professors, and other experts, and have seriously considered my own experience as a psychotherapist, always pondering what would be best for the patient. I concluded that based on my clinical experience, my narrative could be of benefit to Latinx who identify with similar vicissitudes of their own. Similarly, I am very aware that my experiences and struggles are not unique to me and that is precisely why they provide me a frame for understanding my patients. I also had a fabulous role model in my first psychotherapeutic treatment with a Cuban psychiatrist, who was another great mentor on the importance of culture in psychotherapy. His support and self-disclosure served as a catalyst to my decision to become a psychologist and helped me enormously to gain very useful insight into my own dynamics in general.

The College Years and Beyond

My marriage to Hector Vazquez opened up a series of experiences in the New York world in particular. He was thirteen years my senior and fully developed professionally when we met. As the first Puerto Rican appointed to the Board of Education, he became an advisor to John Lindsay, mayor of NYC at the time. Within this role, we attended dinners at Nelson Rockefeller's apartment with his wife, Happy, and we visited the White House to eat breakfast with President Richard Nixon; although Hector was a democrat, visiting the White House was perceived as helpful in his role at that time to help the community he was representing. We also participated in governor inaugurations in Puerto Rico, all advantageous experiences that facilitated my involvement in social issues and in the political world of New York. By the time we became a couple and seriously contemplated marriage, I had been executive secretary for the editor of the newspaper *La Prensa* and worked for the Norwich Pharmaceutical Company, an international company where people from the entire world were represented. I had already visited many places in Europe and other countries, and my acculturation process was moving along very smoothly. Hector and I shared the same values: the family was first, and primarily the woman's responsibility, but I still wanted economic independence and insisted on continuing to work as a bilingual executive secretary.

I remember my decision to go back to school started during a dinner with a vice president of Chase Manhattan Bank that I attended with Hector. During this meal, I was asked what college I had attended, and my response – "I have not attended college" – made me realize I was missing something. Education was always a very important component in my home as we were growing up. Although while very young I used to say that I wanted to be a physician or an explorer, my mother always opined that such professions were too demanding for a woman and would interfere with the proper bringing up of my family; yet there was no question that I was expected to attend the university. On the other hand, I was aware that my brother Abelardo had been told since he was at my mother's breast that he was destined to be a physician, and indeed he became a very competent and well-respected neurosurgeon.

When I lecture and mention my undergraduate education, primarily to a college population, I am often asked with curiosity how I managed to obtain a doctoral degree with a general diploma. I must confess that I feel pride in telling this part of my story, but the most fulfilling aspect of my narrative is when it can impact any one of my listeners in a positive manner. It is with the same objective that I will proceed to narrate the beginning of my college education; I was enrolled in a program at Queens College, New York, named "Open Enrollment," which unfortunately is no longer functioning. In order to become matriculated in this program, a student was required to obtain an average of "B" or higher upon attainment of eleven credits. I attended college while pregnant with my youngest son, Miguel, who was born in April. His birth coincided with the Spring Break, which allowed me not to miss classes and prompted my teacher to say, "Oh – you were not fat; you were pregnant?" My son Jaime was six years old when I started attending college, which reminds me of the shock in the face of a classmate, who was at least fourteen years younger than I was, when at some point I could not accept an invitation to eat pizza because I had to take Jaime to karate class.

I was attracted to Hector because he was intellectually curious and an avid reader with a very sound sense of fairness for women and equality. He encouraged and supported my going back to school; nonetheless, he was also a traditional Latino man, and it was clear that my taking care of the home and family held high priority. I had to be *la dueña de la casa* (the housewife in charge of the house). My family has always been my priority, even when we had help. One of the memories that come to mind, among many that could elucidate this philosophy of mine, is of typing a paper for a college class while my two-year-old son Miguel was climbing on my back, and there I was simultaneously holding a frankfurter in my mouth. This memory seems hilarious now, and there are many others to illustrate the path through school, including when Miguel at the age of three asked me, "Mommy what is the superego?" He heard me practicing a lecture while he was sitting on the floor at my feet playing with his toys, and I was simultaneously practicing a lecture on a recorder.

So this is how it all happened – graduating with honors while bringing up two children, taking them to karate class, orthodontist appointments, piano lessons, and doctors' visits, going on school trips, going to the park, attending birthday celebrations, running a home, having a married life, sharing time with extended family, and managing to have some fun. These experiences were exhausting at times, but also great. I also wanted financial independence and for a while continued working as a secretary. In that position I was exposed to demeaning experiences such as being asked to bring coffee and lunch for my bosses, particularly while working as a temporary secretary, and being summoned to my boss' office to lick a stamp that needed to be placed on an envelope (in those days, stamps were not self-adhesive). I refused to lick the stamp and once more I was fired, though by then my financial situation was different to when I was working at Woolworth.

Becoming a Psychologist

I was lucky to have wonderful supervisors/mentors during my formal training at CUNY, where I obtained a doctoral degree in clinical psychology. Through these teachings, I learned that respect and application of theory does not exclude the cultural reality of the patient. My very first patient, a Dominican woman, brought me a blouse as a gift during the Christmas season. I knew that she was following a normal practice in our culture, but I was also aware of the ethical and clinical guidelines to be followed with gift giving from patients and was concerned about crossing an ethical line (Brown and Trangsrud, 2008; Zur and Lazarus, 2002). Yet following my own understanding of the Latino culture, I decided not to explore her motives and simply said, "Thank you." Then I was faced with a big conundrum, reinforced by my formative years combining a Catholic background, growing up as a girl in a traditional society, and living for sixteen years under a dictatorship. How could I be a good follower of the theoretical teachings I was learning and simultaneously follow my therapeutic instinct that has served me so well? During supervision with a wonderful supervisor, A. J. Franklin, I presented him with my plight: "A. J., the patient gave me a blouse as a Christmas gift – What should I do?" A. J.'s response has stayed with me all my life. He said, "Wear it." Of course he then proceeded to help me understand the ethics and relevant dynamics, but he also validated the importance of cultural values, corroborating the relevance of culture while also applying ethical and effective interventions. Validation of my cultural understanding as being "normal" was a great gift given to me by A. J., which I pass on to my supervisees and patients whenever it is appropriate. I also adhere to the usefulness of understanding and validating gift giving/receiving within the appropriate context. In some instances, I have refused a gift from a patient because, clinically speaking, my understanding of the dynamics was that my act of accepting the gift would not have served the patient well; but this differs from not following cultural values. During my training years, I struggled with the relevance of culture and society. In fact, I remember one of my professors scolding me because I voiced objection during a presentation in class, insisting that the description of an undocumented patient who was afraid of people wearing uniforms should be seen within her undocumented context, not just as "paranoia." My professor simply did not understand the Latinx reality. As the years went by, I eventually developed a solid belief in the importance and relevance of culture in understanding a patient's experience, and the importance of sharing this information with my students.

The Professional Years

My first job as a psychologist was at an alcoholism clinic in the South Bronx. The experience gained at the South Bronx clinic initially included rejections from the counselors since I was the only psychologist in a time and place where it was believed that only ex-alcoholics could help and understand people with alcohol problems. But that initial rejection quickly disappeared, and this position offered me a very exciting, albeit challenging, period of learning. A constant joke in my family was my saying, "Oh my God, what a day I had at the alcoholism clinic – I need a drink." A few of the incidents that come to mind include one of the clients scratching my hand with a bread knife while telling me he had something to show me. Naturally, I was quite alarmed, particularly as the clinic director was not present that day and I was the person in charge. I must have remembered my mother's confrontation of Trujillo's guard and my training in the inpatient units working with acute psychotic patients during an internship at Nassau Medical Center, where I learned to provide structure in a peaceful and calm manner during the treatment of patients in an acute phase of their illness. With a stern voice that masked my fear, I said to the patient, "This will never happen again," allowing the treatment subsequently to progress well. On another of those memorable occasions, one of the clients attending the clinic was not allowed to come in because it was evident she was intoxicated, and one of the cardinal rules was not to allow the clients in the clinic while inebriated. Again, this happened on one of those days when the director was absent; hence, I was asked to intervene when the patient was found lying on the floor outside the entrance of the clinic, and she decided to masturbate in front of the staff and patients. What did I do? I told the alarmed staff, "Close the door." These experiences served as a solid basis for me to thrive professionally later on at Bellevue Hospital Psychiatric Center, the teaching hospital for New York University School of Medicine where I worked for over 25 years, first as a staff psychologist in an inpatient unit and then as director of internship training, founder of a clinic for the treatment of Latinx, supervisor, teacher, and researcher.

The Bellevue Years

During my first years at Bellevue providing services as a staff psychologist in an inpatient unit, I faced difficult challenges and many forms of micro- and macroaggressions. The unit I was assigned to work in as a staff psychologist had never been served by a psychologist, let alone a Latina with an accent. The model at that unit was primarily medical. I conducted daily groups with psychotic patients who were experiencing an acute and disorganized phase and required the least possible disruption so as not to dysregulate further. In order to maintain the necessary structure for the treatment and to provide respect for the patients and my profession, my rule was that interruptions from the staff were not allowed once the group started. Adherence to this rule and changing the disruptive behavior of the staff required a great deal of effort and assertiveness on my part. During daily rounds, I was constantly called "Mrs. Vazquez." Correcting this incredibly disrespectful and unbelievable behavior on a daily basis during rounds required a combination of determination, patience, maturity, courage, and assertiveness. I clarified to the team that in my children's school I was "Mrs. Vazquez," but at the psychiatric unit I was "Dr. Vazquez," especially given that all the other professionals were addressed by their professional titles.

Additionally, my professional input during daily rounds, where different disciplines presented the patients' functioning, was not considered valid and had to be forcefully presented. There were many examples of this, but one in particular involved the discharge of a psychotic patient who was attending the group I led. I strongly opposed her discharge because it was clear to me that she was suicidal and actively psychotic. My strong professional opinion and apprehension about releasing the patient was confronted with, "Mrs. Vazquez, if you are so concerned about the patient, why don't you take her home?" I naturally shared my strong disapproval of such an unprofessional statement in a very forceful manner, but the patient was discharged nonetheless. She cut her wrists outside the hospital within a short period of time after being discharged and was brought back to the unit. Life has a way of providing us with just vindication if we have patience and persistence. I felt very bad for the patient, but the relevance of the profession of psychology became evident in the unit. After that incident, I became "Dr. Vazquez." At this point in my career, finding my voice became quite exciting, and I feel strongly that witnessing my mother's behavior during the Trujillo years and working at the South Bronx alcoholism clinic fresh out of graduate school provided me with the appropriate tools to handle these situations. One of the results of finding my voice was the development of a bilingual clinic and program dedicated to the promotion of wellbeing and mental health of unacculturated Latinx, where research, training, and leadership opportunities were offered.

The Bilingual Treatment Program (BTP) Clinic

Founding the Bilingual Treatment Program (BTP) Clinic at Bellevue Hospital in 1985 provided a great opportunity for me to help both patients and students navigate a smoother sailing than the one I had experienced in my own flesh. At that point, being called a "paraprofessional" or being vehemently opposed with statements such as "over my dead body" did not deter me from my purpose. On the other hand, it was baffling to get such strong opposition to the idea of opening an inpatient unit at the hospital, the main purpose of which was to benefit Latinx patients, given that we had been allocated external funding to open such a unit.

Acknowledging that the time was not "right" to have a Latina head an inpatient unit, the next step was to develop a specialized outpatient clinic. This shift marked the beginning of BTP. The primary mission of the program was the provision of state-of-the art, as well as culturally and linguistically competent, psychiatric care to the large Latinx population, utilizing evidence-based practices specifically geared to help the Hispanic population. At the same time, the program received grants and ample support to conduct research and training.

Besides providing services to a Latinx population in a culturally competent manner, the program was expanded to provide services to the Latinx community within the hospital's different clinics. We provided treatment to patients suffering severe and persistent mental illness with concomitant medical problems, psychosocial traumas and stressors relating to immigration, acculturation, and undocumented legal status. The dedicated faculty, virtually all Latinas, provided training to students from the areas of psychology, psychiatry, and social work who were interested in gaining experience in the treatment of a Latino population. Training was provided in an environment that was both supportive and inspirational, emphasizing through mentoring the development of leaders and culturally competent mental health professionals, who are today helping other Latinx. There were a number of excellent Latinas who supported me in the development of this project and not only contributed their talents and professional experience, but dedicated their best energy to the success of this program. The satisfaction for me was tremendous given that we shared the same passion to work with Latinx. Today, these Latina Psychologists are not only my colleagues, but also my very dear friends, including Yvette, Maria G., Nettie, Alina, and Dinelia. Later on, Maria P., Alejandra, and Juana Elena also formed part of the staff. Ruth, who is not a Latina, provided supervision to the students and offered her wonderful and supportive friendship.

The program became an excellent functional family. Our cultural input throughout the hospital was of great value in the provision of mental health services and research efforts addressing Latinx issues, which were successfully achieved, as well as through the application of cultural practices, such as celebration of the feast of the Tres Reyes (Three Kings Day, or Epiphany) and other important holidays celebrating and fostering a cultural pride in the Latinx culture. The students, who represented most areas of Latin America, found a place where their cultural values were celebrated and honored while at the same time learning culturally relevant therapeutic applications and opportunities for research. The ten plus years that I directed this program contributed significantly to the continual development of my professional self as a Latina Psychologist.

When I retired from Bellevue in 2005, the program's main leadership was under the very capable hands of Dr. Yvette Caro, my very first trainee at Bellevue, who was a pillar of strength in the successful expansion of the clinic, and who is my dear friend. Yvette expanded not only the services but also the population being served, adding an Asian component. I continued my involvement in the program as a supervisor and mentor. Unfortunately, the program was dismantled in 2011, producing great sadness in me that required years of psychotherapy treatment in order to resolve the anguish I was experiencing. The dismantling of such a competent program again represented a major loss of my culture and my family, a separation, and an affront to my identity as a Latina

Psychologist. To this day, the reasons for ending such a viable and successful program are quite difficult to comprehend. It is painful to be reminded of the loss sustained by the patient population and by the trainees, who were deprived of much-needed mentorship, training, and research opportunities, that could in turn be applied to help the Latinx population. I was humbled by the understanding that wars cannot be fought without soldiers and supplies.

Once the grieving process was accomplished, what became very clear was that the years invested in the creation and furtherance of this program had not been in vain. BTP has served as a conduit for the development of a significant number of Latinx, and others who became part of the BTP family, who now have sensitivity for the culturally relevant understanding of gender-specific conflicts and make a solid contribution through their research efforts and continued input to this area of mental health. Presently, it is gratifying to see that many of the psychologists trained at BTP have moved on to develop other projects. One such project involves helping high-risk Spanish-speaking pregnant women, recognizing the importance of providing support during the stressors of pregnancy while simultaneously going through acculturation stress. These Latinx psychologists have continued contributing to the advancement of psychology work with Latinx. Their enthusiasm has softened the void I felt when BTP was forcefully dismantled.

The Grieving Years and Beyond

The sense of family that existed at BTP extended to most areas of my life, and this became most evident to me when Hector was diagnosed with prostate cancer and died thereafter. Most of the staff had been my trainees at the clinical internship I was directing, but there were other Latinx practicing at the hospital who, to the fortune of the patients and my own, became part of the BTP family. These wonderful mental health providers afforded me solace during my grief, became part of my extended family, and made my grieving process much more bearable, and I am eternally indebted to them. My grief experience also included losing my father and subsequently my therapist, Isabel, while still in treatment, and then my mother. The BTP experience allowed me to understand the grieving process in the Latino culture and prompted the writing of my book *Grief Therapy with Latinos: Integrating Culture for Clinicians* together with my former supervisee and colleague Dinelia Rosa, PhD (Vazquez and Rosa, 2011).

As the process of grief moved on and resolved, I met a wonderful man, Martin Juvelier, who has been my husband for the last eighteen years. Through Martin, I once again experienced love and joy of life as well as a supportive force full of enthusiasm for my professional goals that has fueled my desire to contribute to the development of a Latina Psychology. We share professional endeavors, such as presentations in conferences in different parts of the world and publications in addition to fun activities including playing tennis, traveling, visiting museums, enjoying gourmet food, love of good wine, cooking, and gardening. Martin is not Latino, but is very enamored of the Latino culture. Through him, I also gained a daughter, Oriana, who has enriched our lives by seeing her progress from a typically difficult adolescent to a very kind and successful businesswoman; and through me, Martin gained two wonderful sons, Jaime and Miguel.

Changing my philosophy of life to include the motto "tomorrow we are dead" has been added to the many gains defining my personal and professional growth. This philosophy is fueled by an awareness of my mortality and vulnerabilities. In fact, I learned this way of thinking from Martin. Seeing today as the last day of my life enables me to let go of certain unpleasantness that I cannot change and to have more patience in general to truly accept people's differences while also embracing my own individualism. This is not always easy to accomplish, but most people who have experienced significant losses in their lives tend to report growth after experiencing trauma. People who have experienced the death of a child or relative, chronic illness in themselves or their loved ones, military combat, accidents, sexual assault, or loss of a job tend to report growth after their trauma (Calhoun and Tedeschi, 2001). This way of thinking is not morbid in any way; it is a reminder to live life to the fullest on a daily basis and to share with others. In this regard, I experience fulfillment and joy, being able to help those that come to my private practice and mentoring/supervising psychology graduate students. I equally enjoy being a representative of the American Psychological Association (APA), an NGO at the United Nations (UN), where I work alongside a group of inspiring and wonderful colleagues. Naturally, practicing yoga, doing Pilates, walking, reading, and playing tennis are very helpful activities for my wellbeing.

Momentarily Wrapping Up

Once again, my story and what has transpired across the trajectory of my life to this day is not necessarily unique to my person. On the other hand, it is precisely how and why my story and development as a Latina Psychologist could serve as a frame of reference for those helping Latinx patients. It is this resemblance, albeit with a certain degree of uniqueness, that sharing my story hopes to achieve. I see an analogy between my life and that of a tree or a plant that has been uprooted and transplanted with good results, producing good fruits and shade for others to enjoy and benefit from. It just dawned on me that the reason I adore flowers and gardens is because I see a resemblance between my life and the cycle of plants. This is clearly why I love gardening, and visiting botanical gardens everywhere I travel. In particular, the symbolism of the garden is always present in my mind when I visit the New York Botanical Garden in the Bronx, which I do often. There, I always like to go through the different climate zones, which depict different vegetations that are unique to tropical areas, wetlands, desert zones, and rainforests. I marvel at how they all have adapted to the challenges they have faced in their transplantation and have thrived, looking magnificent in their differences. My fantasy is that just like me, these plants have been brought to the Bronx from distant places and all have thrived in their new environment. I would like to close this chapter with that beautiful thought for all the Latinx that struggle with their differences and vicissitudes in the cultural borderlands of their lives.

Note

1 From an interview with Julia Alvarez by The National Coalition Against Censorship, January 29, 2008 (http://ncac.org/blog/interview-with-julia-alvarez). Copyright © 2008 by Julia Alvarez. By permission of Stuart Bernstein Representation for Artists, New York, NY. All rights reserved.

References

Alvarez, J. (1994). *In the Time of the Butterflies*. Chapel Hill, NC: Algonquin Books of Chapel Hill.

Berg, H., Antonsen, P., and Binder, P.-E. (2016). Sediments and vistas in the relational matrix of the unfolding "I": A qualitative study of therapists' experiences with self-disclosure in psychotherapy. *Journal of Psychotherapy Integration*, 26(3), 248–258.

Berry, J. W. (1990). Psychology of acculturation: Understanding individuals moving between cultures. In W. R. Brislin (Ed.), *Applied Cross-Cultural Psychology, Vol. 14, Cross-Cultural Research and Methodology* (pp. 232–253). Newbury Park, CA: Sage.

Berry, J. W. (2009). A critique of critical acculturation. *International Journal of Intercultural Relations*, 33(5), 361–371.

Brown, C., Trangsrud, H. B. (2008). Factors associated with acceptance and decline of client gift giving. *Professional Psychology: Research and Practice*, 39(5), 505–511.

Calhoun, L. G. and Tedeschi, R. G. (2001). Posttraumatic growth: The positive lessons of loss. In R. A. Neimeyer (Ed.), *Meaning Reconstruction and the Experience of Loss* (pp. 157–172). Washington, DC: American Psychological Association.

Crockett, L. J., Iturbide, M. I., Torres Stone, R. A., McGinley, M., Raffaelli, M. and Carlo, G. (2007). Acculturative stress, social support, and coping: Relations to psychological adjustment among Mexican American college students. *Cultural Diversity and Ethnic Minority Psychology*, 13(4), 347–355.

DeAngelis, T. (2009). Unmasking "racial microaggressions". *Monitor on Psychology*, 40(2), 42–44.

Farber, B. (2006). *Self-Disclosure in Psychotherapy*. New York: The Guilford Press.

Henretty, J. R. and Levitt, H. M. (2010). The role of therapist self-disclosure in psychotherapy: A qualitative review. *Clinical Psychology Review*, 30(1), 63–77. http://dx.doi.org/10.1016/j.cpr.2009.09.004

Herer, Y. and Ofra, M. (2000). Emotional and social adjustment of adolescents who show role-reversal in the family. *Megamot*, 40(3), 413–441.

Mendoza, M. M., Dmitrieve, J., Perreira, K. M., Hurwich-Reiss, E. and Watamura, S. E. (2017). The effects of economic and sociocultural stressors on the well-being of children of Latino immigrants living in poverty. *Cultural Diversity and Ethnic Minority Psychology*, 23(1), 15–26. http://dx.doi.org/10.1037/cdp0000111

Moghaddam, F. M. (2013). *The Psychology of Dictatorship*. Washington, DC: American Psychological Association.

Rosenthal, L. (2016). Incorporating intersectionality into psychology: An opportunity to promote social justice and equity. *American Psychologist,* 7 1(6), 474–485.

Sue, D. W., Capodilupo, C. M., Torino, G. C., Bucceri, J. M., Holder, A. M. B., Nadal, K. L. and Esquilin, M. (2007). Racial microaggressions in everyday life: Implications for clinical practice. *American Psychologist,* 62(4), 271–286. http://dx.doi.org/10.1037/0003-066X.62.4.271

Vazquez, C. and Rosa, D. (2011). *Grief Therapy with Latinos: Integrating Culture for Clinicians.* New York: Springer Publishing Company.

Wachtel, P. L. (1977). *Psychoanalysis and Behavioral Therapy: Toward an Integration.* New York, NY: Basic Books.

Wachtel, P. L. (1997). *Psychoanalysis, Behavior Therapy, and the Relational World.* Washington, DC: American Psychological Association. http://dx.doi.org/10.1037/10383-000

Wachtel, P. L. (2014). *Cyclical Psychodynamics and the Contextual Self: The Inner World, the Intimate World, and the World of Culture and Society.* New York: Routledge.

Ziv-Beiman, S. (2013). Therapist self-disclosure as an integrative intervention. *Journal of Psychotherapy Integration,* 23(1), 59–74. http://dx.doi.org/10.1037/a0031783

Ziv-Beiman, S., Keinan, G., Livneh, E., Malone, P. S. and Shahar, G. (2016). Immediate therapist self-disclosure bolsters the effect of brief integrative psychotherapy on psychiatric symptoms and the perceptions of therapists: A randomized clinical trial. *Psychotherapy Research* (published online February 3). http://dx.doi.org/10.1080/10503307.2016.1138334

Zur, O. and Lazarus, A. (2002). Six arguments against dual relationships and their rebuttals. In A. Lazarus and O. Zur (Eds.), *Dual Relationships and Psychotherapy* (pp. 3–24). New York: Springer.

3

CONNECTING WITH SPIRIT IN THE CULTURAL BORDERLANDS

Lillian Comas-Díaz

> My whole struggle in writing, in this anticolonial struggle has been to … connect up the body with the soul and the mind with the spirit.
>
> *Gloria Anzaldúa (2000, p. 11)*

"Your daughter will be mentally retarded," a nurse told my mother soon after my birth. "*Ya veremos*" (We'll see), my mother said to herself.

This anecdote is etched on my flesh as a psychological tattoo. My mother was a strong, spirited woman who faced adversity with resilience and perseverance. In this *testimonio* I share my journey of connecting with Spirit. I focus on how adversity, trauma, and oppression shaped my living in the cultural borderlands.

A Wounded Voice

I was born with a cleft palate and a Nevus Flammeous (port wine stain) on my right hand and arm. Doctors at the Women and Children's Hospital in Chicago feared that I had a congenital syndrome that included mental retardation. Mami prayed for divine intervention. My parents were born into extreme poverty in Puerto Rico. Mami grew up in a barrio outside of Yabucoa, a small town on the southeastern coast of the island. "I used to walk barefoot several miles to school, carrying the single pair of shoes I owned and only wearing them in the classroom," Mami used to say. Similarly, Papi grew up hungry: "I joined the United States Army to have enough to eat." After his Army tour Papi moved to New York, where he found unskilled work at a postal office. Without a doubt, my parents taught me about scarce financial resources early in my life.

During the 1940s and 1950s, Puerto Rico experienced high unemployment. To address this problem, the government sponsored a massive migration to the continental United States. My parents were among the thousands who migrated in search of work. They met in New York, and it was love at first sight. "I serenaded your mother the first time I saw her at the post office," Papi told me when I was a girl. Out of the kitchen Mami added: "Your father's beautiful voice enchanted me. We named you Lillian after Lily Pons, his favorite singer." Ironically, named after a singer, I inherited a wounded voice.

After marriage, my parents decided to move to California in search of a better life. I often wonder if that was the real reason for their decision. My father's dark skin in contrast to my mother's fair complexion marked them as an interracial couple before *Loving v Virginia* – the Superior Court case that invalidated laws prohibiting interracial marriage. On their way to California, my parents stopped in Chicago and were delighted to find factory jobs. Like many Latinx (im) migrants, Mami and Papi each worked two full-time jobs. After learning English, my mother, a Puerto Rican trained nurse, secured a job at the University of Illinois Hospital.

David, my only sibling, was born; and to my parents' relief, he was healthy. Moreover, he was physically different from me – a mixed-race girl with a speech disability. In addition to being able-bodied, David's skin was the color of alabaster and his hair grew blond with beautiful soft curls. David was such a stunning baby that my mother enlisted him in a Carnation Milk baby contest. Paradoxically, the son of an interracial Puerto Rican couple won a contest to represent the American healthy baby. According to Mami, the winning prize was free Carnation milk for a year. This event accentuated a dynamic embedded in my family – and for that matter, in many Puerto Rican families. The preference for whiteness over darkness and for maleness over femaleness are characteristic of a colonized mentality. A colonized mentality refers to an internalized oppression where the colonized feels inferior to the colonizer as a consequence of colonization (David & Okazaki, 2006). Since the island has always been a colony, first by Spain and now as a U.S. territory, many Puerto Ricans suffer from a colonized mentality.

When I was four years old, Mami discussed my clinical case with the doctors at the hospital where she worked as a nurse. They offered my parents a free-of-charge experimental surgery to repair my cleft palate. I underwent the surgery and the doctors declared the operation a success. But Mami knew better – she declared the operation a divine intervention. Notwithstanding the medical success, it took many years for my wounded voice to heal. To assist my parents during my recovery after the operation, Antonia, my maternal grandmother, boarded a plane for the first time and flew to Chicago. She brought a special gift, one that I only understood years later.

La Isla del Encanto (The Island of Enchantment)

Due to Puerto Rico's political colonial status and the easy travel between the island and the continental United States, many Puerto Ricans engage in circular migration (Ramos, 1992). When I was six years old, my parents participated in circular migration, and we moved to Puerto Rico to live with my maternal grandparents in Yabucoa. Abuela Antonia and Abuelo Mato lived in a two-story house at the end of a cul de sac. We occupied the downstairs and Aunt Paulina and her family lived upstairs. Cousins Alberto, my age, and Elba, two years older, became my constant companions. We played, ate, studied, and, more importantly, dreamed together. During that time, I developed a taste for storytelling. Elba and Alberto patiently listened to my wounded voice, smiled at me lovingly, and asked for more after I finished each story. This was a magical time in my life. Everything in Puerto Rico was enchanting. I lived in the midst of musical sounds, vibrant colors, pungent scents, luscious food, and loving people. I became Alicia in *La Isla del Encanto.*

Circular migration interrupted my enchantment. For financial reasons, my parents moved back to Chicago and took my brother with them. I was left behind with my grandparents. At the airport, tears in her eyes, Mami told me, "You like to study and Alberto will be in school with you." Even though leaving children behind with relatives is a common practice among Latinx (Hurtado-de-Mendoza, Gonzales, Serrano, & Kaltman, 2014), my parents' departure left a vast emptiness in my young heart. However, something unexpected happened: Classmates at school confided their distress to me. Even my teachers trusted me with their problems. My pain began to hurt less. At an early age, I found that helping others helped me. My wounded voice turned me into a good listener. I decided to become a psychologist. Looking back, I believe that my wound opened up an empathic intuitive space that allowed me to connect with people's pain.

With this new awareness, I began to feel that our house was full of spirits. When I mentioned this to Abuela, she confirmed it. Moreover, she encouraged it. I was confused because Abuela was a pious Catholic. However, her devotion was primarily to the Virgin Mary and female saints. She gave me a wonderful gift: a female-centered spirituality. "We are spiritual beings and connecting with Spirit is essential to our development," Abuela taught me many times. Moreover, such spirituality was informed by animistic and magical realism elements. "Everything has spirit, including animals, land, rivers, mountains, and stones," Abuela affirmed. Additionally, she talked about spirit guides, *ánimas en pena* (confused ghosts), and *despedidas* (when the recently departed says goodbye to loved ones) (Comas-Díaz, 2006b). Likewise, she asserted that spirits communicate with humans through dreams, visions, *celajes* (partial visions), possession, intuition, and other metaphysical means. "We all have the capacity to connect with spirits; you just have to be receptive," Abuela explained. Many years later, this knowledge allowed me to examine the similarities between *espiritismo* (Puerto Rican spiritualism) and psychotherapy (Comas-Díaz, 1981). What is more, Abuela taught me the importance of developing my *don* (the spiritual gift of intuition). Interestingly, Anzaldúa (1987) identified this sixth sense as *la facultad*, an intuition that moves ordinary functioning to a deeper unconscious state. Today, I use *la facultad* to *feel* what my psychotherapy clients feel. *La facultad* facilitates my *holding space*, a state of witnessing clients' pain with empathy, compassion, and non-judgment.

My parents and brother returned to Puerto Rico when I was nine years old. This was both a blessing and a curse. Of course, I was very happy to be reunited with my nuclear family. However, my parents bought a house and we moved with my grandparents away from Aunt Paulina and cousins Elba and Alberto. It was painful leaving my playmates behind. We moved again during my adolescence. This time, we relocated to a small farm outside Yabucoa, while my grandparents remained in town. This was not surprising to me. My father and Abuela Antonia, his mother-in-law, never got along.

Life went on, but my voice remained wounded. During my senior year in high school, I realized that I needed to heal my voice before entering college. Due to stammering, I frequently pretended to not know the answer when teachers asked questions in class. I had to change, because my strategy wouldn't help me in college. To this end, I found out how the Greek orator Demosthenes overcame his stammer by placing pebbles in his mouth while practicing oratory. I followed his example, but added a cultural adaptation. In other words, I placed small acerola berries in my mouth and recited poems in front of the mirror (Comas-Díaz, 2017). After long years of pain, suffering, and shame, I conquered the stammer. This accomplishment deepened my commitment to become a psychologist.

Pigmentocracy and Racial Consciousness

I attended college during *independentismo* (a political pro-independence movement) fervor at the University of Puerto Rico. Cousin Elba and I roomed together and we became politically active. As I read liberation literature, I became disappointed with the *independentismo*'s lack of inclusion. In my opinion, the movement excluded women and Blacks. I noticed that at the university cafeteria, the Black students sat together on one side and the *blanquitos* ("White" Puerto Ricans) at the opposite side. Puerto Rican racism entails a relationship between race and class where the higher your social class is, the whiter you are. Indeed, the Puerto Rican racial DNA is a mix of Taíno Indians, Europeans, and African slaves. The colonial Spanish system imposed a racial hierarchy on the island, designating individuals according to their racial characteristics. Within this racial system, I am classified as a *jabá* – mixed-race female with high yellow skin and kinky hair (*pelo malo*). Moreover, colonial mentality breeds internalized racism. Without a doubt, pigmentocracy is alive and well in Latin America, particularly in Puerto Rico. This concept describes societies where skin color determines wealth and social status (Telles, 2014). Moreover, research has documented that Puerto Ricans in prosperous socioeconomic classes tend to be light-skinned, while dark-skinned individuals predominate in the lower classes (Lynn, 2008).

Racism is painful for mixed-race Latinx, but it is harder on females. For example, a study found that young Latinas with darker skin in the continental

United States felt less attractive, had negative self-perceptions, and wanted their skin color to be lighter (Telzer & Vazquez-Garcia, 2009). In addition to the class-color correlation, there is a complex female attractiveness-color association. Namely, Black Latinas are perceived as unattractive and sexually available. Even when these women are considered attractive, they are not seen as desirable marriage material (Comas-Díaz, 1994). In contrast, White women are seen as attractive (in the colonial mentality) and, thus, desirable marriage partners *adelantar la raza* (to improve the race and, thus, to have offspring with lighter skin).

I carry a heavy heart with regards to race. Needless, to say, I have no doubts that my Abuela Antonia loved me. However, instead of engaging in positive hair combing interactions (Lewis, 1999), she inflicted gendered racial microagressions on me. Every time Abuela combed my hair, she exclaimed "*Este pelo!*" (This hair!), exasperated at brushing my kinky, course hair. As a result, I painfully embodied a racist injury. To cope with this pain, I compartmentalized Abuela's racism in one part of my heart, far away from her love for me. Fortunately, as I matured, I forgave Abuela and allowed her love to occupy my entire heart.

The Black is Beautiful movement reached Puerto Rico during my college years. As a result, I became racially conscious. I proudly began to wear an Afro, à la Angela Davis, as a political manifesto. I sat on the Black side of the university cafeteria. Even though Elba and I were cousins, we were physically very different. Elba's skin was the color of alabaster and her blond hair could be in a shampoo commercial. Indeed, elementary school teachers frequently chose Elba to play the Virgin Mary during Christmas plays. In contrast, I was never asked to participate – not even as a shepherdess. Despite the fact that Elba was a beautiful *blanquita*, she sat next to me in the university cafeteria. To this day, I remain grateful for Elba's sisterhood.

As a mixed-race woman, I have suffered multiple racial microaggressions. However, the worst insult was my father's angry words regarding my Afro: "Why do you want to look Blacker than you are?" Papi's question cut me like a machete. A mulatto, Papi was a victim of internalized racism and, thus, projected racism onto his daughter. The exposure to gendered racist microaggressions nurtured my racial consciousness, one that helped me years later to become a social justice psychologist. Moreover, my experiences with racism led me to coin the term LatiNegro/a. I developed this concept to raise AfroLatinx consciousness. Many members of the mainstream society, as well as numerous Latinx, perceive AfroLatinx as being solely Black, stripping them of their Latinx ethnicity (Comas-Díaz, 1994). Therefore, I coined the term LatiNegra/o to facilitate AfroLatinx's mixed-race self-designation. By placing the Latinx ethnicity in front of the Black identity, LatiNegra/os can choose to maintain their mixed-race identity without being assigned a single one to the exclusion of the other. The concept of LatiNegra/o resonated with many Puerto Ricans. Many years later, this work led to my inclusion in the list of "10 Afroboricuas Everyone should Know" (http://larespuestamedia.com/black-boricua-10/).

Saudade and Ethnocultural Archeology

I engaged in circular migration after completing a master's degree in clinical psychology. I landed in Connecticut to direct a small mental health community for Latinx. New England welcomed me with racism, xenophobia, sexism, elitism, and linguistic terrorism – an attack for speaking English with a Spanish accent (Anzaldúa, 1987). At the Clínica Hispana de Evaluación y Orientación (CHEO), I encountered first-hand the plight of the Latinx community in the continental United States. Notwithstanding my work on behalf of Latinx mental health, I experienced excruciating pain during that period in my life. I did not know how to negotiate the cultural borderlands as an ethnic minority woman. Consequently, I suffered severe culture shock, lost my cultural anchor, and developed *saudade*. A Portuguese word, *saudade* refers to a profound nostalgia; in my case it was a yearning for Spirit (Comas-Díaz, 2013). To cope with *saudade*, I indulged in Puerto Rican food. As I became overweight, I gained another status to my intersecting oppressive identities – I became a fat, mixed-race Puerto Rican woman. During that time, Delia Lebrón, a friend from college, got divorced and moved to Connecticut. We supported each other – Delia eased my *saudade*, and I *witnessed* her grief. Additionally, we practiced mutual care by exercising regularly, eating healthily, and practicing yoga. Fortunately, I lost the extra weight. However, I still experienced cultural melancholia. So, I engaged in ethnocultural archeology; in other words, I dug deep into my Latinx roots to relieve my nostalgia. Out of this process, I developed a cultural awareness initiative. Specifically, I offered cultural training to mental health professionals, trained Latinx parents on child development, and appeared on local TV discussing Latinx issues. Through these activities, I connected with other Puerto Rican psychologists, and we founded the Puerto Rican Psychological Association of Connecticut (Comas-Díaz, 2012). We acted as *promotora/es* (promoters) advancing education, health, and cultural pride in the Puerto Rican community.

To further alleviate my cultural melancholia, I reconnected with Abuela Petra, my paternal grandmother. As a young woman, Abuela divorced my paternal grandfather and migrated to New York, leaving her only child with relatives in Puerto Rico. She established herself as a professional psychic in New York's El Barrio. Abuela Petra was successful in her profession, and, thus, became financially independent. Unlike many women of her era, she divorced several times before she became a widow. Like Julia de Burgos' (1967) poem, "*Yo misma fui mi ruta*" (I was my own path), Abuela Petra was the architect of her destiny. More importantly, she exerted a lasting influence on me.

Abuela Petra nurtured my spiritual development. Like Abuela Antonia, she practiced a female-centered spirituality. Abuela Petra initiated me, her only granddaughter, in her profession. First, she taught me to read *La Baraja Española* (Spanish Tarot cards). Moreover, she taught me how to meditate and to connect with spirit guides. Even more, Abuela Petra taught me to cast blessing spells.

According to her, blessing others functions as a spiritual boomerang; in other words, when you bless someone, you also receive a blessing. My connection with Abuela Petra was so strong that when she died, she announced her death to me in a spiritual *despedida*. In other words, Abuela Petra communicated her death to me before my parents called me with the sad news.

I have been blessed having two *abuelas* as my spiritual teachers. In fact, Latina grandmothers are spiritual bridges to ancestral knowledge, teaching spiritual and healing traditions as a means of empowerment and liberation (Norat, 2005). Thanks to my *abuelas* and my mother, I continue to be committed to my spiritual development. In this process, I have attempted to connect psychology with Spirit. As a spiritual seeker, I have completed training in several psychospiritual practices, such as bioenergetics, shamanism, meditation, creative visualization, Silva Method, and numerous other mind/body/spirit healing approaches.

After a few years of working with a master's degree, I decided to complete a doctorate in clinical psychology. I enrolled at the University of Massachusetts in Amherst and was fortunate to find empowering mentors. For this reason, I consider Bonnie Strickland, a White lesbian psychologist, and Castellano Turner, an African American psychologist, as my psychology parents.

Dionysus' Daughter

After obtaining my doctorate, I secured a clinical internship at Yale University Department of Psychiatry. Upon completing my training, I was offered a faculty position and I accepted it. In this new role, I supervised clinical interns, conducted research, and delivered psychological services to inner city populations. Once more I was fortunate to find mentors such as Robert Washington, Stephen Fleck, Boris Astrachan, Myrna Weissman, and Behnaz Jalali. During my New Haven chapter, I became the assistant director of a Yale School of Medicine community mental health clinic. Most of my clients were low socioeconomic class African Americans and Whites. This work taught me valuable lessons in negotiating the cultural borderlands. Even though supervisors, colleagues, and supervisees taught me a lot, my greatest life lessons came from my clients/patients. They showed me how to endure adversity and cultivate hope.

Years later, I became the director of the Yale University Hispanic Clinic. This mental health clinic had an alcohol and drug treatment component. I was insecure about managing the addiction program, because I had no experience in substance abuse. Or so I thought. Working with addicted clients opened up a buried wound: My father was an alcoholic.

Being mulatto and poor in Puerto Rico was very difficult for my father. Due to his color, he was rejected by family, bullied during his military service, and subjected to many racial indignities. I still remember an incident during a beautiful sunny afternoon when my father, my brother David, and I were enjoying a walk in town. Holding our hands, Papi was flanked by his two children. All of a sudden, a man on the street shouted, "That girl looks like your daughter, but that blond boy is not your son!" Papi squeezed my hand hard, tensed his face, and said nothing. I stared at my father's face. I can still feel his pain today.

When I was young I thought I had two fathers. One father was loving, intelligent, charming, talented, and hard-working. My "other" father was a violent man under the influence of alcohol. Although Papi was a caring father, he exorcized his demons on his loved ones. Needless to say, the effects of alcohol on my father terrorized my whole family. Ironically, Mami was an intelligent, beautiful, successful, and loving woman who created her own path. I did not understand why my mother endured Papi's addiction. I shared my concern with her. To my surprise, I did not understand Mami's response: "Prayer and love are the best healers."

To reconcile my two fathers, I told myself that Papi was Dionysus, the Greek god of wine who, in ecstasy, lost his mind. As a child, I consoled myself by saying that I was Dionysus' Daughter. Many years later, when I had grown up, I realized that my version of Dionysus' Daughter was an Adult Child of an Alcoholic (ACOA). During my tenure at the Hispanic Clinic, I engaged in personal therapy to address the trauma of my father's alcoholism. Paradoxically, my father's illness helped me to survive in the cultural borderlands. Using psychology, I cognitively reframed Papi's illness as a teaching tool. For example, I used to "get out of my father's line of fire" by paying close attention to his moods. Like many ACOA individuals, I learned to read my father's body language and emotional state. The skill of "mind reading" has been extremely helpful in my work as a psychologist. Sadly, Papi never healed from his illness. However, I recovered from being Dionysus' Daughter. Fortunately, while exorcizing my own demons, I developed compassion towards my father. Moreover, I deepened my connection with Spirit.

Dancing with the Spirit

Towards the end of my New Haven chapter I married Fredrick Jacobsen, and we moved to Washington, DC. I became Director of the Office of Ethnic Minority Affairs at the American Psychological Association (APA). In this position, I met many psychologists of color who became my friends/siblings. Together we worked to establish APA Division 45 – the Society for the Psychological Study of Ethnic Minority Issues. During my APA tenure, I participated in a joint APA and American Psychiatric Association mission to Chile to investigate the human rights abuses under the Pinochet dictatorship (Comas-Díaz & Padilla, 1990). I met with Chilean victims of political repression and the psychologists working with them. This experience was transformative. I renewed my interest in trauma psychology and my commitment to psychotherapy as a means for liberation.

The lack of clinical work in my APA position led me to another professional journey. I became a full-time private practitioner and co-founded with Fred, my husband, the Transcultural Mental Health Institute in Washington, DC. Additionally, I became a Clinical Professor at the George Washington University

Department of Psychiatry and Behavioral Sciences. To this day, I work in my psychotherapy practice with people of color; immigrants; lesbian, gay, bisexual, transgender, and queer (LGBTQ) individuals; women; internationals; and people with cross-cultural experiences. Several years ago, I noticed the absence of a publication on the psychology of culture and ethnic minority issues. Out of this concern, I founded *Cultural Diversity and Mental Health*, a journal published by John Wiley and & Sons. Years later, the APA Division 45 acquired the journal and renamed it *Cultural Diversity and Ethnic Minority Psychology*. I was deeply honored when the division's board of directors asked me to become the journal's founding editor-in-chief. As a multicultural feminist psychologist, I continue to infuse spirituality into my work. Consequently, I incorporated two spiritual feminist identities; namely, *nepantlera* and *mujerista*.

Nepantlera

Gloria Anzaldúa (2002) acknowledged the central role of spirituality in her borderlands theory. This model describes Latinas' experiences living betwixt and between cultures. You can read a full description of Anzaldúa's borderlands theory in the Introduction of this edited book. Toward the end of her life, Anzaldúa developed the concept of *nepantlera* from the Nahuatl (Aztec) word *nepantla*, meaning in-between (see Keating, 2006). She defined *nepantlera* as a specific Latina identity that does not require external forms of identification. Rather, *nepantleras* are boundary-crossers, thresholders who, similar to priestesses, initiate people in rites of passage. Anzaldúa (2002) described *nepantla* as a precarious space in constant displacement, leading Latinas to disorienting identity dissociation. Paradoxically, living in *nepantla* opens up a shamanistic power for women's healing and transformation. In this way, *nepantleras* connect with the pain of oppression, and become aware of their fragmented self. Such awakening helps Latinas to examine their psychological Shadow, resulting in the development of an alternative vision of the world, one that nurtures the integration of the traumatized self. Interestingly, Anzaldúa (cited in Roman-Odio, 2013) recommended creativity and expressive narratives such as *autohistoria* (assemblages) to facilitate this development.

As contemporary shamans and *curanderas, nepantleras* heal and liberate through psychospirituality. Moreover, they become visionary cultural workers who use *la facultad* to promote radical social changes. In other words, *nepantleras* engage in spiritual activism – the practice of spirituality, especially spiritual vision, to promote social justice (Anzaldúa, 2002; Keating, 2006). Although *nepantleras* inhabit conflicting worlds, they respect differences within and among groups, and they embrace solidarity towards all oppressed individuals. However, this orientation exposes *nepantleras* to being misunderstood, rejected, and accused of disloyalty (Keating, 2012). Even though *nepantleras* face adversity, ultimately, they are blessed with psychospiritual rewards.

Needless to say, the concept of *nepantlera* resonates with me. I must confess that as a child, I wanted to be a priest – not a nun, but a priestess. I still remember my arguments with the catechism instructor as I questioned why women could not be Catholic priests. Years later, I realized that being a psychologist is similar to being a priestess. Both attend to the soul, given their common roots in Psyche, the Greek goddess of Soul. In other words, both priestess and psychotherapist engage in what Jung (1965) termed the "cure of souls," where the helper goes beyond healing clients' distress to assist them in achieving self-realization. Based on this foundation, I believe that the source of healing is the connection with the inner feminine divine (Medina, 2014). Without a doubt, spirituality enriches my psychotherapy practice. Likewise, my "outsider within" status (Collins, 1986) facilitates the development of creative ways to produce a multicultural feminist spiritual psychology. I call this practice Dancing with the Spirit – an integrative and holistic healing. To illustrate, I find inspiration in the Latinx culture for my therapeutic work. I share two examples below. They are *comadre* and *duende* therapies.

Comadre (co-mother) therapy is based on the relationship between the mother and the godmother of a child. Born out of a Latina reality, this therapy is relationally oriented, measuring women's progress by their ability to utilize relationships to heal, develop, and grow. Indeed, empirical findings indicate that female relationships heal (Taylor, 2002).

In addition to facilitating healing, I nurture women's thriving by helping them obtain support from a positive female bond (Comas-Díaz, 2013b). Similar to indigenous healers, I *accompany* clients on their liberation journey. Being a *comadre* healer helps me to step out of the "blank screen" therapist persona, allowing me to gain clients' information through *la facultad*. In this role I foster my clients' resilience, assertiveness, agency, and empowerment. Moreover, I help them to awaken their inner freedom fighter through the promotion of decolonization, social justice action, and solidarity with all oppressed individuals (Comas-Díaz, 2013b). Finally, I assist my clients in psychologically giving birth to themselves.

Another culture-specific healing approach is *duende* therapy. As a girl, I loved to watch flamenco (originated by Gypsy or Romani people) movies with Abuela Antonia. She used to shout "*tiene duende*" (to have *duende*) during flamenco fiery dances. García Lorca (1933) asserted that *duende* loves pain and, paradoxically, it heals the wound that refuses to heal. Evocative and powerful, *duende* dances at the edge of life and death, affirming and intensifying life (Lopez-Pedraza, 1990). Therefore, according to Abuela, *tener duende* means to connect with Spirit. "Everyone has the potential to connect with *duende*," she said. "Summon your *duende*," she urged me. I did not know what she meant by that until I suffered from cultural melancholia. To assuage my *saudade*, I searched for a family album. Suddenly, a photo of a mixed-race girl dressed in a flamenco dress struck me. She wore a radiant smile on her face. It took me a while before I realized that I was the girl in the picture (Comas-Díaz, 2013a). Needless to say, I summoned my *duende*.

As a trauma psychotherapist, I invite clients to summon their *duende* only when I intuit that they are receptive. However, most traumatized clients navigate spiritual storms during their journey. Since *duende* intensifies life, it infuses a life-affirming meaning into pain. This new meaning imparts wisdom that helps clients to alchemize suffering into liberation. Indeed, *duende* is similar to good psychotherapy because both promote people's empowerment and liberation (Elkins, 2009).

Mujerista

Long before the term *mujerismo* existed, all of my female ancestors were *mujeristas*. I learned *mujerismo* through a gendered cultural osmosis. Notably, it was not until my middle age that I named myself *mujerista*. Ada M. Isasi-Diaz (1996), a former nun, coined the term *mujerismo* (from the Spanish word *mujer*, meaning woman) to designate a Latina womanism. *Mujeristas* consider healing, social justice, and love as inseparable. Rooted in liberation theology, *mujeristas* subscribe to a psychospiritual, emancipatory, and transformative process. However, due to liberation theology's lack of gender inclusion, *mujeristas* become dissident daughters. In other words, they promote a racialized gender identity as they struggle against oppressive structures (Comas-Díaz, 2017). Specifically, *mujeristas* focus on inclusion, decolonization, activism, and a global geopolitical struggle. Guided by these principles, Thema Bryant-Davis and I organized a group of African American and Latina Psychologists to develop womanist and *mujerista* psychologies (Bryant-Davis & Comas-Díaz, 2016). In this project, we emphasized women of color's resilience, strength, gendered gifts, solidarity, creativity, and Spirit.

Ironically, the term *mujerismo* bears negative connotation among several Latin American feminists (Aquino, Machado, & Rodriguez, 2002). Similar to mainstream White feminism, Latin American feminism tends to exclude indigenous, LatiNegra (AfroLatina), and poor women (Bryant-Davis & Comas-Díaz, 2016). In contrast, *mujeristas* practice inclusion, recover their disowned *sabiduría* (wisdom), and share their *conocimiento* (ancestral knowledge) with their community. Accordingly, they commit to service humanity through fostering love, compassion, and mutual care. The *dicho* (proverb) *Haz bien y no mires a quien* (Do good and don't look at who it is for) illustrates such *mujerista* values.

As a mixed-race Latina from a low-income background, I gravitate towards *mujerismo*. Consistent with this orientation, I commit to a lifelong spiritual development. Therefore, I commune with the *mujerista* value of honoring Spirit in *lo cotidiano* (daily life). Given that Catholicism was the colonizing religion imposed on our Latinx ancestors, *mujeristas* frequently express their spirituality through Catholic forms. For instance, growing up in Puerto Rico, I fondly remember my female relatives invoking the sacred in daily blessings, such as: *Que la Virgen te accompañe; Dios te bendiga*; and *Prenderé una vela y rezaré por tí*. Since Latin American Catholicism echoes the vestiges of colonization, *mujeristas* reappropriate Catholic icons as symbols of resistance, empowerment, and liberation.

As an example, the Virgin of Guadalupe is a Latina feminist icon of struggle against oppression (Castillo, 1996). She is a transnational symbol for the human rights of women, (im)migrants, LGBTQ, indigenous, and the environment (Roman-Odio, 2013).

Mujeristas integrate indigenous cosmologies into healing. Likewise, I subscribe to a secular syncretistic *mujerismo* based on an integration of Eastern practices and indigenous and African beliefs into psychotherapy (Comas-Díaz, 2014). Within this framework, I use *la facultad*, magical realism, and animism as spiritual vehicles. To illustrate, I combine, visualization, meditation, *espiritismo*, Eye Movement Desensitization Reprocessing (EMDR), shamanism, and energy work into psychotherapy. Interestingly, such a holistic approach is similar to the Comprehensive Resource Model (CRM) (Schwarz, Corrigan, Hull, & Raju, 2017), a method for treating complex trauma through a combination of psychology, spirituality, neurobiology, and shamanic power animals.

Mujerismo reignited my creativity. After baptizing myself *mujerista*, I rescued my childhood storyteller. In this fashion, I began sharing cultural stories with my nieces to help them connect with their Latinx ancestry. Consider the following anecdote: Soon after my mother's death, I embarked on a scheduled trip. While in India, a thousand miles away, my oldest niece *announced* her birth to me in a dream. This experience led me to process my mother's death and her first granddaughter's birth in my personal story – "In Search of the Goddess" (Comas-Díaz, 2006a). Another painful loss made me re-examine my life-work balance. Elba, my *hermana del alma* and spiritual companion, succumbed to cancer. Once more, I resorted to cultural creativity to process grief. I celebrated Elba's life in a story. The publication of "A *Coquí* Serenade" (Comas-Díaz, 2013c) opened up new vistas for me. The editor of SageWoman online invited me to write a blog. "An Invitation" (http://witchesandpagans.com/sagewoman-blogs/an-invitation.html) became a canvas for stories about multicultural feminist psychospirituality. In the spirit of *familismo*, I invited my husband Fred and my brother David to add their creativity to the blog. As a result, Fred's photos and David's paintings grace "An Invitation."

A Promise and a Wish

> I am a feminist because a lot of amazing women have made me the woman I am today.
>
> *Salma Hayek*

As I reflect on my journey, I realize that I have used *la facultad* for important life decisions. For instance, I intuitively chose not to have biological children, fearing that they would inherit my congenital syndrome. Moreover, I extended this worry to my brother's children. To illustrate, when David and his wife, Holly, got pregnant for a second time, I consulted an international expert on cleft palate about my concern. The doctor declared that if I had children, they would not be as fortunate as I was. She said, "It took many years after your experimental operation for doctors to develop a successful cleft palate repair." Tears in her eyes, the doctor added, "Your operation was a divine intervention" (Comas-Díaz, 2010, p. 162). At that moment, I remembered my mother's words: "Prayer and love are the best healers."

The decision not to have biological children helped me to exercise generativity with relatives, friends, clients, colleagues, students, and others. To paraphrase Salma Hayek, I am a *mujerista* because a lot of amazing *mujeristas* made me the woman I am today. Needless to say, I owe a loving debt of gratitude to my women ancestors. They entrusted me with an inspiring legacy. My women ancestors were traumatized and blessed, wounded and healed, oppressed and liberated, despised and loved. In spite of these paradoxes (or maybe because of them), my women ancestors flourished. To honor them, I promised to thrive.

Below, I offer you some suggestions to connect with Spirit (Comas-Díaz, 2017). They are the outcome of my desire to connect the body with the soul and the mind with the spirit. Since these suggestions are based on my lived experience and circumstances, I urge you to consult your *facultad* and examine how these apply (or not) to you.

Suggestions for Connecting with Spirit

1. See yourself in the Other.
2. Embrace the sacred in *lo cotidiano* (daily life).
3. Practice mutual care.
4. Cultivate *la facultad* (intuition) and other spiritual gifts.
5. Share your *conocimiento* (ancestral knowledge).
6. Cast blessing spells.
7. Heal and liberate yourself by healing and liberating others.
8. Summon your *duende.*
9. Engage in spiritual activism.
10. Alchemize adversity into thriving.

Finally, I leave you with a wish: May you find happiness as you thrive in the cultural borderlands.

References

Anzaldúa, G. E. (1987). *Borderlands/La Frontera: The new mestiza*. San Francisco: Aunt Lute.

Anzaldúa, G. E. (2000). *Interviews/Entrevistas*. Ed. A. L. Keating. New York: Routledge.

Anzaldúa, G. E. (2002). now let us shift ... the path of *conocimiento* ... inner work, public acts. In G. E. Anzaldúa & A. L. Keating (Eds.), *This bridge we call home: Radical visions for transformation* (pp. 540–570). New York: Routledge.

Aquino, M. P., Machado, D., & Rodriguez, J. (Eds.). (2002). *A reader in Latina feminist theology: Religion and justice*. Austin: University of Texas Press.
Bryant-Davis, T., & Comas-Díaz, L. (2016). *Womanist and mujerista psychologies: Voices of fire, acts of courage*. Washington, DC: American Psychological Association.
Castillo, A. (Ed.). (1996). *Goddess of the Americas/La Diosa de las Américas: Writings on the Virgin of Guadalupe*. New York: Riverhead Books.
Collins, P. H. (1986). Learning from the outsider within: The sociological significance of Black feminist thought. *Social Problems*, Special Theory Issue, 33(6), S14–S32.
Comas-Díaz, L. (1981). Puerto Rican espiritismo and psychotherapy. *American Journal of Orthopsychiatry*, 51(4), 636–645.
Comas-Díaz, L. (1994). LatiNegra: Mental health issues of African Latinas. *Journal of Feminist Family Therapy*, 5(3–4), 35–74.
Comas-Díaz, L. (2006a). In search of the goddess. In M. L. Tompkins & J. McMahon (Eds.), *Illuminations: Expressions of the personal spiritual experience* (pp. 64–67), Berkeley, CA: Celestial Arts.
Comas-Díaz, L. (2006b). Latino healing: The integration of ethnic psychology into psychotherapy. *Psychotherapy: Theory, Research, Practice, Training*, 43(4), 436–453.
Comas-Díaz, L. (2010). On being a Latina healer: Voice, consciousness, and identity. *Psychotherapy: Theory, Research, Practice, Training*, 47(20), 162–168.
Comas-Díaz, L. (2012). *Multicultural care: A clinician's guide to cultural competence*. Washington, DC: American Psychological Association.
Comas-Díaz, L. (2013a). Duende: Evocation, quest, and soul. In M. Hoyt (Ed.), *Therapist stories of inspiration, passion, and renewal: What's love got to do with it?* (pp. 50–57). New York: Routledge.
Comas-Díaz, L. (2013b). Comadres: The healing power of a female bond. *Women & Therapy*, 36(1–2), 62–75.
Comas-Díaz, L. (2013c). A *coqui* serenade. *Crone: Women Coming of Age*, 6, 23–28.
Comas-Díaz, L. (2014). La Diosa: Syncretistic folk spirituality among Latinas. In T. Bryant-Davis, A. Austria, D. Kawahara, & D. Willis (Eds.), *Religion and spirituality for diverse women: Foundations of strength and resilience* (pp. 215–231). Santa Barbara, CA: Praeger/Greenwood.
Comas-Díaz, L. (2017). Healing: Reclaiming my ancestral legacy. In J. M. Casas, L. Suzuki, C. Alexander, & M. A. Jackson (Eds.), *Handbook of multicultural counseling* (4th ed.) (pp. 88–95). Thousand Oaks, CA: Sage.
Comas-Díaz, L., & Padilla, A. (1990). Countertransference in working with victims of political repression. *American Journal of Orthopsychiatry*, 60(1), 125–134.
David, E. J., & Okazaki, S. (2006). Colonial mentality: A review and recommendation for Filipino American psychology. *Cultural Diversity and Ethnic Minoirty Psychology*, 12(1), 1–16.
de Burgos, J. (1967). *Antología poética*. San Juan, Puerto Rico: El Coquí.
Elkins, D. (2009). *Humanistic Psychology: A Clinical Manifesto: A Critique of Clinical Psychology and the Need for Progressive Alternatives*. Colorado Springs, CO: University of the Rockies Press.
García Lorca, F. (1933). Teoría y juego del duende (Theory and play of the *duende*; translated by A. S. Kline). Retrieved from www.poetryintranslation.com/PITBR/Spanish/LorcaDuende.htm
Hurtado-de-Mendoza, A., Gonzales, F. A., Serrano, A., & Kaltman, S. (2014). Me mandó atraer: Weak "strong ties" in Latina immigrants' social networks. *Journal of Community Psychology*, 42(4), 479–494. doi: 10.1002/jcop.21623
Isasi-Diaz, A. M. (1996). *Mujerista theology: A theology for the twenty-first century*. Maryknoll, NY: Orbis Books.

Jung, C. (1965). *Memories, dreams, reflections.* New York: Random House.

Keating, A. L. (2006). From borderlands and new *mestizas* to nepantlas and nepantleras: Anzaldúan theories for social change. *Human Architecture: Journal of the Sociology of Self-Knowledge*, 4(3), Special Issue, 5–16.

Lewis, M. L. (1999). Hair combing interactions: A new paradigm for research with African-American mothers. *The American Journal of Orthopsychiatry*, 9(4), 504–514.

Keating, A. L. (2012). Making face, making soul: Spiritual activism and social transformation. In K. M. Vaz & G. L. Lemons (Eds.), *Feminist solidarity at the crossroads: Intersectional women's studies for transracial alliance* (pp. 205–219). New York: Routledge.

Lopez-Pedraza, R. (1990). Reflections on the *duende.* In *Cultural Anxiety* (pp. 55–78). Einsiedeln, Switzerland: Daimon Verlag.

Lynn, R. (2008, Summer). Pigementocracy: Racial hierarchies in the Caribbean and Latin America. *The Occidental Quarterly (University of Ulster)*, 8(2), 25–44.

Medina, L. (2014). *Nepantla* spirituality: My path to the source(s) of healing. In E. Facio & I. Lara (Eds.), *Fleshing the spirit: Spirituality and activism in Chicana, Latina, and Indigenous women's lives* (pp. 167–186). Tucson: University of Arizona Press.

Norat, G. (2005). Latina grandmothers: Spiritual bridges to ancestral lands. *Journal of the Association for Research on Mothering*, 7(2), 98–111.

Ramos, F. A. (1992). Out-migration and return migration of Puerto Ricans. In G. J. Borjas & R. B. Freeman (Eds.), *Immigration and the workforce: Economic consequences for the United States and source areas* (pp. 49–66). Chicago: University of Chicago Press.

Roman-Odio, C. (2013). *Sacred iconographies in Chicana cultural productions.* New York: Palgrave Macmillan.

Schwarz, L., Corrigan, F., Hull, A., & Raju, R. (2017). *The comprehensive resource model: Effective therapeutic techniques for healing complex trauma.* New York: Routledge.

Taylor, S. E. (2002). *The tending instinct: How nurturing is essential to who we are and how we live.* New York: Holt.

Telles, E., & Project on Ethnicity and Race in Latin America (PERLA). (2014). *Pigmentocracies: Ethnicty, race, and color in Latin America.* Chapel Hill: University of North Carolina Press.

Telzer, E. H., & Vazquez-Garcia, H. A. (2009). Skin color and self-perceptions of immigrant and U.S.-born Latinas. *Hispanic Journal of Behavioral Sciences*, 3(3), 357–374.

PART III

Scholarship/Research

4

STAYING WOKE AT THE INTERSECTIONS

Melanie M. Domenech Rodríguez

> To be woke / is not just a political ideology, / It is an unretractable existence / A contradictory remedy of healing and pain. / The cultivation of a deep and necessary consciousness of survival / that slices white patriarchal supremacy / and wounds the heart – opening minds. / Our eyes never shut. Our voices never seize. / We are courageous, we are fierce, we are exhausted. / And yet we persist. We are Alive. We are here. / We are WOKE.
>
> *Ashlee, Zamora, & Karikari, (2017, p. 89)*[1]

My 12-year-old recently stumped me with this riddle.

> A father and son were driving when they got in a terrible accident. The father died. The son was rushed to the hospital and wheeled into the operating room. The surgeon rushed in to perform and operation, stopped, and said "I can't operate on him. He's my son."
>
> Who is the doctor?

My response? "He had two fathers so his other father was the doctor." I was a little smug about my tip of the hat to marriage equity. My child chortled in delight. "No mama! The doctor was his mother!" !*No hay peor ciego que el que no quiere ver!* My inner voice wailed: Stay woke! Damn. It is hard to stay woke. This light skin. I turned 12 again for a moment. I could see the elder women in my family: *Estamos mejorando la raza contigo* said nobody out loud and everybody in all the subtle ways in which cultural programming is instilled in the young. According to cultural beliefs, I was brought up to believe that I had been "blessed" with light skin. And over the course of my life, I worked diligently to erase any trace of an accent and become fully bicultural with mainstream US culture. Little did I know all the forces had collided to position me for complete invisibility in a culture and context poised to reject me. The blessing was also a curse.

My Developmental Narrative

I was born in 1971 in Santurce, Puerto Rico. When I was growing up, the Beatles were playing on my parents' record player and so was Juan Manuel Serrat. There was salsa and merengue on the radio, but that was for *cocolos*. Cocolos were other Puerto Ricans, or maybe Dominicans, typically darker skinned, who listened to salsa and merengue blaring from their low-riders, and who, for these displays, were considered unrefined. Cocolo, in my time, was a close relative of *cafre*, another word of African origin used to denigrate people, typically those with dark skin and of low socioeconomic status, whose behavior reflects that economic status. Cocolo does not appear in the dictionary of the Real Academia de la Lengua Española (RALE), thus it is particularly susceptible to variability in meaning and use. The meaning of *cafre* is an inhabitant of Cafrería, a former South African English colony; later meanings point to barbaric, cruel, rude, and lacking social graces (Real Academia de la Lengua Espanola, 2017).

Growing up, I did aerobics with Richard Simmons, wore a neon orange skinny tie, and, once I was able to afford one, took my Walkman everywhere. I made mix tapes. At my grandmother's house, I ate rice and beans, and at home, we ate *fiambreras* [home-delivered meals] as a sanity-management strategy of my hard-working parents. I was very excited when we finally had cable TV in the 1980s, and I thought that *I Dream of Genie* was a brand-new series when I saw it for the first time. I did not know then that the show had ended filming before I was born. I certainly did not recognize the colonial nature of these experiences until years later. The sights, sounds, and smells of my youth were voices full of cultures and histories: oppressor, oppressed, colonizer, colonized. The music, food, movies, jargon, fashion, technology all carried culture and (trans)formed mine.

Like many children in Puerto Rico in that time period, my family was the central socialization unit. I was born within a generation following the major social and economic shift on the island from an agrarian to an industrial society (Ayala & Bernabe, 2007), which also transformed families and family functioning. My mom was a first-generation Cuban immigrant/refugee; my biological father was Puerto Rican. I was born and raised in Puerto Rico, speaking with a hybrid Cuban-Rican accent and learning about my own biculturalism through confusing, if often humorous, experiences. During a holiday gathering, a vociferous Cuban man was telling a story of being assaulted by a very big *bicho*. I was horrified; my parents were laughing merrily. My father was an academic and I was able, unlike many of my same-age peers, to ask questions when confused. "Papi, why are you laughing? He said a bad word." In Puerto Rico, a *bicho* is a crude word for male genitalia; but in Cuba, it used to describe an insect. In my family microcosm, I was learning early on to question the assumptions underlying my judgments of people's behaviors and to temper my reactions. Language was fluid. Location and cultural background were critical contexts for my development.

My biological father and mom divorced when I was still an infant, and my mother remarried Papi, my father. Papi is a proud Puerto Rican. He always celebrated my *puertorriqueñidad*. Papi is also a socialist. I grew up with books by Marx and Engels on the shelf and during my senior year in high school read *The Communist Manifesto* for fun. I learned about national/ethnic identity, pride, and political positioning from him. I saw from an early age that science was political and that those in authority maintained their power through well-crafted narratives intended to shape the thoughts and feelings of entire communities. Imagine my delight when, years later, I became acquainted with the writings of scholars who clearly and directly addressed these issues (e.g. Gloria Anzaldúa, Lillian Comas-Díaz, Jorge Duany, Ignacio Martín Baró, Martiza Montero).

My mother, Mami, is the quintessential West Indian woman, strong of character and resolve, in charge, and unapologetic; a matriarch. When Mami left Cuba with her family, her studies were interrupted. Rather than persuing her architect career in Cuba, she found herself working an assistant job to make ends meet and help her family of origin. She married Papi when I was an infant. Between 1973 and 1976, my parents moved to New Haven from Puerto Rico so Papi could finish his doctorate in Sociology. I remember Mami telling stories of being the wife of a doctoral student and suffering through his dissertation as if it were her own. These stories resonate with me years later as I mentor my students and see their significant others tackle theses and dissertations as family tasks. My mother completed a bachelor's degree while in New Haven. I don't remember being cognizant of her studies then. We returned to Puerto Rico in time for me to enroll in kindergarten. By the time I was in elementary school, Papi had encouraged Mami to enroll in law school. She and I studied together at the dining table. From Mami, I learned that it was never too late to pursue a goal. I remember Mami hosting her colleagues at our house for study sessions where everyone gathered, ate together, and collaborated toward a common goal. I listened to intellectual conversations that I could barely follow but which deeply shaped me. Today students come to my house for *café con leche*, and we work together towards common goals; my students also become de facto aunties and uncles to my children, who are more well-versed in social justice concepts and advocacy than most college students. My parents delivered this gift to my children through me.

Time and gratitude have a way of making the past sound idyllic. My childhood was real. My parents worked, and I spent time at home alone with my brother after school. When alone, we had epic fights. From my brother, I learned I could deeply affect another's emotional state to the point of physical action. I also learned to run like hell. During one of our many altercations, I used my words to drive him into a frenzy. This was typical. I was short and slight and could not physically overwhelm him. I saw the shift in his eyes, the curl of his fists, and I ran to my parents' bedroom and locked the door. It was the only room in our 20th-floor apartment that had a lock. My brother punched a hole through the door with his bare fist. I was scared for a moment, but empowered for the rest of my life. I developed a strong sense of efficacy in my ability to influence others into action through my words, and I knew to be cautious for the strengths of those responses could cause harm to myself or others.

Beyond my nuclear family, extended family had an important role in my cultural programming. My maternal grandfather was a business owner who left Cuba on a homemade raft to seek economic opportunity in the US. When he arrived in Puerto Rico, he built a successful business and found love anew. But for the fact that he was already married, it would be a romantic tale of migration. My mother, aunt and uncles, and maternal grandmother left Cuba by airplane in 1966 after my grandfather was established in Puerto Rico. The family had been well off in Cuba. My mother, a light-skinned Cuban child, had been raised with dark-skinned Cuban helpers who did everything from cleaning and cooking to childrearing that involved breastfeeding, grooming, and general caring. When she arrived in Puerto Rico, the family started anew, as many immigrants do, and lived with limited means for quite some time. Mami lived within limited means longer than others in my extended family because Papi was a hippy graduate student in sociology, and he was extremely sensitive to socioeconomic disparities. Our economic limitations were real, but also temporary. The experience of temporary poverty and the accompanying resilience it can afford has been captured in other testimonies (e.g. Bernal, 2017).

During our years in New Haven, my parents struggled with protecting us from serious discrimination. My brother was pelted with rocks by kids claiming he did not belong "here," and neighbors refused to open the door for me, "that little spic," on Halloween. After our return to Puerto Rico, our positionality shifted dramatically. We moved to a building in Rio Piedras. It was a very modest area. There I met Fernandito, my first real friend. As I recall it, my friendship with Fernandito was not entirely well received. I was confused by the unspoken but palpable apprehension toward this friendship. There were prompts to play with other children. I should play with children more "like me." I don't recall by whom or when these messages were transmitted or what signals in the environment led me to see that particular reality. Over the years, as I made sense of other interactions, I assumed the apprehension was fueled by Fernandito's blackness; not just skin color, but facial features and hair texture as well as family history and cultural practices and values. In the Puerto Rican context, blackness seemed more normative, but in the Cuban context, there was clear push for separation of Black and White. In cutting-edge academic lingo, I was experiencing *colorism* (Chavez-Dueñas, Adames, & Organista, 2014) from a position of privilege. Colorism is the expression of prejudice based on skin color and other physical characteristics that suggest African or Indigenous heritage. Back then, I was growing up in two worlds, navigating different expectations and values that I associated with my parents' differing national origins. It is important to me to honor my parents' claim; they recall a different story that did not involve colorism. Yet the veracity of the story is perhaps irrelevant as these personal narratives shaped me personally and professionally; I was not shaped by an objective reality but by my interpretation of it.

I do remember being explicitly taught the difference between Blacks and Whites because I had difficulty seeing racial differences as a child. It was an informal and jocose training based on my parents' discovery, by some forgotten coincidence, of my inability to correctly categorize people as Black or White. I suspect my difficulty was not related to any personal characteristic, but to the reality that there were many shades of brown in Puerto Rico and a simple "black and white" dichotomy is nearly impossible to adhere to when categorizing people who live on the island. Is Daddy Yankee Black or White? Does the answer change if he is compared to Ricky Martin? What about when compared to Celia Cruz? These early experiences trained me to present my current students with questions to challenge their assumptions. Rich programs of research on prejudice, discrimination, and, especially, implicit attitudes served to validate my experiences as a child. Implicit attitudes or biases "are thoughts and feelings that often exist outside of conscious awareness, and thus are difficult to consciously acknowledge and control" (Hall et al., 2015, e60). Implicit attitudes tend to be automatically expressed without ill intent on the part of the actor; these are the result of years of socialization as part of a particular cultural group. As the years progressed, I noticed how many adults were participating in my socialization as a cultural being, programming my biases.

Power of the Matriarchs

Two women were instrumental in my development and in my getting woke. My biological paternal grandmother, Abuela Toña, and my maternal great-grandmother, María Luisa, "Ita." To this day, I carry symbols that remind me of their continued presence in my life. I wear Abuela Toña's wedding ring on my left (dominant) hand, and I named by eldest daughter after Ita. I keep pictures of both of them in my home and workspaces. They live in me. Their love has never left me.

Abuela Toña was a petite woman, skin a light *café con leche, azabache* hair that was straight as a pin, and a "native" nose and forehead. She was a quiet Puerto Rican woman. One of my vivid memories of her is a vine-style gesture over her lips as if closing a padlock. She would lock eyes with me and, with a swift gesture, remind me that silence was a choice made in the service of larger goals. When she spoke, it was powerful, memorable. She chided me every time I returned from the beach with a tan: "you are wasting the gift you were given," referring to the fact I was darkening my light skin. I would roll my eyes internally, the way my students now report they do when they are home with their "racist" families. But I did not speak up or challenge her. I was silenced by my love for her and my desire to behave in ways that communicated that love respectfully. Yet once I saw that cultural socialization, I couldn't unsee it.

Abuela Toña was not the only strong woman that I both deeply loved and, on occasion, disagreed with. Ita, my great-grandmother, was another powerful force in my life. She raised my mother and grandmothered me. She was loving, smart, strong. She was an elder, so when I began seriously dating someone at 17, I brought him to meet her. My joy quickly withered when she pinched me, pulled me to her kitchen, and growled, "How dare you bring THAT into my house?!" "That" was my first real boyfriend. I thought he was quite the catch, a handsome college student that was the son of a judge. "*¡Es un negro!*" [He's Black!]. I refocused my eyes and looked again. Medium-dark skin, tight curly hair, wide-set nose, thick lips, and so on. OK. "*¿Pero qué tiene?*" [So what?] The only response: "*¡Es un negro!*" That was sufficient explanation and I should understand.

These women that I love were products of their social context. Their strength of character may have been a liability, perhaps locking in biases. To their credit, they were able to hold complexity, and they taught me that also. Ita's son, my great-uncle, is a brilliant mathematician and educator. He is a gay man whose handsome features made him particularly vulnerable to the mockery of men and women in Cuba in the 1940s and 1950s. Men and women both likely agreed that his good looks were "wasted" on a gay man, and he became a target of explicit discrimination. My great-grandmother did not approve of his sexual orientation, but she also loved him profoundly and protected him from the physical harm that family and community members wished they could have inflicted upon him. They lived together until she died in the late 1980s, and he feels her loss as an open wound to this day. I understood families are complex and so was love, even maternal love.

Just as time and gratitude have a way of making the past sound idyllic, telling specific stories can make the past fit neatly into one simple box. There was pain in these moments and these stories, and I share them to uncover my own cultural socialization, to push myself to see, to stay woke. And these two women, along with Mami, taught me about strength, personal power, love, humility, dignity. They made me feel loved and safe in the world. They were not perfect. Neither am I. They were valuable and love-worthy. These stories are not to vilify them. These stories were moments, the firepits lighting up in the vast cave of my consciousness. Our closeness allowed the fire within me to kindle. With enough light, I started to get woke. By the time I was a college-bound adolescent, I was well programmed to see class, race, sexual orientation, and gender as important factors in personal, interpersonal, and social dynamics. I understood many of my privileges, yet I had yet not awoken to how I was embedded in a colonial context. I had to physically leave the colony to "see" the colony.

Cultural Programming

These family stories have made their way into my classroom teaching as I attempt to engage students in their own learning journeys. Over the years, teaching on diversity and multiculturalism, I have found myself grasping for a term that would capture the passive and pervasive ways in which individuals are shaped by their environments and that result in our unchecked implicit attitudes and biases. I call this *cultural programming*. I use this term as an instrument in teaching. I have learned that pointing to external forces that exert their influence on individuals' behaviors seems to allow students to engage with an honest exploration of privilege and identity in a manner that invites reflection rather than resistance.

Cultural programming is complicated. Parents, grandparents, aunt, uncles, family, friends, and neighbors can all be tasked with socializing children. The task is to culturally program youths for optimal success in our society as we know it. Families use stories to pass on histories and enculturate their young into these and other value systems (Imada & Yussen, 2012). Storytellers build on their own experiences to provide warning and guidance so their young do not make the same mistakes. Families transmit *consejos* [advice] and also shape the listening behaviors of children by providing attention, a warm lap, or other loving contexts. After all, *el que no oye consejo, no llega a viejo* [Those that do not listen to advice do not reach old age]. As I grew older, and perhaps wiser and more woke, I learned to listen beyond the message. Abuela's chiding for tanning was not necessarily a message about rejecting others; her voice carried the pain of her own rejection. Her Taína physical features earned her the spot as the ugliest of eight siblings and some hurtful nicknames. *My* light skin was *her* evidence of a legacy for a better life for me. The layers of cultural programming were many and textured.

The ability to observe my cultural programming has been a lifelong process. Clarity appears sometimes at unusual moments. By 17 years of age, I was well-trained to notice skin color, lip thickness, hair texture, eye shape, and nose shape; others' and my own. Some lessons registered a bit more slowly. For example, all my life and into my thirties, my mother would chase me around with hairbrushes in an attempt to smooth out my curls. I often looked like a meme of Frankenstein's bride. I resolved to let my hair grow out, which was wonderfully cis-female and socially accepted, and for many years, I wore it in a ponytail or with a headband and just submitted to the hair brushing, at times even enjoying it. That stopped suddenly in my thirties when a hairdresser asked me why I was using a hairbrush. "Doesn't everyone use a hairbrush?" She matter-of-factly said, "Not people with curls like yours." Here was a piece of cultural programming exposed. How I could participate in this cultural process and not know it? We are never done growing up, exposing cultural programming, learning, waking up.

Negotiating the pieces of cultural programming that I wanted to keep and those I did not was challenging. There were many moments in my childhood that I remained silent. I didn't challenge Abuela when she frowned upon my tan.

I didn't call my great-grandmother racist when she did not approve of my boyfriend's blackness. The silenced voice of my younger self has made itself heard through my life's work. As a psychologist I know there isn't one simple explanation for my silence. It was partly fueled by cultural prescriptions of respect toward authority figures, especially parents and grandparents. How could I possibly call my family out on racism, sexism, homophobia? It was partly fueled by my confusion and lack of words for what I was experiencing. My silence was partly fueled by constant reminders that *los niños hablan cuando las gallinas mean* [children speak when hens pee]. Speaking up would be disrespectful, and I was *una niña bien educada* [a properly socialized child].

My silence was perhaps the result of others' silences. When my great-grandmother and great-uncle resolved to not address his gayness so as to avoid conflict, there was silence. For many years, the word "gay" would not even be uttered, and when it was, it only appeared in hushed tones. After my great-grandmother mother died, my great-uncle's gayness was somehow more accepted, more open, but not fully so. I learned that one person's disapproval can be powerful enough to silence a whole family. Those that supported my uncle's sexual orientation were affected by those whose conditional love demanded silence on the issue. I learned that disapproval was not an all-or-nothing proposition. Those who were supportive of my uncle while Ita was alive said later, "I don't mind that he's gay; I just don't need to have it rubbed in my face all the time." Shedding bias can take generations (Clement, 2015).

Seeking Understanding in Scholarly Pursuits

In my work, I have sought to understand cultural context broadly, and families in their cultural context specifically. When I look at my career, seemingly coincidental and accidental bits come together into a coherent whole. As a graduate student, I spent a summer working at the Mexican Institute of Psychiatry (IMP) through a Fogarty International Center fellowship. That experience marked the beginning of what has now been an almost 20-year collaboration with colleagues at the IMP. That collaboration afforded me the first opportunity to publish scholarly work in Spanish. I had acculturated to the US mainland, and it was time to enculturate. Publishing in Spanish was an act of resistance toward intellectual colonization. Imagine the heartbreak when I realized that Spanish is also a colonial language. There are cages within cages.

Early work on adolescents, substance use, and media messages helped me understand the importance of developmental context in examining outcomes. I learned that US-born Latinx adolescents responded positively to beer advertisements in English but responded negatively to beer advertisements in Spanish; teens verbalized that the pairing of the beer with cultural symbols and activities was a "diss" of their culture (Domenech Rodríguez, 1999). I also learned that some theories could explain behaviors across groups. In my dissertation, I examined the utility of Primary Socialization Theory in predicting marijuana use among Mexican American and White adolescents. Primary Socialization Theory states that so-called antisocial behaviors like substance use and deviance are learned in three contexts – family, school, and peer clusters – and the impact of these three clusters varies by developmental stage (Oetting, Donnermeyer, & Deffenbacher, 1998). For Mexican American and White youths, parental disapproval, peer disapproval, and school success predicted lifetime and 30-day use of marijuana. But the variables did not predict equally; school success was a stronger predictor of marijuana use for White than Latinx youths. The experiences of Latinxs in US schools turned out to be more complicated than I had imagined. In working with adolescents, I realized I wanted to work with younger children to truly be able to engage in prevention, and working with younger children de facto meant working with parents.

Latinx children and families are a population, not an area of expertise. I progressed to deepen my knowledge and struggled to understand the places and spaces in which I *wanted to* and in which I *could* support productive social change. I became involved with the Family Research Consortium III, a national network of postdoctoral research fellows and mentors, through which I was lucky to be placed at the University of Washington under my first Latina mentor, Ana Mari Cauce. Ana Mari helped me grow as a Latina scholar and taught me how to be ferocious and unapologetic in my academic pursuits. She gave me a beautiful office, a lifetime of stories, and the freedom to follow my passions and develop my expertise during my fellowship. My postdoc was not the indentured servitude that others experience. When my first child was born, Ana Mari took the initiative to ask me about my plans for childcare and encouraged me to bring María Luisa to work with me. Up until that time, I had navigated a male-dominated academic context. Her acknowledgement and celebration of womanhood and motherhood shaped my development as a teacher and a mentor.

During my postdoc, I met Marion Forgatch. Marion taught me about evidence-based interventions and, not just allowed, but *encouraged* my pursuit of cultural adaptations to her treatment manuals. Because of her, today there are cultural adaptations of the Parent Management Training – Oregon Model (Generation PMTO™) intervention for Latinx families in Mexico, Michigan, Oregon, and Utah. My mentees, colleagues, and I have secured multiple grants to promote this work, and we have met with great success in serving families in need in ways that are appropriate for their cultural context. We have told the tale in many publications and have significantly contributed to pushing forward a national and international agenda on cultural adaptation of evidence-based interventions. I have learned how to tinker with manualized interventions to balance fidelity to the treatment while properly addressing cultural fit. My colleagues and I have wrangled with the notion of culturally adapted vis-à-vis culturally grounded treatments and whether the former are warranted or are just expressions of intellectual colonization. We checked ourselves often. We pushed for many adaptations. I learned from Marion, the original developer of GenerationPMTO, that manualized interventions are written on paper, not stone tablets, and they are organized in three-ring binders because they are *supposed to be flexible*; they are *meant to be adapted* (Forgatch & Domenech Rodríguez, 2016). Marion helped me see the obvious: treatments are developed in the service of helping families, not in the service of promoting of our academic agenda and ourselves. Her advice perfectly aligned with Liberation Psychology (Tate, Rivera, Brown, & Skaistis, 2013). She put a beating heart into my operational definition of science.

In many ways, my postdoctoral experience was a process of academic "deprogramming." For example, in the process of culturally adapting GenerationPMTO, I asked people in communities to be research partners. I developed relationships with amazing people in my community and learned a great deal about what I didn't know about working with Latinx families. While I knew my family, and we were "Latinos," my experience as a Latina in the US was dramatically different than that of the families we were serving in the Cache Valley, Utah. Even though I had substantial experience working in Mexico City, the families that migrated to the US didn't look like those of my colleagues and collaborators in Mexico. The families that migrated to the Cache Valley had particular characteristics that warranted careful examination and care. As a Latina scholar working with Latinx families, I was absolutely working cross-culturally. There were poignant moments in which my privilege was revealed, especially related to economic status and citizenship.

The intervention work in Utah laid part of the foundation for strengthening and extending collaborative relationships with treasured colleagues such as Marion Forgatch, Ana Baumann, Rubén Parra-Cardona, Nancy Amador-Buenabad. My graduate students played a significant role in service delivery – Melissa Donovick, Elisaida Méndez, and Jesús Rodríguez helped deliver the intervention trial in Logan (Domenech Rodríguez, Baumann, & Schwartz, 2011). We served 87 families, some during the traumatic local Immigration and Customs Enforcement raids (Baumann, Domenech Rodríguez, & Parra-Cardona, 2011). These students are now all doctors in their own right. In 2010, Ana and I packed our bags to train therapists in Mexico City. Nancy was waiting for us with open arms and Sipatkli, our Mexico-based intervention team, was born. In that trial, 87 more families were served in Mexico City (Baumann, Domenech Rodríguez, Amador Buenabad, Forgatch, & Para-Cardona, 2014). That same year, I conducted training in Michigan with Rubén Parra-Cardona to deliver GenerationPMTO to local Latinx families. In Michigan, 103 Latinx families were served (Parra-Cardona et al., 2017). Rubén has been a pioneer in learning how to engage Latino fathers, with truly amazing results.

Preliminary findings of the Mexico City randomized controlled trial (RCT) showed excellent acceptability and strong movement in child externalizing behavior as well as parental depression. In Mexico, we delivered the culturally adapted GenerationPMTO intervention, focusing on adaptations to the existing lessons. In one of the RCTs in Mexico, families saw improvements in parenting and child outcomes compared to control families (N = 202; Amador et al., under review). In Michigan, we studied the adapted intervention and compared it to a different cultural adaptation where cultural content, such as immigration struggles and biculturalism, were added. Findings from the Michigan implementation showed significant change in parenting practices and excellent acceptability (N = 103; Parra-Cardona et al., 2017). We learned that parents enjoyed the cultural content in the sessions, and they also reported a great sense of urgency about their children's wellbeing. Sessions were organized to prioritize skills development, and the cultural content augmented the benefits of the intervention, suggesting both additive and transformative cultural adaptations were warranted (Bernal & Domenech Rodríguez, 2012).

Intervention work is slow and effortful. Parallel lines of research in cultural adaptation led to a meta-analysis, an edited volume, and a special issue. My work in cultural adaptations was motivated by theoretical and ethical considerations. Over time, we documented the importance of cultural adaptations empirically. Culturally adapted treatments work, and more adaptations result in better outcomes (Smith, Domenech Rodríguez, & Bernal, 2011). When I was personally challenged at a conference by treatment providers about the feasibility of culturally adapting treatments, I sought to understand what providers were doing in sessions, and we learned that they are making adaptations "on the fly" that very much matched what the cultural adaptation models recommend (Koslofsky & Domenech Rodríguez, 2017). Our findings were giving me confidence in the utility of cultural adaptations.

Professional and Personal Blend

In the midst of all this work, I was experiencing profound personal transformations. In 2001, I gave birth to my best teacher in parenting. My eldest daughter, María Luisa, was my first and best parent trainer. She was born at the time when I was engaging the first set of translations for the original GenerationPMTO parenting manuals. I was ready to be a perfect parent! I was trained in an evidence-based parenting intervention, after all. She has been a fierce woman from the get-go, challenging me at every step to live by my words. She uttered her first sentence as toddler: "I do it!" This was not the triumphant exclamation of a toddler that has figured something out, but rather the frustrated admonishment of a toddler whose overly attentive mother insisted on buckling her car seat despite her child's desire to do it herself. And with that statement, she made me question whether I was truly embracing a maieutic or Socratic approach to teaching. Was I teaching her to be her own woman? Empowered and self-efficacious? I was not. I was doing for her what she could do for herself. As the years progress, I find that my interactions with her are where I most clearly see the clash between my multicultural/feminist orientation and incongruent behavioral prescriptions of my Latinx cultures. The behavioral prescriptions for *respeto* often are in direct opposition to any form of liberation. María Luisa's lessons have been critical in uncovering my vulnerabilities as a teacher and mentor. In the power structures of academia, my mentees seldom "call me out" on my incongruences, so I have worked to uncover them myself and name them in the course of our work together. My fearless daughter has been instrumental in serving as a mirror for me to see my pedagogical practices.

As I started feeling a sense of increased efficacy in parenting, my second child was born. My Baby Dragon arrived and everything I thought I knew about parenting and parent training evaporated into thin air. My Baby Dragon has a mild and sweet temperament. There are no frustrations, no struggles for control and autonomy. They have been happy to love and be loved. Their challenge for my growth has been one of advocacy. My Baby Dragon identifies as pansexual and nonbinary. Their disclosures have put into sharp relief my need to consistently confront discrimination. The notion that I may remain silent until I could figure a "right" or "therapeutic" way to confront discrimination has been directly challenged, and this has led me to wonder if some of my silences have been tied to avoidance and privilege, wrapped in eloquent academic discourse. With their realization that they are attracted to people across the gender identity spectrum, an awareness grew in the core of my being that silence was no longer an option. It is not an intellectual response; it feels like a moral imperative. In addition, their generosity in sharing their sexual orientation and gender identity with me has also pushed me more fervently toward incorporating intersectionality and social advocacy in my work.

These two young people taught me perhaps one of the most powerful lessons about delivering evidence-based interventions, and the stuff that is hardest to capture in training or intervention manuals: that emotions play an enormous role in what we do and how we do it. Love, anger, frustration, confusion, embarrassment. I am much more mindful of emotions in my clinical work, teaching, and mentorship. My teaching, clinical practice, and supervision have shifted from "telling what to do" to a collaborative stance, a dialogic orientation. A dialogic orientation is

> expressed in the need to incorporate the cultural knowledge and the people's voices. The need to understand that everything happens within social relationships, and that the other in those relations has to be not only acknowledged, but also heard and answered. A dialogue implies another person, an Other, who needs to be accepted not as a subject, but as a social actor, who must be respected, who constructs knowledge, who has a history. So, there must be mutual respect. In those relationships, both the human actors and the very relationship changes. As consequence, the Other is conceived as an active person, not a passive entity, a mere reacting being.
>
> *(Montero & Sonn, 2009, p. 2)*

Interestingly, there is empirical evidence that a collaborative approach reduces resistance in psychotherapy (Patterson & Forgatch, 1985), and my own experience is consistent with those findings. The collaborative approach is also fundamentally consistent with a multicultural/feminist stance.

Paying It Forward

Thus far, it might seem as though I could have carried out my work anywhere and met success. I think the truth is far from that. My longer-term academic home, Utah State University (USU), has been critical to my success. At USU, I have been surrounded by social justice advocates and scholars who provided me a community to grow in. These scholars were academic mothers and sisters. Two senior colleagues showed me many ropes and provided a stable and loving "academic home" for my academic sister and I to belong. I have also been fortunate to belong to important professional homes like the Society for the Psychological Study of Culture, Ethnicity, & Race (APA Division 45) and the National Latina/o Psychological Association (NLPA). NLPA in particular has provided me with the community of Latinx psychologists who supported my socialization by way of content (e.g. liberation psychology) and process knowledge (e.g. *liderazgo*; Miville et al., 2017).

My leadership activities with NLPA have been particularly transformational. In my time on the leadership council, I had the privilege of experiencing the power of collective commitment. Discussions at leadership council meetings and at NLPA conferences about important social problems resulted in real actions that included academic and policy reports, networking with other organizations to lobby for policy changes, and developing resources to provide direct support to Latinxs, whether through mentoring initiatives for students or development of informational sheets for use in communities. NLPA has provided a surprisingly safe space for easy and difficult conversations alike. Prior to my arrival on the leadership council, my colleagues discussed their collective sociodemographic privilege, and this awareness led to the development of Orgullo, a special interest group focused on advancing LGBTQI+ issues within NLPA. During my presidency, Orgullo's efforts were so notable that they received a presidential citation at the 2016 NLPA conference. More recently, we have developed a professional ethics guideline document that articulated a Latinx-centered perspective of ethics in psychology (NLPA, under review). Through concerted collective action, we have worked to transform psychology in ways that will be evident well into the future.

The highlight of my career has been the ability to mentor and support students, who begin their journeys as my academic "children" and eventually become my professional brothers and sisters. Every student I have mentored has provided me opportunities for growth and learning. Some have helped me uncover pieces of my cultural programming, and in so doing, they have modeled great ways for educating others. I will never ever forget the day a graduate student called me out on using a slur in Spanish. Much of my professional training has occurred in an English-speaking context. I have great mastery of the English language and its metaphors, at least in the US context. But we were speaking in Spanish, and I was happily wading in my comfort zone when I let out a joke about a person that I described as *mongólico*. The literal definition of *mongólico* is a person from Mongolia. The popular use in Puerto Rico is a denigrating slur used to refer to someone with limited intellectual abilities. Research has found that people exhibit fewer biases when making decisions in a foreign language than in their native language, which might be due to the increased psychological distance and the reduction of emotional reaction associated with a foreign language (Keysar, Hayakawa, & An, 2012). I had never stopped to consider the word until I was invited to do so by Elisaida, a former mentee. It was part of the landscape of my language. Awareness led to shame. I also felt gratitude for Elisaida's courage in correcting me. I am grateful to have had enough humility at the time to recognize that and thank her for the gift she gave me. Eventually, I was able to share that story more widely through a TEDxUSU talk about failures in multicultural exchanges (Domenech Rodríguez, 2014). Many students have benefited since from my increased humility and incorporation of this lesson to my training.

Early on in my career, I developed a mentoring statement to ensure that students and I engaged in a process of consent for the mentor-mentee relationship. The latest version can be found here: www.domenechrodriguez.com/mentorship-statement/. Most of my relationships with advisees have included a strong personal connection. Thankfully, colleagues have written about mentoring relationships between faculty and students of color to provide guidance and validation for the personal nature of these relationships (e.g. Castellanos, Gloria, Besson, & Clark Harvey, 2016). I have experienced profound joys at the many successes including graduations, marriages, births and adoptions, professional appointments and awards, and – perhaps most satisfying – "lives well lived" full of travel, laughter, and meaningful engagement with the world. I have also experienced challenges and profound sorrows. Challenges have varied tremendously. Some relationship disruptions have been painful; being called "a sellout" for pursuing a tenure-track appointment or being told my privilege got in the way of my understanding. The longevity of my relationships with students with whom I've experienced challenges is my best evidence that we negotiated those impasses successfully. I am grateful for the risks they took. Mostly, external forces led me to witness pain and experience it vicariously, from rushing a student to the emergency room during conference travel to accompanying others through psychiatric hospitalizations, relationship dissolutions, domestic violence, and family woes. I have witnessed homelessness and overuse of substances. I have witnessed the devastation from sexual harassment and assaults. I have walked besides students when they have experienced denigration by community members and police officers. Staying woke is "both a defeating and empowering praxis of existence" (Ashlee et al., 2017, p. 98). I am grateful to be able to bear witness and to join in, and it is enraging and exhausting to constantly witness injustice and inequity.

In these journeys, I have nourished hope with the realization that we are living life together, and like family, our bonds go beyond moments. Building community helps shield us all against the negative effects of prejudice, discrimination, and stress (Hope, Hoggard, & Thomas, 2016). The challenges are opportunities to build our strong, lifelong ties, and the good times give us stories to tell and laugh about in the future. Recently, however, this comfort was shattered when a doctoral student who had joined my research lab a mere two months prior completed suicide. The student, an international student with multiple marginalized identities and a significant trauma history, was experiencing a poor fit in her research lab. Her multicultural and feminist interests were a great fit for mine, so I had invited her to join our lab family. I was hopeful we would all bond and she would thrive. But the broader dynamics that led to her distress had not yet been fully addressed. It is difficult to put into words the impact of this event as it is still fairly recent. I have considered it a profound failure of mentorship and have had to actively fight my "flight response" to stop mentoring students. The parallel process is not lost on me. The complexities of experiencing and honoring my own grief, supporting students in theirs, and navigating departmental dynamics surrounding this tragedy have been overwhelming.

The classroom, usually an extension of my mentoring realm, will soon be a welcome retreat. I typically take a mentoring approach to classroom teaching. In my seminars, I use my knowledge about cultural programming, cultural adaptations, and effective interventions. Right after my promotion to Full Professor, when I was officially free to take risks, I taught Multicultural Psychology with a team of graduate and undergraduate students of color, and we made a big change from my typical instruction. We told students at the outset: "We are looking to change you: your attitudes, your beliefs, and your values. If this does not sit well with you, you may want to drop this class." Nobody dropped the class. In fact, the course was over-enrolled. We gave the students measures of colorblind racial attitudes, ethnocultural empathy, and professional beliefs about diversity during the first week of classes and at the end of the semester. Over the course of two years, we saw colorblind attitudes decrease and ethnocultural empathy and professional beliefs about diversity significantly increase from the beginning to the end of the semester. Perhaps most satisfying of all, these shifts were not tied to the students' final grades, suggesting that their attitude shift was not contingent upon grades (Patterson, Papa, Reveles, & Domenech Rodríguez, in press). We are now tasked with finding out if these changes hold over time.

Pulling Pieces Together

As I reflect on this narrative, I notice a pattern of being surrounded by powerful women from birth – mother, grandmother, great-grandmother – through my professional career – mentors, colleagues, students, friends. I also notice an intrinsic drive to understand the world around me and to make sense of it, but also to change it in the service of justice and equity. While I have clarity in my values, I also understand that humans are fallible and that I can fail to execute my values in a way that leads to my desired outcomes. Using scientific methods to examine key questions can provide evidence for utility of specific initiatives. I trust my humanity to be fallible, so I employ science to keep myself in check. I have learned that science too is fallible, so I engage collaborations and multiple methods in the hopes of reducing those fallibilities. I engage this work because I feel a deep sense of responsibility to leave a legacy for my children and my mentees that is both personal and social. I hope for them that they may walk in the world always feeling my love right at their backs, like a warm Caribbean breeze, sustaining them and lifting them up to do good work and to live a plentiful life in which struggles are learning opportunities and successes are the result of collective effort. I am humbled that I can witness the growth and development of my children and my students. I am often awed by their potential, and I treasure the opportunities to learn from them.

I would love to be able to conclude that I am now a wise Latina, but I'm still on my journey. In my childhood, I learned about the power of skin color and my personal privilege in having light skin, temporary poverty, highly educated parents, and a heterosexual orientation. I owe a debt of gratitude to writers and scholars that have helped me get woke. I feel a delectable pleasure in reading Willie Perdomo's (1995) "Nigger-Reecan Blues" and also the brilliant writing of scholars like Hector Adames and Nayeli Chavez-Dueñas (2017). Their words validate my experiences and give me energy to continue asking questions and learning the answers.

The most powerful movement toward staying woke has come from interpersonal interactions, especially with people that I love and trust. I am still learning about the impact of colonization on the thinking and feeling of individuals and society. I got woke to the fact that Spanish is a colonial language, that judging other Latinxs for their bilingualism, or lack thereof, was simply participating in my own oppression (Pyke, 2010). I have learned to see colonial mentality in a de facto "drop of white blood" rule, where any indications of roots from Spain are highlighted and all others are obscured. I am becoming immersed in mujerista psychology (Bryant-Davis & Comas-Díaz, 2016), which resonates with me deeply. There is much work yet to be done. Staying woke is a constant act of rebellion.

Note

1 Reprinted with permission

References

Adames, H. Y., & Chavez-Dueñas, N. Y. (2017). *Cultural foundations and interventions in Latino/a mental health: History, theory, and within-group differences*. New York: Routledge.

Amador Buenabad, N. G., Sánchez Ramos, R., Díaz Juárez, A. D., Guitiérrez López, M. L., Ortiz GallegosA. B. … Villatoro Velázquez, J. A. (under review). Efectividad del modelo Huellitas-CAPAS-Mx para la prevención de conductas de riesgo a partir del desarrollo de habilidades sociales y de prácticas de parentalidad positiva en niños y sus cuidadores. [Effectiveness of Huellitas-CAPAS-Mx for the prevention of risky behavior through development of social skills and parenting skills in children and their caregivers].

Ashlee, A. A., Zamora, B., & Karikari, S. N. (2017). We are woke: A collaborative critical auto ethnography of three "womxn" of color graduate students in higher education. *International Journal of Multicultural Education*, 19(1), 89–104.

Ayala, C. J., & Bernabe, R. (2007). *Puerto Rico in the American century: A history since 1898*. Chapel Hill, NC: University of North Carolina Press.

Baumann, A. A., Domenech Rodríguez, M., Amador Buenabad, N., Forgatch, M. S., & Para-Cardona, J. R. (2014). Parent Management Training – Oregon Model (PMTOTM) in Mexico City: Integrating cultural adaptation activities in an implementation model. *Clinical Psychology: Science and Practice*, 21(1), 32–47. doi: 10.1111/cpsp.12059

Baumann, A., Domenech Rodríguez, M., & Parra-Cardona, J. R. (2011). Community-based applied research with Latino immigrant families: Informing practice and research according to ethical and social justice principles. *Family Process*, 52(2), 132–148. doi: 10.1111/j.1545–5300.2011.01351.x

Bernal, G. (2017). Multiculturalism – The final frontier: Resistance is not futile. In J. M. Casas, L. A. Suzuki, C. M. Alexander, & M. A. Jackson (Eds.), *Handbook of Multicultural Counseling* (4th ed.) (pp. 60–70). Los Angeles, CA: Sage.

Bernal, G., & Domenech Rodríguez, M. M. (Eds.). (2012). *Cultural adaptations: Tools for evidence-based practice with diverse populations*. Washington, DC: APA Press. doi: 10.1037/13752-000

Bryant-Davis, T., & Comas-Díaz, L. (Eds.). (2016). *Womanist and mujerista psychologies: Voices of fire, acts of courage*. Washington, DC: American Psychological Association.

Castellanos, J., Gloria, A. M., Besson, D., & Clark Harvey, L. O. (2016). Mentoring matters: Racial ethnic minority undergraduates' cultural fit, mentorship, and college and life satisfaction. *Journal of College Reading and Learning*, 46(2), 81–98. doi: 10.1080/10790195.2015.1121792

Chavez-Dueñas, N. Y., Adames, H. Y., & Organista, K. C. (2014). Skin-color prejudice and within-group racial discrimination: Historical and current impact on Latino/a populations. *Hispanic Journal of Behavioral Sciences*, 36(1), 3–26. doi: 10.1177/0739986313511306

Clement, S. (2015, April 7). Millennials are just about as racist as their parents. *The Washington Post*. Retrieved from: https://www.washingtonpost.com/news/wonk/wp/2015/04/07/white-millennials-are-just-about-as-racist-as-their-parents/?utm_term=.316b34678849

Domenech Rodríguez, M. M. (1999). Marijuana use among Mexican American and White, male and female adolescents: A practical application of Primary Socialization Theory. PhD thesis, Colorado State University.

Domenech Rodríguez, M. M. (2014, October). No way but through. USU TEDx. Retrieved from: https://www.youtube.com/watch?v=2orqr-nOIPk

Domenech Rodríguez, M. M., Baumann, A., & Schwartz, A. (2011). Cultural adaptation of an empirically supported intervention: From theory to practice in a Latino/a community context. *American Journal of Community Psychology*, 47(1–2), 170–186. doi: 10.1007/s10464–10010–9371–9374

Forgatch, M. S., & Domenech Rodríguez, M. M. (2016). Interrupting coercion: The iterative loops among theory, science, and practice. In T. J. Dishion & J. Snyder (Eds.), *The Oxford handbook of coercive relationship dynamics* (pp. 194–214). New York: Oxford University Press.

Hall, W. J., Chapman, M. V., Lee, K. M., Merino, Y. M., Thomas, T. W., Payne, K., … Coyne-Beasley, T. (2015). Implicit racial/ethnic bias among healthcare professionals and its influence on health care outcomes: A systematic review. *American Journal of Public Health*, 105(12), e60–e76. doi: 10.2105/ajph.2015.302903

Hope, E. C., Hoggard, L. S., & Thomas, A. (2016, June). Becoming an adult in the face of racism. *Monitor on Psychology*, 47(6), 35–38. Retrieved from: www.apa.org/monitor/

Imada, T., & Yussen, S. R. (2012). Reproduction of cultural values: A cross-cultural examination of stories people create and transmit. *Personality and Social Psychology Bulletin*, 38(1), 114–128. https://doi.org/10.1177/0146167211421938

Keysar, B., Hayakawa, S. L., & An, S. G. (2012). The foreign-language effect: Thinking in a foreign tongue reduces decision biases. *Psychological Science*, 23(6), 661–668. https://doi.org/10.1177/0956797611432178

Koslofsky, S., & Domenech Rodríguez, M. M. (2017). Introduction to special issue: Cultural adaptations to psychotherapy: Real world applications. *Clinical Case Studies Journal*, 16(1), 3–8. doi: 10.1177/1534650116668273

Miville, M. L., Arredondo, P., Consoli, A. J., Santiago-Rivera, A., Delgado-Romero, E. A., Fuentes, M. A., … Cervantes, J. M. (2017, Online First). Liderazgo: Culturally grounded leadership and the National Latina/o Psychological Association. *The Counseling Psychologist*. doi: 10.1177/0011000016668413

Montero, M., & Sonn, C. (2009). About liberation and psychology: An introduction. In M. Montero & C. Sonn (Eds.), *Psychology of liberation: Theory and applications* (pp. 1–10). New York: Springer.

NLPA. (under review). Ethical Guidelines: National Latina/o Psychological Association. *Journal of Latina/o Psychology*.

Oetting, E. R., Donnermeyer, J. F., & Deffenbacher, J. L. (1998). Primary socialization theory: The influence of the community on drug use and deviance III. *Substance Use & Misuse*, 33(8), 1629–1665.

Parra-Cardona, J. R., Bybee, D., Sullivan, C. M., Domenech Rodríguez, M., Dates, B., Tams, L., & Bernal, G. (2017). Examining the impact of differential cultural adaptation with Latina/o immigrants exposed to adapted parent training interventions. *Journal of Consulting and Clinical Psychology*, 85(1), 58–71. doi: 10.1037/ccp0000160

Patterson, C., Papa, L. A., Reveles, A. K., & Domenech Rodríguez, M. M. (in press). Undergraduate student change in cultural competence: Impact of a multicultural psychology course.

Patterson, G. R., & Forgatch, M. S. (1985). Therapist behavior as a determinant for client noncompliance: A paradox for the behavior modifier. *Journal of Consulting and Clinical Psychology*, 53(6), 846–851. https://doi.org/10.1037//0022-006X.53.6.846

Perdomo, W. (1995). Nigger-Reecan blues. In R. Santiago (Ed.), *Boricuas: Influential Puerto Rican writings – an anthology*. One World: New York.

Pyke, K. D. (2010). What is internalized oppression and why don't we study it? Acknowledging racism's hidden injuries. *Sociological Perspectives*, 53(4), 551–572. doi: 10.1525/sop.2010.53.4.551

Real Academia de la Lengua Espanola. (2017). Cafre. Retrieved from: http://dle.rae.es/?id=6bsxzJj

Smith, T., Domenech Rodríguez, M. M., & Bernal, G. (2011). Culture. In J. Norcross & M. J. Lambert (Eds.), *Psychotherapy relationships that work: Evidence-based practices* (2nd ed.) (pp. 316–335). Cambridge: Oxford University Press.

Tate, K. A., Rivera, E. T., Brown, E., & Skaistis, L. (2013). Foundations for liberation: Social justice, liberation psychology, and counseling. *Interamericanan Journal of Psychology*, 47(3), 373–382.

5

HEAD OVER HEART

Hortensia de los Angeles Amaro

> Set your life on fire. Seek those who fan your flames.
>
> *Rumi*

Driving to work, through the loud speakers of cars, stores, and street vendors, the *rancheras* of Chavela Vargas and Pedro Infante, *corridos* of Los Tigres del Norte, and Celia's *salsa* beat make their way to my CuChiRican heart (Cuban-born, raised among Chicanos in Los Angeles, and lived with Puerto Ricans in Boston). That's me, a CuChiRican refugee, psychologist, advocate, and scientist, back in Los Angeles, for now.

The Beginning – *La Tierra de Los Tinajones,* the Land of the Jars

The decade my family and I lived in Camagüey was one of great beauty, exciting adventure, and imprinting trauma. It shaped me absolutely. Being born a Catholic Cuban girl in Camagüey Province in 1950 meant obedience, modesty, and feminine limitation. All things I came to question.

Do you know Camagüey? Most tourists skip it, deeming it unremarkable. For me, though, it was home and had its own kind of magic. Lost at sea, Cristóbal Colón stumbled upon Cuba in 1492, encountering Siboney, Guanahatabey, and Taino inhabitants with established communities. Few survived the onslaught of disease, mass suicides, and death due to Spanish exploitation. Two decades later, just around the time that my home town was founded, the mass importation of slaves began. By 1886, when Spanish Queen María Cristina abolished slavery in Cuba, there were about a million slaves, but de facto slavery, exploitation, and social inequities did not end then. Laws under Spanish rule had cemented clear social inequalities regarding race, gender, and sexual honor, which remained

(Arvey, 2012). The history of race in Cuba is complex and full of contradictions, evolved in distinct ways compared to the United States (Nodal, 1986). As early as 1880, José Martí, the Cuban poet, national hero, and revolutionary leader against Spanish rule, argued against slavery and promoted racial equality (Nodal, 1986). Although Cuba's 1940 constitution established equality based on race, gender, and class and while people of African ancestry have played critical roles in Cuban society throughout history, there is considerable debate about if and how the vestiges of slavery and discrimination continue to be evident in Cuba's socioeconomic hierarchy (Arvey, 2012; Clealand, 2013; de la Fuente, 1998).

Camagüey, Cuba's third-largest city, is halfway between the capital of Havana to the west and the seaport Santiago de Cuba to the east. My inland colonial town has been referred to as *La Ciudad Confusa*, the Confusing City, for its extremely labyrinthine layout. Built to perplex pirates and other invaders from centuries past, it features blind alleys everywhere and winding, snaking streets, some so narrow that only passers-by and those on bicycles can navigate them. Also, everywhere are *tinajones*, enormous earthenware jars, roughly the size and weight of a Smart car. *Tinajas*, as they're called in Spain, are round and have a large hole in the middle, like an open mouth, to capture and store rainwater. The medieval Moors introduced them to Andalucía, whose conquering sailors continued the tradition in Cuba. This is why Camagüey is also known as *La Tierra de Los Tinajones*, the Land of the Jars. There's an old saying: "The one who drinks water from the *tinajon* will remain forever in this place."

In this place, the whole world for nearly the first ten years of my life, there are green parks and Spanish public squares, lovely churches and cathedrals, and houses with wrought iron windows and inner patios. And beyond those, beneath swollen white cumulus clouds, cattle farms roll on and on and spiky sugar cane fields reach all the way to the azure horizon.

Do you see? Magic.

Mi Familia

As a middle-class family, we had what most in rural areas considered luxuries: running water, indoor plumbing, electricity, a refrigerator, plenty of food, a telephone, a television, a car, and parochial schools (Álvarez, 2004). My ultimate luxury was a surfeit of angels. Angel Amaro, my loving and handsome father, worked in the communication tower at the Camagüey airport, using Morse code – because of the telegraph key sound made when operated, we came to call it "*tiqui-tiqui*" – that his father, my *abuelito*, El Cabo Amaro, had taught him as a child. My grandfather, a lifelong telegrapher for the Cuban armed forces, was a figure of authority in his town – he was often seen in uniform riding his army horse through town. While not a wealthy man, Abuelito was respected and perceived as an intellectual among local folk, and he was a member of La Orden de Los Caballeros de la Luz (the Order of the Knights of Light) in his town of Florida.

My Abuelita Maria, El Cabo's wife, had a fourth-grade education. She was a typical *guajira*, a woman of the countryside. Together with my father, uncles (Alejandro, Luis, and Antonio), and godmother (Carmela), they lived on a modest plot of land where they harvested crops for household use, including coffee and *fruta bomba*, what you would call papaya. (We never said "papaya" out loud because it's slang for vagina.) They lived in what had been a small countryside train station – Abuelito had been the station master – previously operated by the Cuban armed forces. During the Cuban uprising against Spanish rule, the government created a railroad system throughout the island as a supply route for the armed forces to control the revolt. A humble, hard-working, and unpretentious woman of few words, Abuelita Maria was down to earth and a great cook. Like many other Cuban women of her era, she suffered Abuelito's infidelity and the financial and emotional diminishment caused by his having a parallel family in *la casa chica* – a well-known family "secret" Mami shared with me after his death.

Although poor by the standards of most city dwellers, Papi and his family made do. They lived in a rural neighborhood in Florida, a tiny town 25 miles northwest of Camagüey. When he was 14, Papi began taking crates of the homegrown *fruta bomba*, every weekend, on his bicycle to Florida's center to sell. He was earning centavos and dreaming of a better life. Imbued always with a strong sense of justice and democracy, Papi longed to become a lawyer. Patient, even-tempered, thoughtful, and logical, Papi was a *caballero*, a gentleman – and lean and strikingly handsome. But after high school, such a white-collar higher education was financially out of reach. Although university education was free, the cost of 30 pesos for housing in a *casa de huespedes* was beyond reach – my grandfather earned 30 pesos a month. Papi went to work at the *tiqui-tiqui* – officially as a telegrapher, first in the Cuban air force and then at Cubana Airlines at the Camagüey airport. When I did not have school, he would often take me to work with him at the air traffic control tower, and we would climb up the narrow spiral stairs that led to the glass-lined room where he did *tiqui-tiqui* and I watched the planes taking off and landing.

Hortensia Nodarse Amaro, my beautiful mother, after whom I'm named, earned her teaching degree tuition-free – after passing an arduous exam – from La Escuela Normal Para Maestros, the Normal School for Teachers. It's located in Santa Clara, the capital city of Villa Clara Province, almost exactly in the middle of Cuba. Afterward, Mami taught kindergarten in the town of Florida and later at a local public school in Camagüey – where she often took me to join her class before I was kindergarten age. A Florida native like Papi, Mami too had a challenging childhood, though for different reasons. Her father was Luciano Nodarse, whose family came from San Sebastián in northeastern Spain. They originally lived in Santa Clara – hence Mami's educational connection to that city – but moved to Florida when it was developing as a new town. Luciano built a whole block of wooden houses on the main street, which he rented to businesses. Initially, he made his money as a trader and later invested in real estate. I never knew him. He died at age 40 of a massive brain haemorrhage, when Mami was just a young girl.

A *viuda* – a respected status at the time, my Abuela Leonela Nodarse raised four children on her own after my grandfather's sudden early death. Abuela made sure that her children took advantage of the free higher education, resulting in two teachers, my mother and Aunt Lucia, and a pediatrician, my godfather, Rafael. My Aunt Ofelia (Ofe), who became a multilingual executive secretary for the president of the Cuban workers' union, studied in upstate New York, sent there by my grandmother, who knew the challenges a young woman with polio, like Ofe, would face in Cuban society. Mind you, Abuela did not have the advantage of higher education.

Abuela even took over Luciano's business and flourished, periodically moving with her brood from Florida to Havana to get Ofe medical treatment for polio. I tell you, Abuela was one tough and smart Cuban woman. A dignified fighter. Outspoken and stern, she overcame the challenges of being a woman head of household with no man to "protect them" – a concern Mami often mentioned to me. No wonder it took Papi two years of being confined to speaking to my mother through the front wrought iron window of Abuela's house to convince Abuela that he was a worthy suitor for Mami. You definitely didn't want to cross Leonela.

So whenever I think of Leonela's daughter, my mother Hortensia, as I often do, my mind always goes to her strength. Mami believed in women's rights when most women were not employed in the formal sector and did not drive a car, as she did (Arvey, 2012). Mami didn't refer to herself as a feminist, but her views were consistent with those of the Cuban feminist movement that in the 1920s and 1930s advocated for women's right to vote, for women's and children's rights, and for more equitable gender relations (Arvey, 2012). She spoke her mind and was as kind as she was demanding. It was important to her that all her children be *encaminados*, or settled and able to provide for and take care of ourselves.

We Were All Angels

My brother Rafael "Rafa" Angel Amaro, a year my senior, is the firstborn. He was a sort of Cuban Dennis the Menace, and smart, curious, adventuresome, and prone to temper tantrums that would come on strong and then pass like the summer. Rafa became a Harvard-trained internist, a dedicated son and father, and a generous man with an even-handed temperament. Through his career as a physician, Rafa took care of many poor immigrant Latino families, mentored Latino medical students, and helped Latino-serving community health centers improve patient care while transforming their bottom line from red to black. Most lovingly, he has shepherded those in our family who have faced terminal illnesses through the medical care system and ensured their comfort and dignity.

Next came Hortensia de los Angeles Amaro. I was shy, sweet, quiet. I was a "good" girl. But I had my naughty moments – we'll get to those shortly. In my first few years, I was practically bald, and Mami used many techniques with the hopes of spurring hair growth. As I got a bit older, she would take me to the hairdresser, who fashioned curls from an octopus-like contraption with electrical tentacles attached to my hair; this was before chemical perms.

My younger brother, Angel Armando Amaro, nine years my junior, was a beautiful baby and rather awkward teen who grew to be strikingly tall and handsome. He looked like El Cabo Amaro, my paternal grandfather, and unlike the rest of us had Abuelito's tan skin tone. He was gentle and funny, sensitive, and creative. More on Armando later.

Lucille "Lucie" Amaro, my baby sister, was born 14 years after me and 3 years after we fled Cuba. She was smart from the start – testing in the gifted category in third grade, a rebellious artiste who eventually turned into a mellow artist and therapist, meditation practitioner, and mother par excellence. Named after the social worker who helped us in the United States, Lucie was the only one among the Amaro children not to have "Angel" in her name, but her namesake was prophetic as Lucie went on to become a mental health clinician for recently arrived refugees from the Congo, Bhutan, Nepal, Iraq, and Syria. Surely that qualifies her.

A Girl's Red Schwinn Bicycle

Like most Cubans prior to 1959, we were a Catholic family. Not deeply devout, mind you. Papi was an agnostic. Mami, however, was a believer – not so much in the Church as an institution, of which she was critical, but in the teachings of Jesus, especially those of love and compassion. She kept a small prayer card on her bedroom dresser, that I saw every day – El Sagrado Corazón de Jesús. We celebrated La Pascua de Resurrección, Easter; Navidad, Christmas; and of course El Dia De Los Reyes Magos, Epiphany.

My 1958 Epiphany was particularly rewarding. That January, Los Reyes (i.e. my parents) brought me a girl's red Schwinn bicycle. Oh how I loved that *bicicleta roja*! Its bright candy apple red color stood out and made me feel special. Papi taught me how to ride it, and once I'd mastered that, I wanted to go everywhere and see everything. But I was a girl. I was not to stray past our street. Ever. Our house was three houses away from a dirt road lined with ramshackle dwellings. No well-brought-up White Catholic Camagüey girl had any business wandering over there. And yet, I yearned to see what lay beyond. One Saturday in spring, when the weather is especially wonderful (warm but not humid), we were eating our typical, and my favorite, breakfast. I sipped my sugary *café con leche* and dragged a torn chunk of freshly baked Cuban bread across a big plate of warm olive oil and garlic. That's when it came to me. I knew what I must do.

After breakfast on Saturday mornings, my brother Rafa and his guy friends often met up to go exploring on their bikes. They left behind the city parks and public squares, the mysterious, snaking streets, the churches and shops to ride out to the vast expanse and brightest sunlight of *el campo*, the countryside. I decided I would join them. Everything about my secret plan was forbidden. How many times was I told never to ride my bike past our block? A hundred times? A thousand? More? But I ached to go. How come Rafa, only one year older, got to go and not me? Was it because a few years earlier I had been seriously ill with hepatitis A and bedridden for what seemed like forever at my young age, or because my mother didn't want me to get my frilly dresses dirty, or because I was a girl? I believed it was the latter. So unfair! Even at 8 years old, I had ballsy ideas that made my heart beat nearly out of my chest. So what would it be? My head or my heart?

My red bike was kept in the garage, which gave me easy access and a quick way out. I slipped in there, got on the black seat, and raced away before Mami could notice and stop me. My wheels hit pavement and then dirt. I stopped suddenly on a mound, breathless and terrified. Dropping my head back, I looked heavenward. The sky was as blue as the sea, with low-hanging white cotton-candy clouds. Presently my curiosity outweighed fear of the forbidden. It was not lack of fear or disregard for how I was expected to behave that propelled me, but rather the thrill of exploration and self-determination – I would not allow fear to keep me from a path to discovery. So I pedaled on, a boat against the current, where only boys were allowed.

I never did find Rafa and his friends. I did, however, find one slice of my country in its urban *campo* essence: an endless landscape carpeted in beige cracked soil with royal palms in the distance. A cow carcass crowned by circling vultures. Not at all what is described in the traditional country song "*El Carretero*," the Cart Driver, which goes, "*el campo es el edén, más lindo del mundo entero,*" the countryside is Eden, the most beautiful in the entire world. I had seen that song's countryside in my father's extended family *bohio* and small *finca* in El Tomeguín, Matanzas. But just blocks from my house, that is not what the city's countryside offered. And as I witnessed with fear and anguish that day, one block away from my house on the dirt road under my bicycle wheels, the street was lined with shanty housing, outside of which played barefoot Black and mulatto children next to open filthy *zanjas* – drainage ditches covered in green muck. And so it was. My homeland was full of contrasts and inequities I would later come to understand. I rode home. It was the most thrilling day of my Cuban life. That bike ride and its psychological complexities would prove emblematic of the journey ahead.

The Immigration Ordeals

Being the eldest daughter of refugee parents is no *fiesta*. Actually, neither is being an immigrant, period. My family fled Cuba on a Sunday. To be even more precise, we fled on November 20, 1960 – 1 year, 10 months, and 20 days after Fidel Castro's *revolución*. It was just a month after the United States declared the first of several embargos on all American products to Cuba except for medicine and food and the arrest of Martin Luther King Jr. in Atlanta along with 280 students for the historic lunch counter sit-in. Why did we flee? Because my parents witnessed the failure to hold promised elections; to protect freedom of speech, enforced in part at the block level under the watchful eye of the *comites de la revolución*; and to ensure due process. Television images showed thousands of citizens having sham trials and being executed by the *el paredón* firing squads that had also killed previous Batista officials and others deemed enemies of the state. Initial supporters of the ideals espoused by the Sierra Maestra *barbudos*, my parents became disillusioned with the *revolución*'s failed promises. They forecasted dictatorship, and the idea of loss of freedom filled them with foreboding.

That October was the month that Soviet leader Nikita Khrushchev, in a fit of rage at a UN General Assembly debate, pounded his shoe on the table; a Cuban air force fighter plane buzzed the USS *Balao*, a US Navy submarine, in international waters for 37 minutes; and a Milwaukee woman splashed a whiskey-filled tumbler at Democratic candidate John F. Kennedy as he rode by in an open convertible. Politics which we had nothing to do with and even less control over would change our lives and our very identities. Instead of being Cuban, now we were Cuban refugees. We lost our paradise and were now *gusanos*, worms, for the sin of wanting to be free.

We were about to become Cuban exiles in need of asylum. Papi, Mami, Rafa, Angel Armando, and I were permitted one suitcase each at the José Martí International Airport, then known as the Rancho-Boyeros Airport, outside of Havana. Papi had tucked 500 American dollars inside the lining of a piece of our luggage, all the money he had. We did not know our future. As I clutched my beloved oversize, hard-plastic, bald baby doll against my chest, fearing she would be taken from me, we were put in *la pecera* – a glass-walled waiting room that served as the last homeland memory for hundreds of thousands of Cubans. My parents had not revealed the reason for our departure, but I knew this was no vacation trip. How did I know? The secrecy under which we packed and, before sunrise, left our home in Camagüey *en la madrugada* for Havana – not Camagüey airport, which was much closer; the load of soldiers with machine guns that surrounded us with despising looks; the drama of crying families inside and outside the *pecera*; the various times my father was taken into a secluded room for interrogation. And then, finally, we walked the long steaming tarmac to the gray metal passenger boarding stairs leading to the two-propeller Cubana de Aviación plane to Miami. Passengers hardly spoke.

Relief finally came – wheels hit US territory at the Miami International Airport. For a week – or was it a day? – we lived in a small hotel room and on Campbell's tomato soup – it was cheap and nutritious, sort of – that we heated up on a burner and ate with saltines. To this day, I don't much care for Campbell's tomato soup. Though I was only 9 years old – my birthday is in December – I grasped that this was the end of something. In my mind's eye, the view was the reverse of Dorothy's in *The Wizard of Oz*: It went from brilliant color to drab black and white. I felt fragmented and disoriented. We were in survival mode. All the innocence, beauty, and stability of my old life had vanished in a single flight that detached me from my *bicicleta roja* and our extended family, although most would eventually join us. I don't remember all the details of this period. My previous life is much more vivid. Maybe I had to tune out this time.

My parents found work in Miami factories. We moved to a one-bedroom apartment in the northwest, and Rafa and I were enrolled in public elementary school. The American children and teachers didn't speak Spanish. They didn't even try. Assigned a seat in the back of the fourth-grade classroom, I felt diminished, bewildered, comprehending nothing and unable to say anything. Gone were the slow-paced Cuban schooldays of walking home for lunch and a siesta before returning to school. All I could do now was follow the English-only herd heading to the cafeteria.

After school, a pack of older boys would routinely shadow Rafa and me, taunting and laughing at us – maybe just "normal" kid bullying. I had no idea what their words meant, but I didn't require translation. One day, a few boys started punching Rafa. Something came over me and I started punching one of them as hard as I could, right in the gut. The next thing I knew, I was on the ground with excruciating pain in my left eye – his blow was faster than mine. But I was OK with a black eye as the price for standing up for myself and my brother; it was worth it.

A Change of Pace

Physical violence was one way to defend myself, but it did not prove useful. The indisputable way forward was to learn English. Papi spoke a little English; Mami did not. Papi taught us some basic words and phrases – "apple," "hello," "how are you?" "thank you" – but I knew I needed fluency to make it through this change. Having command of English meant what the *bicicleta* had meant: the means to explore uncharted territory, and personal independence.

Five months later, around the time of the Invasión de Playa Girón (Bay of Pigs), we moved to California via the Cuban Refugee Resettlement Program (Mitchell, 1962). A decade earlier, Congress had passed legislation providing refugees from communist countries special admissions channels that facilitated immigration (Haines, 2015). Authorized by President Eisenhower in February 1961 in response to the mounting number of Cubans fleeing the Castro regime, by 1962, some 2,000 Cubans were arriving weekly in Miami. This federal program provided many forms of assistance, including up to $100 a month per family, employment, food, college student loans, retraining programs for professionals, child welfare services, medical care, and relocation assistance. Public and private sectors and religious and philanthropic organizations pitched in. Never before in US history had this nation become the country of first asylum for such large numbers of displaced persons (Mitchell, 1962). Referring to the US stance on Cuban refugees, the Commissioner of the Social Security Administration noted, "From the beginning the refugees have been considered not as intruders but as friends. Efforts in their behalf have been regarded not as burdens but as opportunities for service to fellow Americans, to be given with understanding and generosity" (Mitchell, 1962, p. 5). This was seized by Presidents Eisenhower and Kennedy as "an opportunity to demonstrate this country's humane dynamics, competence, and capacity for constructive social action" (Mitchell, 1962, p. 8).

During those early asylum years, Cubans were generally described as educated, resourceful, proud, courageous, and grateful people from every walk of life (Mitchell, 1962), and we were received with warmth and given opportunity to stand on our own two feet. A letter sent to the head of the Cuban Refugee Assistance Program by my dear friend Ana Anders (1961) – a Cuban refugee social worker who, from her arrival, joined efforts to help other Cuban refugees – expressed what my family felt and the spirit that should be applied toward other groups:

> Through persons like you, we learn to understand and love the people of this country. It is not only the financial help given to the refugees that counts, but the feeling of warmth, of friendship, of brotherhood. … It should be the same with Chinese, or African negroes.
>
> *(Para. 4)*

A One-Way Ticket Odyssey

On April 1961, with a one-way ticket, we arrived in Los Angeles and were greeted by Lucille Richards, the social worker assigned to us by the Cuban Refugee Relocation Program. Also at the airport were our sponsors, two American families from St. Mary's Episcopal Parish. They had arranged for a three-bedroom apartment and helped us settle in. We'd almost run through those $500 in our suitcase linings, and we needed help.

Toward the end of our Cuban life, we'd left the Catholic Church and joined the small community of Episcopalians. It was all because of a frilly white *sayuela*, a petticoat, Mami had given me to wear under my party dresses. I loved that short *sayuela*. One morning I impulsively pulled on my prized *sayuela* under my staid Catholic school uniform. On schooldays, I wore a crisp white cotton short-sleeved blouse with a Peter Pan collar, a gray-and-blue plaid jumper, white anklets, and profoundly hideous orthopedic booties whose inserts were supposed to help my flat feet. It was a look. A look begging for a little cha-cha-cha. Well, the nuns were scandalized. One took me by the hand to the chapel down the hall. I was led to the altar, where a ceramic Baby Jesus with a cherubic expression sat in a miniature straw manger. On the left side of his tiny chest was a red valentine cloth pincushion heart. The nun handed me a palm-full of glass-head straight pins and told me, "*Hazlo*" (Do it). Perplexed and ashamed, I knelt before the Baby Jesus and pierced his puffy heart over and over with the pins, murmuring for forgiveness – not for wearing the *sayuela* but for this symbolic act of violence. Mami enrolled me in the American Episcopal school the next day.

This is why, when we left Miami for California, St. Mary's Episcopal Parish near Culver City, rather than a Catholic congregation, sponsored us. St. Mary's is seven miles east of the Pacific Ocean and ten miles west of downtown Los Angeles. Our apartment was in Mar Vista Gardens, a disingenuously named Del Rey public housing project for low-income families about two miles from the church. We were given a 30-day supply of groceries – no tomato soup, mercifully – and jobs for my parents. Periodically, we received goods from the government food surplus program; this included unfamiliar foods we had no idea what to do with, like huge cans of peanut butter; but Abuela concocted a recipe for peanut butter candy that we fought for. Papi initially worked the swing shift at the downtown Bank of America as a verification teller in a vault 30 feet underground. Mami assembled transmitters in an electronics factory. Later, Papi got a day-schedule job in the cargo department at National Airlines.

And I became a virtual second mother to my younger brother, Angel Armando, and later to my younger sister, Lucie. That assignment was in addition to regular public school attendance and academic achievement. Because Rafa was the eldest son, his duties were limited to taking out the garbage and helping Papi mow the lawn. But as the eldest daughter, after school I babysat, refereed sibling conflicts, changed Lucie's diapers, cleaned the house, washed the dishes, did the laundry, and helped Papi prepare dinner. My parents had made great sacrifices, and each balanced two jobs and English classes to provide for our family and *encaminarnos* so our family could gain sound footing in this country.

Understanding the Disconnect

Yes, I was often overwhelmed with family responsibilities. But I was also proud to have such an important role in the family. And I liked Stoner Avenue Elementary School. And my English was improving. I was grateful and relieved that my fourth-grade teacher spoke a bit of Spanish. She took me under her wing and let me to do my homework in Spanish until I'd completely conquered English. But she couldn't shelter me from everything. There was a day when my fourth-grade classmates and I were presented with yellow No. 2 pencils and a booklet full of words and tiny blank circles next to them. What was I supposed to do? Looking around, I saw everybody filling in the circles, so I did the same. It was an IQ test or achievement test.

Flash forward to junior high school, where I was excited to be entering seventh grade. Mami had bought me a brand-new dress, a fresh notebook, and a No. 2 pencil. I arrived ready to learn. First period was math. The teacher asked us to figure out the sums for 1 + 1, 1 + 2, and 1 + 3. It had to be a joke, I thought. It wasn't. That night at home, I told my parents what had happened and made my case for why they should speak to someone at the school about why I was being asked to perform first-grade arithmetic. After a bit of coaxing, Papi agreed to take a day off work and speak to the school counselor. I was given a new test and placed in top-level college preparatory courses.

Where was the disconnect? English. Or rather, no English. I didn't know I'd been placed into classes for low-achieving students based on the results of the test given to me back in fourth grade when I did not speak English. I graduated from Marina del Rey Junior High with honors. By the time I got to Venice High School, I knew I would pursue a college degree.

All the while, Mami and Papi kept me on a tight leash. When I was in tenth grade, one sunny summer Saturday afternoon, after I'd finished my household chores, I asked Mami, for the millionth time, to let me go out with friends to Santa Monica beach. Her consistent reply: "*Ya veremos*" (We'll see). "I'm going to the beach," I finally told her. I got my stuff, walked to the bus stop, and went to the beach. I was dizzy and nauseated on that bus ride; it was like that moment on the mound in Camagüey on my *bicicleta roja*. Except this time I wasn't concealing my intentions. I was openly acting on them. California made me feel free.

Coming of Age in a Time of Social Turmoil

After high school, Papi taught me how to search for jobs in the local paper's Help Wanted ads. Two weeks later, I was thrilled with my first full-time job. I began working the 7 a.m.–3 p.m. shift as a waitress at the House of Pies near our house, and one month later was given a promotion to head waitress; now, I was in charge. That fall, I enrolled in evening classes at El Camino Community College, where, in my first psychology course, I decided to become a psychologist. It was all because of a field assignment at a local elementary school where I was assigned to tutor a newly arrived 10-year-old Cuban boy refugee. In his shyness and lowered gaze mixed with anger, I recognized his confusion, disorientation, and sense of diminishment. I realized that my lived experience was an inner source of knowledge, strength, and insight – the field of psychology would allow me to discover it more fully and put it to good use. Later, I would learn that being myself in my chosen field would take outrageous courage and constant grounding.

Within one year, my daily dumping of tip coins at the local Bank of America deposit counter resulted in enough savings to buy a used car and get my own apartment – not too close to my parents' house. Papi had taught me how to budget and poverty had taught me to be frugal, and so I recruited one of my waitress friends as a roommate and managed to eat all my meals at work for no cost. I soon saved enough money for a \$5/day summer trip to Europe with my high school sweetheart. Moving out of my parents' house and then that prenuptial trip caused havoc in my family. Once again, I was going against Cuban gender norms. Eventually, my parents' unconditional love and well-practiced ability to adapt to things foreign prevailed. To their relief a couple of years later, I married the young man they had previously accused of dishonorable intentions – all was forgotten. My marital status would bring them short-lived satisfaction.

Two years later, with encouragement from my psychology professor at El Camino, I applied and was accepted to UCLA with financial aid and a scholarship. Like El Camino, UCLA was a hotbed of social change. My scope broadened along with continued and emerging movements – civil rights, Chicano, women's, and something called gay pride. Protests against the Vietnam War were daily news items, women burned their bras, and men burned their draft cards. Television news broadcasts showed images of police officers beating, handcuffing, and killing people who were peacefully marching for their rights and in opposition to the war, including students at Kent State. I felt compelled to be part of that change. I wondered how to effect it. Do you sneak out through the garage on a red bike? Head over heart? Do you physically fight? Acquiesce to bullies or get a black eye? Or do you just take it? Get on a bus and go?

Here is what I did. I started a summer bilingual-bicultural preschool. Along with four other UCLA Latino undergrads, we recruited and enrolled 150 beautiful, eager, and loving monolingual (Spanish-speaking) children from the low-income Pico Union neighborhood and ran the program for several years at Magnolia Avenue Elementary School. Together we put our lived experience and knowledge about early childhood gained from our UCLA education to work. It was both the worst-paid and the best job I have ever had.

When One Door Closes, Another One Opens

During many, many late nights studying in my UCLA cubicle, I eventually decided that knowledge was the best weapon to combat ignorance and bring forth change. An informed voice armed with facts might diminish social injustice, police brutality, racial and gender discrimination, and societal suffering. You actually think that way when you're in college. I became convinced that there was a way to the heart through the head.

After earning my BA with honors in 1975, I applied to the UCLA doctoral program in clinical psychology. I received a reply stating that I was not "a good fit" for the program. Later, I found out that only one Latino student had ever been accepted into the program. My 3.8 GPA, high GRE scores, publication in a major journal, significant community service work, and interest in family dynamics – a key interest among the clinical faculty members – did not persuade them. But my father's often-repeated adage, "When one door closes, another one opens," served me well. I applied and was accepted into the UCLA School of Education's early childhood development doctoral program. Then a new Latino psychology professor, Amado Padilla, encouraged me to apply to the doctoral program in developmental psychology; I was accepted and decided to also minor in social psychology.

My consciousness raised, as the saying went, by the social and political changes all around me, I became a constant questioner. I questioned why in my social psychology course we didn't include institutionalized violence in the study of aggression. I questioned why we weren't focusing on how poverty affects education and the health of the most vulnerable. Not realizing I was touching on a hotly debated topic in psychology, I questioned why our syllabus included highly disputed work by the prominent educational psychologist Arthur Jensen on the genetic basis of race differences in IQ, but not Leon Kamin's scholarship on the science and politics of IQ. These weren't simply academic exercises for me. As a child, I'd lived three doors down from poverty in Cuba. Later, in public housing, I had seen families that, unlike us, were never able to make it out. It troubled me.

Yet, none of my doctoral program professors were talking about or seemed concerned with how psychology could contribute to issues of equality, equity, or social justice. In fact, my Latino doctoral advisor called me into his office to discuss the wisdom of presenting at the 1978 National Coalition of Hispanic Mental Health and Human Services Organization conference in Washington, DC, on an issue I was living just at that time – the coming out process among Hispanic gays and lesbians. He, along with another Latino professor, knew I had been married, and they were "curious" about the nature of my interest in the topic and expressed concerns about "possible negative career repercussions." I was also concerned, actually. But I did it anyway. Head over heart. Or was it heart through the head? My presentation was a triumph. It was standing room only, and the crowd of mental health professionals stood and applauded me and the panel of presenters. I felt encouraged. There seemed to be others who thought that speaking one's truth was of value. One was psychologist Eduardo Morales, the person who had organized the session and invited me; he would become a lifelong friend and colleague. I realized I needed to change doctoral advisors and, *gracias a Dios*, Professor Anne Peplau agreed to be my dissertation mentor.

An important lesson in graduate school was my realization that I was responsible for my own education, so I began the practice of creating a reading list by authors outside mainstream psychology. Their influence would later be evident in my course syllabi as a professor of public health and in my scholarly work, research, and community-based programs on HIV prevention and substance use disorders treatment for women. For example, the investigative work and resulting book by Frankfort and Kissling (1979) inspired my dissertation research on reproductive attitudes and experiences of Mexican American women (Amaro, 1988). Their research revealed that the death of Rosie Jimenez, a young Mexican American community college student (my age at the time), resulting from an illegal abortion was not due to cultural beliefs and shame as had been asserted by the Centers for Disease Control and Prevention. Rather, it resulted from restrictions on Medicaid funding after the 1977 passage of the Hyde Amendment – three years after *Roe v Wade*. Others who inspired and informed my thinking and subsequent research included Martinique-born Afro-Caribbean psychoanalyst and social philosopher Frantz Omar Fanon and his work on the ethnopsychology of discrimination. Also, Brazilian educator and philosopher Paulo Freire. *Pedagogy of the Oppressed*, Freire's 1970 opus, is a foundational text of the critical pedagogy movement. Finally, feminist psychiatrist, clinician, and Bronx native Jean Baker Miller. Her groundbreaking classic, *Toward a New Psychology of Women*, was partly inspired by the feminist movement of the 1960s (Miller, 1976).

The New *Bicicleta*

My real-life treasure chest came in the form of the American Psychological Association's (APA's) National Institutes of Health-funded Minority Fellowship Program (MFP; Jones & Austin-Dailey, 2009). As a member of the third cohort, my MFP family was composed of fellow doctoral students – diamonds in the rough who would become distinguished leaders and pioneers in research, teaching, and service. They included Melba Vasquez, a past APA president, Ana Marie Cauce, the current president of the University of Washington, to name just two. The crowning jewels were the dedicated MFP founders and mentors throughout the country who were a fountain of inspiration, wisdom, and research-savvy. Leading psychologists involved in the MFP were the pioneers of minority psychology. Professors Martha Bernal, Dalmas Taylor, and James Jones opened doors in my mind and professional life. Dr. Nancy Felipe Russo, prominent feminist psychologist and then director of the APA Women's Program Office, was my first mentor and a later coauthor (Amaro & Russo, 1987; Amaro, Russo, & Johnson, 1987; Russo, Amaro, & Winter, 1987). I would turn to this network throughout my career. My dream was no longer elusive. The MFP's aim of advancing psychology to benefit society and improve people's lives finally provided me with an intellectual home aligned with my own goals. I didn't know it then, but this treasure chest was my new *bicicleta*. As a young girl in the United States, I had a recurring dream of discovering a house full of mysterious rooms – one of which was empty except for a treasure chest full of jewels in the center. As I delved into the treasure contents, it would disappear. No matter how hard I searched, I could not find that room again. Then, I would wake.

Who Do You Think You Are?

Jewels in back pocket and newly minted PhD briefcase in hand, I went off to search for my first faculty job. It was 1982, smack in the middle of the Reagan Administration, the 1980s recession, and the devaluation of social science research (Reinhold, 1981; Saiter, 1982; Silver, 2014). Faced with severe cuts to social science research and faculty jobs, I made lemonade of lemons. My graduate school job, working with psychologist Dr. Linda Beckman at the UCLA Neuropsychiatric Institute, led to introductions to Boston-based researchers planning a study on women's drug use during pregnancy. They were looking for a study coordinator. Though not initially a faculty position, it was a good match for my experience based on my dissertation topic on reproductive attitudes and experiences of Mexican American women and my research with Beckman on women's access to alcoholism treatment (Amaro, 1988; Beckman & Amaro, 1986). There, I was confronted with stereotypes in negotiating the terms of my first professional research position. I delivered a presentation, met with team members, and was offered the job. "The salary is the same as I was earning prior to completing the PhD," I told the MD leading the study, and I asked for a higher one. "We don't have that in the budget," he said, so I proposed that for their offered salary, I would work four instead of five days a week. "You sure are a tough negotiator. You don't seem like the typical compliant Latina," he replied. I wanted to say, "You don't know *mi* Abuela Leonela." I got the conversation back on track. He accepted my proposal. I got busy making lemonade.

As the only psychologist and most junior member of the team, I successfully argued for the inclusion of study measures that interested me – race, ethnicity, interpersonal violence, social support, depression, and partner risk factors. It turned out sweet. Using the data, I later published numerous articles that set the course of my research career (Amaro, Fried, Cabral, & Zuckerman, 1990; Amaro, Zuckerman, & Cabral, 1989; Zuckerman, Amaro, Bauchner, & Cabral, 1989; Zuckerman, Amaro, & Beardslee, 1987). A few years later, I joined the faculty as an assistant professor in Boston University School of Medicine's Department of Pediatrics and School of Public Health. This first academic job also led to my first grant from the William T. Grant Foundation – a grant awarded annually to a handful of junior faculty nationally – which funded my time and work for five years as a faculty scholar. Using data from the recently completed Hispanic National Health and Nutrition Examination Survey, in 1990 I published the first article on acculturation and drug use among Latinos using a large representative sample, in the *American Journal of Public Health* (Amaro, Whitaker, Coffman, & Heeren, 1990). It never occurred to me that many years later I would be appointed to the journal's Editorial Board and then serve as one of its associate editors.

Noting the dearth of research on Latino alcohol and drug use, I discussed with my department chair my desire to pursue a study on substance use among Latinos. "It will never get funded. It's a marginal research area – Latinos are a small population," he responded. Shortsighted – we all know how population growth went. I would find my way. No significant personal or professional achievement has ever come easy. From my earliest years, there have been those who told me what I couldn't do. It's nearly impossible to not internalize such messages. I'd regularly question myself, my intelligence and abilities – but not my inspirations and aspirations.

"Who do you think you are that you can do anything?" my Venice High gymnastics teacher asked me, closing her office door behind her. I had been class president in the tenth grade, and the next year, I competed for cheerleader. She was a cheerleading judge, so you know how that turned out. Although the school was demographically diverse, the classrooms, social clubs, and clicks were highly segregated, leaving me as one of the very few Latinas in college prep classes and mainstream social clubs. The interaction left me confused. I did not understand exactly what had transpired. I felt ashamed and told no one. Looking back, I realize how confused I had become in high school by trying to fit in. Though I did not realize it, I was struggling with understanding my own history and place in the world.

Lived Experience Fuels a New Trajectory

The AIDS Epidemic

Remember how in junior college I had learned that my lived experience was a source of strength and insight? Meeting Mary and a personal tragedy would lead me to clarity about who I am and to change my path. It was during the beginning of the AIDS epidemic in the United States. Mary was a study participant I interviewed in the postpartum ward at Boston City Hospital. A 27-year-old African American woman whose years of heroin use and sex work were etched on her face and body. She'd just been told she was HIV positive and was waiting to learn if her newborn was infected. Little information was available on HIV for women like Mary. I'd been progressing in my academic career, publishing, and getting grants – everything I was supposed to do. Meeting Mary made me rethink my direction. She offered me a mirror for self-reflection.

A few weeks later, my younger brother, Armando, a gay man, 27 years of age at the time, working in San Francisco as a graphic artist, was diagnosed with AIDS. This was a painful and tumultuous time – little was known about treatment for people diagnosed with AIDS. Armando and my family struggled with this stigmatizing diagnosis and, at the time, death sentence. I pored over medical journals and called prominent researchers to find an answer that could give us and his doctors a hint of the best course of treatment, something that could provide even a glimmer of hope.

I coped with an unbridled wish to change reality by spending as much time as possible with Armando in Los Angeles, where he had moved to receive care from my parents, and by becoming an academic-community activist. One of my students, Jose Pares Avila, called on me to become an activist in Boston, where the epidemic was sweeping the Latino community and had taken the lives of too many. This was my entrée into the world of putting science to use and to a whole new way of informing my work through lived experience and owning my voice. I joined the board of the Boston AIDS Action Committee and then cofounded the Latin American Health Institute and the Multicultural AIDS Coalition, both of which brought visibility and much-needed program funding for HIV prevention to communities of color. While trying to keep up with teaching and publishing, I had a hectic schedule of national and local speaking engagements. I developed a deep sense of agency and felt energized.

In 1989, two years after his diagnosis, Armando died at the age of 29. It took years for me to transcend the deep sense of loss; therapy was instrumental in my grieving process. Instituting the Armando Amaro Memorial Fund for Latino art students sponsored by my family at Santa Monica City College, where Armando had been a student, was another important step. Witnessing my parents' growth beyond the stigma of AIDS and a gay son as well as my mother's subsequent volunteer work with Mothers of AIDS Patients soothed my aching heart and taught me how grief can lead to transformation. Having been with Armando and helping him during his illness and passing – although the most difficult thing I have ever experienced – served as comfort. Most important was the process of learning to be present. Well-worn on my home library shelf are Stephen Levine's books – classics in the field of death and dying, healing, forgiveness and compassion (see Levine, 1979, 1987; Levine and Levine, 1982) – which Armando and I read together during his illness. Levine's words helped me to be present during Armando's journey. While I was grieving, life went on.

Taking it to the Streets: Programa Mamá

At around the same time, I was offered an auspicious opportunity. Dr. Ken Edelin, who was department chair of obstetrics and gynecology at Boston City Hospital, asked me to replace him as principal investigator for the Boston site on a study on HIV prevention among pregnant women drug users, sex workers, and partners of sex workers. The study was funded by the National Institutes of Health. A tremendous opportunity – offered early in my career by an African American physician and senior mentor. Known as the Mom's Project or Programa Mamá, it transformed me and the direction of my work (Amaro & Aguiar, 1994). Women who walked into our community site's storefront were my best teachers. Their experiences resonated and inspired me to publish "Love, Sex and Power," a seminal critique of HIV prevention with women (Amaro, 1995), to document the role of gender relations in women's drug use and recovery (Amaro & Hardy-Fanta, 1995) and, later, to collaborate with one of my students on the role of relationship power in women's HIV risk (Pulerwitz, Amaro, De Jong, Gortmaker, & Rudd, 2002).

Over the following two decades, along with collaborators from Boston's health department, we developed and implemented multiple HIV prevention and substance abuse disorder treatment programs for inner-city women and men of color living in Boston's most disenfranchised neighborhoods. Key among my collaborators was Rita Nieves, a phenomenal nurse, public health practitioner, and licensed social worker with years of experience developing and implementing public health programs in Boston and Puerto Rico. Our massive programmatic undertaking in Boston became a shared vision that blended her management ingenuity and implementation creativity with my hard-nosed perseverance and focus on documenting outcomes. Through this shared passion, we became and continue to be the closest of friends.

Funded by more than 35 national and state grants, our programs eventually included HIV prevention programs for women of color and all levels of care for substance use disorder treatment. My own life lessons on the importance of agency and my lived experience as a source of wisdom and strength and acquired understanding of the role of culture, gender, and inequities served as essential framing elements for our research, treatment approaches, and practices as well as training and mentoring of clinicians. Our published findings resulted in our Boston Consortium Model of Integrated Treatment for women being approved for inclusion in the National Registry of Evidence-Based Programs and Practices (Amaro, Chernoff, Brown, Arévalo, & Gatz, 2007; Amaro, Dai et al., 2007; Amaro, Larson et al., 2007; Amaro et al., 2005).

I had found a way to become the psychologist I envisioned in my first junior college psychology course. My conclusion during the late-night ponderings while studying at my UCLA cubicle had proven correct. I had learned how the head and heart work together. Witnessing the benefits that women and children gained from our programs satisfied my heart. Contributing to knowledge satisfied my head. Recognitions I have received for my work, including being inducted into the National Academy of Medicine in 2011, serve as an ongoing reminder that an informed voice grounded in facts can make a difference. As a "wise Latina," I invite emerging scientists to consider whether their path reflects their passion, to understand their source of inspiration and their aspirations – whether their chosen path has a heart. For me, answering these questions has required being grounded in my own lived experience and understanding the connections with others who are marginalized by society.

My CuChiRican Heart

In 2012, I moved back to the City of the Angels to join the faculty at the University of Southern California and continue the work I love. Remember that gift that Armando left me through the writings of Stephen Levine's work? It eventually led to my becoming a yoga practitioner and teacher and, later, to developing Moment-by-Moment in Women's Recovery, a mindfulness-based relapse prevention program that we implemented and first tested in our Boston treatment programs (Amaro, Spear, Vallejo, Conron, & Black, 2014). Now I am conducting a randomized clinical trial to test its efficacy in a large and diverse sample of women in treatment, thanks to a grant from the National Institute on Drug Abuse and a most dedicated and talented team of research and clinical collaborators and junior scholars I mentor.

I am fulfilling a career-long dream to live and work in a Latino city with many Latino colleagues. And here I am. Enjoying each instance when I speak Spanish to the postman, grocery store clerk, colleagues, friends, and students, and hear the familiar street rhythms of my CuChiRican life.

Conclusion

Nearly 67 years later, I'm still the girl on the *bicicleta roja* exploring the world – the world of putting science to use, that is – and my curiosity still prevails. Why? Is it because I drank the water from the *tinajon* to remain forever grounded culturally in a place where Spanish is the first language? Because I saw poverty in Camagüey and lived it early in our life here? Because I was blessed with a loving, supportive father? Because my grandmothers, aunts, and mother were the strongest women I've ever known? Because my brothers and I are all named Angel? Or is it because I'm a relentless questioner? I guess that last one is the closest to the truth. All I know is that today, when I drop my head back and look heavenward, the California sky is almost as beautiful as the Cuban one. Almost.

References

Álvarez, J. (2004). *Cuba's agricultural sector.* Gainesville, FL: University Press of Florida.

Amaro, H. (1988). Women in the Mexican-American community: Religion, culture, and reproductive attitudes and experiences. *Journal of Community Psychology*, 16(1), 6–20. doi:10.1002/1520-6629(198801)16:1-6:AID-JCOP2290160104-3.0.CO;2-1

Amaro, H. (1995). Love, sex, and power: Considering women's realities in HIV prevention. *American Psychologist*, 50(6), 437–447. doi: 10.1037/0003-066X.50.6doi:437

Amaro, H., & Aguiar, M. (1994). Programa Mamá/Mom's Project: A community-based outreach model for addicted women. In J. Szapocznik (Ed.), *A Hispanic/Latino family approach to substance abuse prevention* (pp. 125–153). Washington, DC: US Department of Health and Human Services.

Amaro, H., Chernoff, M., Brown, V., Arévalo, S., & Gatz, M. (2007). Does integrated trauma-informed substance abuse treatment increase treatment retention? *Journal of Community Psychology*, 35(7), 845–862. doi: 10.1002/jcop.20185

Amaro, H., Dai, J., Arévalo, S., Acevedo, A., Matsumoto, A., Nieves, R., & Prado, G. (2007). Effects of integrated trauma treatment on outcomes in a racially/ethnically diverse sample of women in urban community-based substance abuse treatment. *Journal of Urban Health*, 84(4), 508–522. doi: 10.1007/s11524-007-9160-z

Amaro, H., Fried, L. E., Cabral, H., & Zuckerman, B. (1990). Violence during pregnancy and substance use. *American Journal of Public Health*, 80(5), 575–579. doi: 10.2105/AJPH.80.5.5doi:75

Amaro, H., & Hardy-Fanta, C. (1995). Gender relations in addiction and recovery. *Journal of Psychoactive Drugs*, 27(4), 325–337. doi: 10.1080/02791072.1995.10471698

Amaro, H., Larson, M. J., Zhang, A., Acevedo, D., Dai, J., & Matsumoto, A. (2007). Effects of trauma intervention on HIV sexual risk behaviors among women with co-occurring disorders in substance abuse treatment. *Journal of Community Psychology*, 35(7), 895–908. doi: 10.1002/jcop.20188

Amaro, H., McGraw, S., Larson, M. J., Lopez, L., Nieves, R., & Marshall, B. (2005). Boston Consortium of Services for Families in Recovery: A trauma-informed intervention model for women's alcohol and drug addiction treatment. *Alcoholism Treatment Quarterly*, 22(2–3), 95–119. doi: 10.1300/J020v22n03_06

Amaro, H., & Russo, N. F. (1987). Hispanic women and mental health: An overview of contemporary issues in research and practice. *Psychology of Women Quarterly*, 11(4), 393–407. doi: 10.1111/j.1471-6402.1987.tb00914.x

Amaro, H., Russo, N. F., & Johnson, J. (1987). Family and work predictors of psychological well-being among Hispanic women professionals. *Psychology of Women Quarterly*, 11(4), 505–521. doi: 10.1111/j.1471-6402.1987.tb00921.x

Amaro, H., Spear, S., Vallejo, Z., Conron, K., & Black, D. S. (2014). Feasibility, acceptability, and preliminary outcomes of a mindfulness-based relapse prevention intervention for culturally-diverse, low-income women in substance use disorder treatment. *Substance Use & Misuse*, 49(5), 547–559. doi: 10.3109/10826084.2013.852587

Amaro, H., Whitaker, R., Coffman, G., & Heeren, T. (1990). Acculturation and marijuana and cocaine use: Findings from HHANES 1982–1984. *American Journal of Public Health*, 80 (Suppl.), 54–60. doi: 10.2105/AJPH.80.Suppl.54

Amaro, H., Zuckerman, B., & Cabral, H. (1989). Drug use among adolescent mothers: Profile of risk. *Pediatrics*, 84(1), 144–151.

Anders, A. (1961, July 26). The Cuban experience in Florida: Revolution and exodus (Letter to the Cuban Refugee Assistance Program). Retrieved from: https://www.floridamemory.com/onlineclassroom/cuban-revolution/sets/anders/

Arvey, S. R. (2012). Sex and the ordinary Cuban: Cuban physicians, eugenics, and marital sexuality, 1933–1958. *Journal of the History of Sexuality*, 21(1), 93–120. doi: 10.1353/sex.2012.0004

Beckman, L. J., & Amaro, H. (1986). Personal and social difficulties faced by women and men entering alcoholism treatment. *Journal of Studies on Alcohol*, 47(2), 135–145. doi: 10.15288/jsa.1986. 47. 135

Clealand, D. P. (2013). When ideology clashes with reality: Racial discrimination and Black identity in contemporary Cuba. *Ethnic and Racial Studies*, 36(10), 1619–1636. doi: 10.1080/01419870.2013.783928

de la Fuente, A. (1998). Race, national discourse, and politics in Cuba: An overview. *Latin American Perspectives*, 25(3), 43–69. doi: 10.1177/0094582X9802500303

Frankfort, E., & Kissling, F. (1979). *Rosie: The investigation of a wrongful death*. New York: Dial Press.

Freire, P. (1970). *Pedagogy of the oppressed*. New York: Herder and Herder.

Haines, D. W. (2015). Learning from our past: The refugee experience in the United States. Retrieved from: https://www.americanimmigrationcouncil.org/sites/default/files/research/learning_from_our_past_the_refugee_experience_in_the_united_states.pdf

Jones, J. M., & Austin-Dailey, A. T. (2009). The Minority Fellowship Program: A 30-year legacy of training psychologists of color. *Cultural Diversity and Ethnic Minority Psychology*, 15(4), 388–399. doi: 10.1037/a0017558

Levine, S. (1979). *A gradual awakening*. New York: Random House.

Levine, S. (1987). *Healing into life and death*. New York: Random House.

Levine, S., & Levine, O. (1982). *Who dies? An investigation of conscious living and conscious dying*. New York: Random House.

Miller, J. B. (1976). *Toward a new psychology of women*. Boston, MA: Beacon Press.

Mitchell, W. L. (1962, March). The Cuban Refugee Program. *Social Security Bulletin*. Retrieved from: https://www.ssa.gov/policy/docs/ssb/v25n3/v25n3p3.pdf

Nodal, R. (1986). The Black man in Cuban society: From colonial times to the revolution. *Journal of Black Studies*, 16(3), 251–267. doi: 10.1177/002193478601600302

Pulerwitz, J., Amaro, H., De Jong, W., Gortmaker, S. L., & Rudd, R. (2002). Relationship power condom use and HIV risk among women in the USA. *AIDS Care*, 14(6), 789–800. doi: 10.1080/0954012021000031868

Reinhold, R. (1981, February 9). Reagan's plans on research cuts are said to aim at "soft" sciences. *The New York Times*. Retrieved from: www.nytimes.com/1981/02/09/us/reagan-s-plans-on-research-cuts-are-said-to-aim-at-soft-sciences.html

Russo, N. F., Amaro, H., & Winter, M. (1987). The use of inpatient mental health services by Hispanic women. *Psychology of Women Quarterly*, 11(4), 427–441. doi: 10.1111/j.1471-6402.1987.tb00916.x

Saiter, S. (1982, November 14). The Reagan effect: Natural scientists gain, social scientists lose. *The New York Times*. Retrieved from: www.nytimes.com/1982/11/14/education/the-reagan-effect-natural-scientists-gain-social-scientists-lose.html

Silver, H. J. (2014, June 20). How Ronald Reagan helped advance social science. *Social Science Space*. Retrieved from: https://www.socialsciencespace.com/2014/06/howard-silver-post/

Zuckerman, B., Amaro, H., Bauchner, H., & Cabral, H. (1989). Depressive symptoms during pregnancy: Relationship to poor health behaviors. *American Journal of Obstetrics & Gynecology*, 160(5), 1107–1111. doi: 10.1016/0002-9378(89)90170-1

Zuckerman, B. S., Amaro, H., & Beardslee, W. (1987). Mental health of adolescent mothers: The implications of depression and drug use. *Journal of Developmental & Behavioral Pediatrics*, 8(2), 111–116. doi: 10.1097/0

6

LIVING IN MULTIPLE WORLDS AS A LATINA PSYCHOLOGIST

Margarita Alegría

> There is no passion to be found playing small – in settling for a life that is less than the one you are capable of living.
>
> *Nelson Mandela (1994)*

The Early Years

Writing about myself is probably hard because reflecting backwards has not been my pattern in life. Quite the opposite; focusing on the future has helped me deal with vast amounts of uncertainty. Yet let me start by briefly saying how my past oriented so much of who I am today, what I value, and my decisions on topics to study as a Latina psychologist. I agree with Justice Sonia Sotomayor that our diverse life circumstances enrich our understanding of the complexity and varied mosaics of life in the US.

I was born under challenging circumstances – my mother got pregnant while on a brief trip to Europe to try to repair her marriage. Once back from the trip, she decided to divorce my father, so pregnancy became a surprising event. With two young children already (ages 4 and 6) and a failed marriage, this was definitively not good news. So as a start, I believe in the implausible chance fate had given me.

Soon after I was born, my mother became seriously ill and was bedridden. I went to live with my aunt and uncle two houses down the road. This event served to transform my world in significant and substantial ways. It lead to three unusual circumstances: I got an incredible amount of love and attention growing up with four rather than two parents; I was exposed to an inconceivable amount of family conflict within the same family unit; and I learned the importance of adaptation to diverse home environments. Crossing from my mother's house to my aunt's house meant moving between dissimilar worlds with different family rituals and customs, even though this was all in San Juan, Puerto Rico. Life could be completely different from one house to the next.

I spent Monday, Wednesday and Thursday with my aunt and uncle, Tuesday with my mom and my stepfather, Sunday with my dad, and weekends alternated between the two families. The predictability of my friends' households became something I craved. I had to draw a family tree to explain to boyfriends, girlfriends and teachers who was who in my family. Yet this brought a rainbow of experiences that catalyzed a desire to understand what leads to a sense of belonging and how it can be formed or destroyed while growing up.

Having this life till the age of 17 was tough, but it built my character. With the constant uncertainty and movement, I focused on the future, aspiring to problem-solve and use my intuition to the maximum. The other great benefit was diversifying my environments while growing up, going from an authoritarian but loving home to an easygoing and indulgent family circle that deeply cared about my happiness. In one family unit, my aunt and uncle could be extremely strict, such that to avoid giving men the wrong message, I could not wear T-shirts without sleeves; nor could I wear black, because it also gave the wrong impression. At the same time, my aunt and uncle were 300% invested in what mattered to me, whether it was constructing a chariot for my class Pep Rally, tie-dying shirts for my class or debating the most inconsequential topics of politics or lifestyle. Being, in effect, their firstborn pushed me to believe that I could be whoever I wanted, giving me extraordinary confidence under high expectations for my future. Going to my mom's house paralleled the tons of attention, but there was greater relaxation with lower expectations and more leniency typically bestowed on the third born. I was able to go out with my older sister's friends and see my boyfriend more frequently without constant supervision, activities that as a teenager you yearn for.

In these different environments, I learned the subtle messaging of inclusion or exclusion that has become central to my professional work. This message could be best framed by seeing Christmas presents that my mother gave to other family members with her name and the names of my stepfather, my brother Jose and my sister Cele (and not me). Why was my name not included? Or seeing how my grandparents from my uncle's side would not incorporate me in family gatherings since I was the one that would be maybe coming but maybe not. Issues of fairness, inclusion and exclusion became paramount to me, possibly because I was trying to work out what behaviors played a role in being a part or being ruled out from being a part of the family.

At the same time, it made me see family life as nuanced and multidimensional. Learning to read people and anticipate events became essential, but it also helped me to learn to put myself in other people's shoes to better predict their behavior. I could see how the same experience could have a dramatically different meaning depending on whether it was my brother Rennie or my sister Myriamcita (both adopted by my aunt and uncle) or me narrating what was happening. I was immersed in moving forward from one house to the next, a junior anthropologist learning about diverse tribes. Going to my grandparents' house on Sundays, to the Alegría family, exposed me to a rich intellectual life and lots of humor but also to the marginalization of girls and favoritism of boys in the family. Being the youngest grandchild (others being 5 to 15 years older) also excluded me from much of the play, but it gave me the chance to scrutinize family dynamics. I saw how men dominated the discussion at the dinner table, how attention and investment was centered on boys, their comments embellished, while the girls were silenced. Observing these interactions made me appreciate being raised in my aunt and uncle's household, where they were interested in what I had to say, encouraging me to have a voice, a strong one, despite how inconsequential or outrageous I probably was then. It also showed me that I did not need to be subjugated to a family where men were more valuable and women were dismissed. In other words, there were other normative scripts and plenty of alternative choices. Not many people have as many choices in family life as I did.

Family conflict was an early dance that I had to master. My aunt and uncle went to family court to restrain my mother from taking me to live with her and her new husband in Scarsdale, New York. The entire family was involved in the decision of what should be done with Maggie. Under such circumstances, you confront what are family alliances, loyalty, familism, affiliative values, all head on. This positioned me in challenging circumstances where family members did not talk to each other or where I faced anger for not making the "right choice" and choosing "my family." All the attention, as stressful as it was, served to remind me that they truly loved me and, thus, allowed me to survive those trying times. My boyfriend Vicen and my sister Cele became my confidants, buffering the pain of instability. But this again helps one grasp the importance of family conflict as central in people's lives, a powerful dimension that I gave attention to in my clinical practice and later in my research.

It was in this drama that encircled the whole family that I thought about what my future should be. On the one hand, being a family lawyer was a potential path to buffer the pain of children to better deal with the chaos and tears of family conflict. On the other hand, being a psychologist or psychiatrist might be a way to heal deep family pain. Which path would be mine? The sisters of Notre Dame and other caring teachers at Perpetuo Socorro (a private Catholic school) had empowered us with the educational foundation to make professional choices.

Getting Enamored with Psychology and Starting my Career

Once my aunt and uncle elected to divorce, staying in an even more multisite family seemed unbearable and made me apply to college during my junior rather than senior year of high school. It was a tough choice because of my close friends and all the work we had done together to prepare for what we hoped to be an amazing senior year. Once I was accepted at Georgetown as a biology major, I decided not to turn back. This was a chance to live a single life, unconstrained by family alliances.

It was at Georgetown University that I became completely seduced by psychology. By incredible luck, I had the benefit of an illustrious teacher, Dr. Daniel N. Robinson, Distinguished Professor Emeritus at Georgetown University. Not even my faulty English dissuaded me from his courses and the struggles that it would entail in terms of writing long convoluted essays. I was mesmerized by his mastery of the discipline but also by the narrative of how psychology encompassed so much of philosophy and ethics, how it was a powerful force in driving human behavior. In this journey at Georgetown, it became clear to me that I should get a graduate degree. My initial plan was to stay in Washington, DC, but love diverted me back to Puerto Rico to get married at age 21, not long after my college graduation. In a matter of weeks, I decided to apply both to law school and to study psychology in Puerto Rico. Trying out law in a summer dissuaded me from that path. I opted for a master's in psychology.

The University of Puerto Rico (UPR) proved to be an intellectual powerhouse with gifted and exceptional teachers including Waldemar Purcell, Jose Bauermeister, Marya Munoz, Agustin Garcia, Laura Leticia Herrans, Edwin Fernandez, Jenny Rodriguez, Joseph Carrol, Irma Serrano, Ilsa Echegarray and many more. The depth of intellectual debate, clinical training and expert supervision was a model that still guides my work. Learning came not only from teachers but also from my brilliant fellow students including Mildred, Mari, Cesar, Norma, Antonio and Santi (you know who you are). It was a testament to the graduate education opportunities that UPR created for all of us. After graduation from UPR, Dr. Jose Bauermeister introduced me to my first research job with a tremendous recommendation to Rafaela Robles, PhD, or Fafy as we all called her. He also offered me a position in his clinical practice as a part-time psychologist. This was a gift since, as the most sought-out child psychologist on the island, he referred many families to my private practice, which blossomed after just a couple of months.

My First Research Job and the Entry into a Different World

Fafy was a role model, an icon who mixed outrageous and creative fashion with scientific rigor and passion for answering the most intricate of social science questions. Eight years working with her in the School of Public Health at UPR opened so many doors. By working in a multidisciplinary context with economists, psychologists, sociologists, health educators, statisticians, medical doctors and health educators, we could explore the problem from different angles. It brought to light the importance of social context, the constraints of poverty, and how narrow one's perspective can be if we only investigate the problem from the perspective of one of those disciplines (Robles, Alegría, Martínez, Vera, &

Muñoz, 1983; Robles, Martinez, Vera, & Alegría, 1987; Vera, Robles, & Alegría, 1988). It also was the time I became aware of how many standardized measures did not necessarily work for some of the people and problems we were researching in Puerto Rico. For example, we quickly figured out that the standard occupations had little meaning in our study of public housing and risk of illegal drug use – a substantial number of people said that none of the occupation categories applied. Once we did cognitive debriefing, new categories emerged, like having a food truck, sheltering gang members and others not to be found on the General Social Survey (Alegría, Takeuchi et al., 2004). Some of the measures of social position were seen as inappropriate or even offensive by our Puerto Rico respondents, who felt education, income and occupation were narrow views of how people acquired social position. The experience reinforced the importance of cognitive debriefing to evaluate whether measures needed to be adapted or modified. It was the time when I realized how small were the sample sizes of Latino participants from which we were trying to generalize to Latinos in general, and Puerto Ricans in particular. The experience also illustrated how Latinos were not a monolithic group; rather, they shared traits, norms and many characteristics but differed in many attributes. This would be a theme that I would come back to later in my career (Alcántara, Chen, & Alegría, 2014; Alegría, Canino, Stinson, & Grant, 2006; Alegría et al., 2007).

Some of the most important work we conducted during 1981–1988 dealt with marginalized populations (e.g. sex workers, the poor, women who used drugs) and the social and health conditions of the oppressed (Alegría et al., 1991; Alegría et al., 1994). During those years, I got a close up view of institutional racism, of how opportunities were constrained not because people were not trying to make meaning of their life, but because those in power did not feel they deserved equal opportunities. For example, sex workers trying to get an education or to find public housing in order to transition out of their occupation had no route open to them.

I felt suddenly aware of what a protected life I had lived and how this protection enabled me and many like me to ignore the suffering of so many on the island. Going to rural houses in the mountains of Puerto Rico to interview participants for our studies opened a window to the daily struggles around food and housing insecurity that the poor suffer. It was while doing the study of Risk for Women's Drug Use in public housing that I was exposed to the persistent violence that was the norm in some public spaces (Alegría, Vera et al., 2004). I witnessed the shoot-out between gangs, a concrete introduction to the constant fear that hangs over those who live without police protection and who have been failed by other institutions as well.

Getting My PhD – the Phantom Student in Philadelphia

Between these studies, Fafy had encouraged me to get my PhD and fulfill my ambition of becoming an independent investigator. But this did not seem feasible given that there was no psychology PhD program in Puerto Rico. By this time, I had two small children, a full-time job and family responsibilities that conflicted with this ambition, including my biological father being quite sick with a serious illness that was not understood. But luck would strike again, with Temple University being willing to run a PhD program for ten UPR professors. They would come to UPR and give us accelerated classes that would cover the material in two or three weeks rather than months. Dr. Sewel and Dr. Blanco, as well as others, came to the island over the course of two years until we completed most of our coursework. This was combined with advanced courses at UPR so as to only require an eight-month internship and some other coursework in Philadelphia. I had the support of my husband (now my ex-husband) and his family.

I rented an apartment in Voorhees township in New Jersey, where I had more space for Antonio (4) and Nicolas (2). Early on, Antonio had a terrible asthma attack that took us to Children's Hospital at 3 a.m. I became extremely frightened that this was a total mistake. My ex-husband and I decided that it was best for the children to remain in Puerto Rico and for me to travel back and forth every other weekend to be with them. The stress and exhaustion of being in two places nearly killed me. I wondered whether trying to have it all – an advanced degree and career along with being a mom – was just too much.

Soon after I started coursework in Philadelphia, two bad things happened, compounding my woes. First, my father was diagnosed with AIDS. This was 1984. He was one of the first recognized cases of this new, not well-understood and frightening disease. This definitively had a toll on my health. I was torn between career and being there for my father, who was suffering the double stigma of HIV and coming out as a gay man. That wasn't the only instance of discrimination that hit me around this time. For the first time in my life, I also became exposed to horrible discrimination in New Jersey and Philadelphia. Something simple, signing up for telephone (or other) services in my New Jersey apartment, required a bigger deposit from a Puerto Rican without a job. Of course, I was a student! This ended up being the era of anger for me, where I could not come to terms with the continuous discrimination: store-owners not accepting checks from Puerto Rico, being followed with one of my friends in high-end stores, or being judged as aggressive because I would call out what I saw as injustice. Having been born and raised as a privileged member of a majority on the island, now becoming a minority cuing others to see me as underprivileged was an eye opening experience. It made me empathetic to the turmoil of African Americans and their cries for social justice, understanding the anger one feels at the daily insults and injustices of everyday life.

It was also a time where I was probably emotionally vulnerable, seeing my father come to terms with being a gay man with AIDS in a macho culture, fearful of this new terrible illness that, in the 1980s, killed fast. The rejection he endured from some of his old friends contrasted with the warm embrace he got from our family (my mom and my sister and brother) and some other great friends (like

Porgy and Gaspar); this taught me how those who love you will always be there for you no matter what. What carried me through this tumultuous time was the support of my family, my work colleagues at the Sociomedical Research Center and the magnificent friends in Philadelphia.

The end result was that I constantly missed classes because of flying back and forth to Puerto Rico, trying to compartmentalize my studies with a chaotic life, becoming a phantom student. The whole experience made me see the price professional women must pay for wanting a career in the context of having a family and extended work. I constantly felt selfish for putting my family, especially my children, through this odyssey so I could advance my career. Even though my professional life was completely put on the back-burner (i.e. I barely published), I felt the stress take some of the fun and joy out of parenting. I became more of an authoritarian, trying to make sure things got done (like science projects, practicing or reviewing for tests or finishing homework) rather than enjoying childrearing.

Eventually, I was able to do my second internship in Puerto Rico at the Children's Psychiatric Clinic, under the supervision of Jose Bauermeister and Hector Bird. This proved incredibly gratifying, learning how to treat severe cases of children's psychopathology. It also connected me with Glorisa Canino at UPR's Medical School, a bond that accelerated my dissertation by years, not months, when she generously offered to let me analyze her epidemiological data instead of collecting my own primary data. Glorisa became not only another significant senior mentor but, eventually, my close friend and colleague in many of the studies we undertook during the next 15 years (Alegría, Canino, Lai et al., 2004; Alegría, Canino et al., 2008; Alegría, Ludman et al., 2014).

My First Independent Research Study

Being in the right place at the right time gave me opportunities to grow into an independent Principal Investigator (PI). The right place was Puerto Rico, where research was scarce, research teams were small, and opportunities to assume responsibilities as a Project Director (with only a master's degree) were common. Fafy believed that if you put yourself to the task, you could do great things, even those you were not necessarily trained to do in school. She was willing to take the risk with me and some other young investigators. Fearing to disappoint her, we went the extra mile, accomplishing more than we thought possible, from self-learning programming to discussing and implementing complex sample designs or advanced statistics. It meant learning while we were doing, a risky proposition. But Fafy's motto was to figure out what you did not know while also finding out who did and then asking that person to consult with you so you could figure out what needed to be done. It was a steep learning curve but one that, in the research world, I accepted and welcomed. Yet the list of my mistakes would fill pages (like erasing a complete data set by inputting the wrong code; luckily, that was soon recovered). To this day I continue to make mistakes, probably more than I realize. But the lesson for me is to acknowledge, as best as you can, your limitations and work with those who complement the skills or knowledge that you lack. There is no question that this approach to team building in research has accompanied me in my career.

Fafy had obtained R01 funding from the National Institute of Mental Health (NIMH) for a study on the Mental Health Needs of the Puerto Rican Poor. Working as co-investigator on this grant with a team of incredible investigators gave me the opportunity to learn how to conduct a complicated data collection effort. This study included two waves of data based on a random household sample of 3,500 poor or near poor Puerto Ricans on the island. Every detail counted, so we gave it our total attention; and it paid off. During our first wave, we were able to get very high response rates, publish some findings and offer some troubling statistics on the need for mental health services on the island (Vera et al., 1998).

Conducting the study of the Mental Health Needs of the Puerto Rican Poor reinforced my admiration for the resiliency of poor people under conditions of extreme duress. Living check to check with almost no institutional supports left the family as one of the few sources of assistance. Families served the multiple roles of providing long-term care for the elderly, childcare services for the young, housing accommodations for extended family, and more. The intergenerational connection and cooperation was the buffer allowing people to move forward, even with slim to no resources. It also made apparent how many people saw their mental health problems as natural suffering with no cure.

Shortly after the first wave of this study was finished, Fafy retired. NIMH consulted the recent site visitors about a leadership change, and they, for reasons I never found out, chose me to finish the data collection and take over as PI. As a requirement, I had to finish my PhD, which meant my dissertation had to be completed in close to eight months. I was pretty sure this was going to be nearly impossible since I was pregnant with my third child and I would need to take my comprehensive exams and finish the dissertation in a short span of time. My grandmother and my father had recently died. As if all of this wasn't enough, I was having complications with my pregnancy and was bedridden for six weeks.

How I pulled this off I don't know. Just before my comprehensive exams, I had my healthy baby, Alejandro, but I got septicemia and became seriously ill. I moved in with my mom and stepfather to help me take care of my newborn while I was studying for my comprehensive exams. So that I would not lose the opportunity to take my comprehensive exams, they tested me at my mother's home while I had a horrible fever from the septicemia. I was grateful not to have to wait another year to take the test. To this day I thank Leticia Herrans, who took it upon herself to give me the test while I was extremely sick.

With access to Glorisa's data, I was able to finish and defend my dissertation in time to become Center Director in 1989. I was 32. Fafy, Glorisa and Milly Vera, my colleague and dear friend, gave me their full support, which enabled me to accomplish these remarkable achievements. Soon after, NIMH invited me to become a member of the Mental Health Services Review Committee, a move that became equivalent to a crash course in reviewing grants and understanding the intricacies of grantsmanship.

Opportunity struck again as the government of Puerto Rico engaged in a monumental policy change, a health reform that was run parallel to the Clinton reform of 1992, which eventually died an unnatural death. The government privatized the public health system. The government created a monitoring and oversight body, but how the new system was or was not working remained unknown. The government claimed the system made enormous advances in improving access and quality of healthcare, while others voiced substantial skepticism about these claims and believed the Medicaid poor were, in fact, being harmed. We as a team submitted my first real R01 proposal and, in the second submission, got it funded. The third wave of the Mental Health Needs of the Puerto Rican Poor was a massive data collection effort, following the same 3,500 participants three to four years after the second wave. Not only was this a mammoth job, that luckily I shared with Milly and a superb team of co-investigators, but it was also one that was taking place in an extremely politicized climate. Our NIMH-funded project became one of the few empirical studies putting these hypotheses of either total failure or great advances in access and quality in healthcare to the test.

Some lessons that I learned doing this work were the importance of scientifically and objectively evaluating policy; the questionable belief that public services might be better than private ones; and the importance of scientific integrity. Our findings showed that the change in policy made no measurable difference – access and quality were unchanged after the policy implementation. It also showed that the private sector with a small capitation could not really improve either access or quality and that the public sector was doing as well as could be expected (Alegría, McGuire, Vera, Canino, Matías et al., 2001). These results led both groups to doubt our research, sometimes coupled with anger and disappointment. I was blindsided by the public reaction to our study results. But negative results they were, and there was no choice other than to stand by them. Publishing was no small feat since this was the era when negative results were unlikely to get published. Luckily, local politicians were not our peer reviewers, and our work was published in several well-respected journals (Alegría, McGuire, Vera, Canino, Albizu et al., 2001; Alegría, McGuire, Vera, Canino, Matías et al., 2001).

Opening the Door to Studies with Mainland US Populations

One of my most significant opportunities came via Ron Kessler, a highly accomplished sociologist and epidemiologist. He asked me if I would be interested in doing a Latino sample for a national study on the prevalence of mental disorders and mental health service needs in the US. This represented my most major professional leap by far. Like he told me, "this is big league." I immediately accepted and thought, why not also collect data from a sample of Asians? My friend David Takeuchi came to Puerto Rico to submit what would become the National Latino and Asian American Study (NLAAS) in 2001. The magnitude, importance and intensity of this endeavor were beyond anything I had previously done. The NIMH budget was approximately 10 million dollars, drawing responsibility and accountability. The review committee recommended that we spent a year doing cognitive debriefing of our measures. Early on, we had received the support of Juan Ramos from NIMH, which funded three meetings over the course of a year to bring the best multidisciplinary team of Latino and Asian investigators to select the constructs and measures.

I would be remiss if I did not say what a challenging and nerve-racking study this was. Having David as my partner PI was instrumental in undertaking this mammoth study. We shared jokes but also our data collection troubles, trusting each other through serious tension. He has been an amazing friend and brilliant colleague and has brought so much wisdom to the table. NLAAS was conducted in five languages, nationally and in coordination with Ron Kessler and James Jackson (Alegría et al., 2004). We also decided to focus on doing sub-ethnic groups, making sure we had sufficient representation of Chinese, Vietnamese, Filipino, Other Asian, Puerto Rican, Cuban, Mexican, and Other Latino participants. Although NIMH was supposed to have a leading role in working with the four PIs, it did not work out that way. After long conference calls and a lot of wrestling, we agreed to all share a minimum core of measures; unfortunately only a few of the interesting constructs (i.e. acculturation, discrimination, gender roles) were shared across the three studies. But we were able to bring issues of immigration, acculturation, loss of social ties, remittances and others to a national study for the first time. Our cognitive debriefing and multilingual translation and adaptation paid off as we were able to include populations that had never participated or been represented in national studies. It deeply convinced me of the importance of approaching participants in their primary language with topics that would resonate for them.

My Move to Harvard Medical School

While conducting NLAAS in 2001, and now with my two oldest kids in college and my youngest in junior year, having divorced and remarried, I decided to start exploring opportunities for moving with my husband, Tom McGuire, who lived in Boston. We had a commuting relationship for six years, three of which we were married. Commuting from Puerto Rico to Boston or vice versa every ten days was taking its toll. So I applied for a job at three universities (Yale, Boston University, and Brandeis), and after meetings and presentations, I was fortunate to have offers from all three. Meanwhile, Jay Burke, Chair of Psychiatry at one of

Harvard's hospitals, heard that I was in the market and invited me to apply to Harvard Medical School. Never in my wildest dreams did I believe that Harvard was on the cards, but I proceeded. I became a Professor in Psychiatry at Harvard Medical School in 2004, after a lengthy promotions process.

Moving from the University of Puerto Rico to Harvard Medical School entailed a transcendental shift in academic culture, expectations, daily routines and pace; it was another world. To start, it meant I had to speak and write in English all the time, to move to a place where a coat, and sometimes a heavy coat, was needed to go outside and to navigate a new city and workplace. To tell you that this really shook my confidence and took me away from my comfort zone is an understatement. I experienced many days of panic and stress. My skill in scholarly writing was not close to par, and probably still isn't. I felt like I had to work harder, working 60 to 70 hours a week and more, to just put in an average performance. Work consumed my life, making me feel isolated and at risk of losing my social ties. Although I traveled every month to Puerto Rico, I missed my family, particularly my sons, mom, uncle and sister, and close social friends more than anything. I also quickly realized how a change of context (from Puerto Rico to Boston) had instantaneously transformed me, in the eyes of others, to a woman of color.

Together with dedicated staff, we started the Center for Multicultural Mental Health Research at the Cambridge Health Alliance (one of the psychiatry department hospitals of Harvard Medical School), with Jay Burke as my boss and seven staff members. With the support of Jay and Norah Mulvaney-Day, we were able to quickly build a unique research group, creating a niche focusing on multicultural populations. The move expanded my professional collaborations and my mentorship role and gave me professional opportunities beyond my utmost expectations. As Harvard faculty, I was invited to the table of several key professional organizations like Academy Health, National Academy for State Health Policy, National Hispanic Research Network and others. Rapidly I was requested to be on several of Harvard's important committees like Faculty Promotions, Psychiatry Research, Faculty Council and others. The exposure to a whole range of premier investigators and colleagues exponentially increased my collaborations and provided me opportunities that would advance my research agenda and my own career.

At that time, there were few research groups concentrating on Latinos or Asians, and given the small sample sizes in national studies, sub-ethnic differences were rarely considered. With the NLAAS data set and the following R01 grants, we were able to consolidate a talented group of young investigators interested in these populations and immigration topics. A lot of persistence was required to transform a site with limited infrastructure for research together with strict policies for hiring personnel and financial requirements to become more aligned to a fast-paced research environment. But coming from Puerto Rico where a similar context of research had been the rule rather than the exception prepared me well.

Jay Burke proved to be a trusted ally, fighting on my side for the institutional changes required to transform the system and giving me the financial support to grow a parallel infrastructure to conduct research within the hospital. Tenacious co-investigators (Norah Mulvaney-Day, Sheri Markle, Ben Cook, Ora Nakash, Chih-nan Chen, Julia Lin, Lisa Fortuna, Jennifer Greene, Kiara Alvarez, Ye Wang, Dharma Cortes) and project directors (Maria Torres, Andrea Ault-Brutus, Nick Carson, Megan Woo, Lizbeth Herrera) together with formidable collaborators from other Harvard departments (Xiao-li Meng, Sharon-Lise Normand, Norma Ware, Richard Frank, Ron Kessler) and universities (Patrick Shrout, Glorisa Canino, David Takeuchi, Naihua Duan, Jeannie Miranda, Ken Wells, Roberto Lewis-Fernandez, William Vega, Bob Roberts, Celia Falicov, Judith Hall, Paco Collazos, Carmela Alcantara, Enrique Baca, Rodrigo Carmona, Javier Escobar, Helena Hansen, Nabila El-Bassel, Kristine Molina and so many others) helped us grow into a haven where we could study the immigrant paradox, the acculturation hypothesis, the social determinants of health and their impact on minority populations. It launched our entry into the disparities research field, now being able to compare and contrast minority groups in terms of behavioral health needs and services (Alegría, Pescosolido, Williams, & Canino, 2011; Alegría, Woo, Takeuchi, & Jackson, 2009). It also opened the field of clinical trials with minority populations based on the adaptation of behavioral health services to their language and better accommodation of their needs (Alegría, Ludman et al., 2014; Alegría, Polo et al., 2008; Jimenez, Reynolds, Alegría, Harvey, & Bartels, 2015; Lucero et al., 2016; Ramos & Alegría, 2014). I spent the next 14 years enamored and completely inspired by the work we were doing, as I still am today.

At the same time, I had started doing more comparative work with other multicultural populations and international projects. Experiencing these changes in my own migratory process led me to investigate differences in outcomes of sub-ethnic groups and of Latinos in different contexts, but also to explore how cross-cultural encounters impacts communication, diagnosis and clinical care. Taking a stab at identifying what might explain clinical uncertainty led our research group to videotape encounters of providers in their first clinical session with mostly ethnic and racial minority patients (Alegría, Nakash et al., 2008). Again, this opened a window into how disparities could take place in the clinical encounter. We saw how providers, without being aware, dominated the clinical conversation with their patients, took a leading role and sometimes disempowered patients by limiting their input into treatment decisions (Alegría et al., 2013).

Meeting Dan Rothstein and Luz Santana of the Right Question Project (Polo, Alegría, & Sirkin, 2012) led us to initiate research on patient activation and what is now the DECIDE intervention (Alegría, Carson et al., 2014; Alegría, Polo et al., 2008; Allen et al., 2017). We also dramatically expanded our Community-Based Participatory Research, collaborating with the Cambridge school project and several other studies, including our Patient-Centered Outcomes Research Institute (PCORI) study. The richness of including the voice of patients, providers and policymakers expanded our horizons, allowing us to visualize the layers of influence that coalesce to enable disparities problems to remain unchanged. It also made me realize how much of our reasoning is driven by our own life circumstances. It further emphasized how having these multiple perspectives at the same table was necessary for obtaining change in disparities outcomes. The collaboration with Nina Wallerstein, Bonnie Duran, Ken Wells, Loretta Jones, Elmer Freeman and many others provided powerful lessons on the importance of cultural humility, healthy partnerships, win-win relationships and sharing of power and budgets (Lucero et al., 2016). This was a paradigm shift from changing patient behavior to changing institutional and provider behavior (Ault-Brutus, Lee, Singer, Allen, & Alegría, 2014), which became the more prominent interest of mine in these five years from 2012 to 2017.

My career journey has now taken me to my position as Chief of the Disparities Research Unit at the Department of Medicine at Massachusetts General Hospital and to have a joint Harvard appointment in both Medicine and Psychiatry. Once more it has been a continuous change of worlds as I learn the lingo of Medicine, the culture of a different institution and navigate different institutional policies, committees, goals and academic environments. Again it is a whirlwind of change that frames and alters your social and academic position and context, and consequently your daily experiences in minute but powerful ways.

The Interpersonal Change of Culture and Minority Status

One of my mentees taught me about the transnational optic, whereby you see the world in which you live differently when you move from one place to the other; in other words, you start living simultaneously in two worlds – the one in which you were born and the one which now hosts you. You start getting cues of how the reactions from others need to be interpreted more carefully because they might not mean the same thing. You get cues that your tone of voice seems "too loud" or "too intense" according to New England standards. You get too close to people and they back off. People look surprised by how much you touch them. But to you, coming from Puerto Rico, you are behaving normally. You dress with more color and maybe edge, and for some the wardrobe is out of sync with what is expected in academic circles.

Having my husband as a go-between (having lived in New England since 1976) was an advantage and significant source of support. He would help craft my message so it could be understood by the receiver, and remind me not to assume that negative reactions were necessarily due to my ethnicity. He sometimes would also edit my writing (taking out the excessive use of adjectives and adverbs). He would help me understand the Anglo humor, which I initially took too literally and failed to enjoy. Many things he saw as normal, I found perplexing, like why people wanted to know about your academic pedigree, why they were unable to give you directions because it would be too difficult to explain the one-way streets in Boston, or why there are three Beacon Streets in the same metropolitan area. These experiences made me aware of the transformation immigrants face as they integrate into the US.

My migration to the mainland also helped to see how emotion recognition can be difficult if you are not from the same ethnic and cultural background. My work in the US included interacting with diverse staff from Asian, Russian, Latino and European countries. Emotions like warmth, anger, disappointment and others could be misinterpreted because the meaning might be so different depending on our ethnic and cultural backgrounds. And to make an accurate interpretation in these cross-cultural encounters required more cognitive demands, attending to every cue or at least asking more questions to make sure you got it right. Under such conditions you become more cautious and reflective, hitting the pause button and thinking how your behavior will be read by others. In a certain way, you have to listen more, speak less and divide your brain between your thinking and translating the cues of what is the thinking, feeling and behavior of the other. I was surprised how much of my interpersonal interactions were done on automatic pilot when living in Puerto Rico compared to Boston, but it has been a positive change.

There are some negative or perplexing changes that also happened. My children saw changes, such as my embraces becoming softer and more superficial, or being less animated in my talk. These changes were so subtle that I had no clue that my behavior or appearance was slightly changing. Puerto Ricans on the plane traveling to Puerto Rico were more likely to assume I was a tourist traveling back to the island, speaking English to me; or taxi drivers in Boston saying they were surprised that I was Puerto Rican because I did not look or talk like that. This saddened me, making me question whether I was changing, becoming different. It is a theme that reverberates in the interviews we have done with immigrants and what they feel they have lost along the way as they try to make a life in the US. It seems like there are great gains and powerful losses with these different worlds and unexpected learning to pave the way.

References

Alcántara, C., Chen, C.-N., & Alegría, M. (2014). Do post-migration perceptions of social mobility matter for Latino immigrant health? *Social Science & Medicine*, 101, 94–106.

Alegría, M., Canino, G., Lai, S., Ramirez, R. R., Chavez, L., Rusch, D., & Shrout, P. E. (2004). Understanding caregivers' help-seeking for Latino children's mental health care use. *Medical Care*, 42(5), 447–455.

Alegría, M., Canino, G., Shrout, P. E., Woo, M., Duan, N., Vila, D., … Meng, X.-L. (2008). Prevalence of mental illness in immigrant and non-immigrant US Latino groups. *American Journal of Psychiatry*, 165(3), 359–369.

Alegría, M., Canino, G., Stinson, F. S., & Grant, B. F. (2006). Nativity and DSM-IV psychiatric disorders among Puerto Ricans, Cuban Americans, and non-Latino Whites in the United States: Results from the National Epidemiologic Survey on Alcohol and Related Conditions. *The Journal of Clinical Psychiatry*, 67(1), 56–65.

Alegría, M., Carson, N., Flores, M., Li, X., Shi, P., Lessios, A. S., … Interian, A. (2014). Activation, self-management, engagement, and retention in behavioral health care: A randomized clinical trial of the DECIDE intervention. *JAMA Psychiatry*, 71(5), 557–565.

Alegría, M., Ludman, E., Kafali, N., Lapatin, S., Vila, D., Shrout, P. E., … Li, X. (2014). Effectiveness of the Engagement and Counseling for Latinos (ECLA) intervention in low-income Latinos. *Medical Care*, 52(11), 989–997.

Alegría, M., McGuire, T., Vera, M., Canino, G., Albizu, C., Marín, H., & Matías, L. (2001). Does managed mental health care reallocate resources to those with greater need for services? *The Journal of Behavioral Health Services and Research*, 28(4), 439–455.

Alegría, M., McGuire, T., Vera, M., Canino, G., Matías, L., & Calderón, J. (2001). Changes in access to mental health care among the poor and nonpoor: Results from the health care reform in Puerto Rico. *American Journal of Public Health*, 91(9), 1431–1434.

Alegría, M., Mulvaney-Day, N., Torres, M., Polo, A., Cao, Z., & Canino, G. (2007). Prevalence of psychiatric disorders across Latino subgroups in the United States. *American Journal of Public Health*, 97(1), 68–75.

Alegría, M., Nakash, O., Lapatin, S., Oddo, V., Gao, S., Lin, J., & Normand, S.-L. (2008). How missing information in diagnosis can lead to disparities in the clinical encounter. *Journal of Public Health Management and Practice*, 14(Suppl), S26–S35.

Alegría, M., Pescosolido, B. A., Williams, S., & Canino, G. (2011). Culture, race/ethnicity and disparities: Fleshing out the socio-cultural framework for health services disparities. In B. A. Pescosolido, J. K. Martin, J. D. McLeod & A. Rogers (Eds.), *Handbook of the sociology of health, illness, and healing* (pp. 363–382). New York: Springer.

Alegría, M., Polo, A., Gao, S., Santana, L., Rothstein, D., Jimenez, A., … Normand, S.-L. (2008). Evaluation of a patient activation and empowerment intervention in mental health care. *Medical Care*, 46(3), 247–256.

Alegría, M., Robles, R., Freeman, D. H., Vera, M., Jimenez, A. L., Rios, C., & Rios, R. (1991). Patterns of mental health utilization among island Puerto Rican poor. *American Journal of Public Health*, 81(7), 875–879.

Alegría, M., Roter, D. L., Valentine, A., Chen, C.-n., Li, X., Lin, J., … Larson, S. (2013). Patient–clinician ethnic concordance and communication in mental health intake visits. *Patient Education and Counseling*, 93(2), 188–196.

Alegría, M., Takeuchi, D., Canino, G., Duan, N., Shrout, P., Meng, X. L., … Woo, M. (2004). Considering context, place and culture: The National Latino and Asian American Study. *International Journal of Methods in Psychiatric Research*, 13(4), 208–220.

Alegría, M., Vera, M., Freeman, D. H., Jr, Robles, R., Santos, M. C., & Rivera, C. L. (1994). HIV infection, risk behaviors, and depressive symptoms among Puerto Rican sex workers. *American Journal of Public Health*, 84(12), 2000–2002.

Alegría, M., Vera, M., Shrout, P., Canino, G., Lai, S., Albizu, C., … Rusch, D. (2004). Understanding hard-core drug use among urban Puerto Rican women in high-risk neighborhoods. *Addictive Behaviors*, 29(4), 643–664.

Alegría, M., Woo, M., Takeuchi, D., & Jackson, J. (2009). Ethnic and racial group – specific considerations. In P. Ruiz & A. Primm (Eds.), *Disparities in psychiatric care: Clinical and cross-cultural perspectives* (pp. 306–318). Baltimore, MD: Lippincott Williams & Wilkins.

Allen, M. L., Lê Cook, B., Carson, N., Interian, A., La Roche, M., & Alegría, M. (2017). Patient-provider therapeutic alliance contributes to patient activation in community mental health clinics. *Administration and Policy in Mental Health and Mental Health Services Research*, 44(4), 431–440.

Ault-Brutus, A., Lee, C., Singer, S., Allen, M., & Alegría, M. (2014). Examining implementation of a patient activation and self-management intervention within the context of an effectiveness trial. *Administration and Policy in Mental Health and Mental Health Services Research*, 41(6), 777–787.

Jimenez, D. E., Reynolds, C. F., Alegría, M., Harvey, P., & Bartels, S. J. (2015). The Happy Older Latinos are Active (HOLA) health promotion and prevention study: Protocol for a pilot randomized controlled trial. *Trials*, 16: 579. doi: 10.1186/s13063-015-1113-3

Lucero, J., Wallerstein, N., Duran, B., Alegría, M., Greene-Moton, E., Israel, B., ... Pearson, C. (2016, Online first). Development of a mixed methods investigation of process and outcomes of community-based participatory research. *Journal of Mixed Methods Research*. https://doi.org/10.1177/1558689816633309

Mandela, N. (1994). *A long walk to freedom*. New York: Little Brown & Company.

Polo, A. J., Alegría, M., & Sirkin, J. T. (2012). Increasing the engagement of Latinos in services through community-derived programs: The Right Question Project–Mental Health. *Professional Psychology: Research and Practice*, 43(3), 208–216.

Ramos, Z., & Alegría, M. (2014). Cultural adaptation and health literacy refinement of a brief depression intervention for Latinos in a low-resource setting. *Cultural Diversity and Ethnic Minority Psychology*, 20(2), 293–301.

Robles, R., Alegría, M., Martínez, R., Vera, M., & Muñoz, C. (1983). Social integration and health among Puerto Rican return migrants. *Puerto Rico Health Sciences Journal*, 1, 119–125.

Robles, R., Martínez, R., Vera, M., & Alegría, M. (1987). Sociocultural factors associated with contraceptive use in Puerto Rico. *International Family Planning Perspectives*, 21(4), 395–404.

Vera, M., Alegría, M., Freeman, D. H., Jr, Robles, R., Pescosolido, B., & Peña, M. (1998). Help seeking for mental health care among poor Puerto Ricans: Problem recognition, service use, and type of provider. *Medical Care*, 36(7), 1047–1056.

Vera, M., Robles, R. R., & Alegría, M. (1988). Sociodemographic, cultural and interpersonal risk factors as indicators of mental health needs. *Puerto Rico Health Sciences Journal*, 7(1), 21–25.

PART IV
Social Justice

7

A JOURNEY TO AND WITHIN THE BORDERLANDS

Courage, Sustenance, and Transformation

Pilar Hernandez-Wolfe

> In my lengthening middle age, I am beginning to understand that writing is a common rite, the daily practice of placing oneself in the position of remembering in order to arrive at something beyond oneself, something not individual to the writer, but which passes through all the ordinary and remarkable of her to arrive at that something in common.
>
> *Cherríe Moraga (2011, p. 93)*

Initiation and Soul Loss

Nothing could have predicted that my life would take a drastically different course on that October morning when I left for school. I was 14 years old; my brother was 12. As I did every day, I woke up and got ready. I don't remember saying goodbye to my parents but vividly remember going to my brother's room to say goodbye. He was still waking up and he mumbled his goodbye. I remember his face and his big beautiful eyes. Later that morning while I was in class, I was called into the principal's office. Two of my mother's friends were there to pick me up. It was shocking to see them there, and I knew that something was very wrong. They said my brother had been in an accident. Our drive to the hospital was quiet; they did not know how to answer my questions, but their silence spoke loudly to me and I thought that my brother's life was at stake. In my young and inexperienced mind, I could not fathom that he had already left us. But he had, instantly, when a military truck hit him while he was trying to cross a street to catch the school bus. When we arrived at the hospital, neither my parents nor my little brother were around. However, all of my other relatives and family friends were there. I felt like I was walking into another time and space, another world. It *was* another world: one without my brother. When I asked to see my brother, I was guided into a room to see his body already resting in a coffin. He was gone. He had been gone since early in the morning. My heart was crushed, opened with a sword, and profusely bleeding. A part of my soul left with him. I descended into a very dark cavern where I spent a long time listening to my pain and the silence his absence left around me. I had to find my way, learning the contours of this cave, touching its walls, listening to the subtle sounds of life that indeed existed there, and later opening my eyes to the tiny torch of light that my grandmother had lit for me all along. Then my dog came along, and we developed a strong and safe bond; he became my companion inside and outside of this cave.

My family was heartbroken and never fully recovered from this loss. I became invisible to my parents and most family members; my younger brother and I were left with a wide age difference between us. He became the focus of attention, and I became invisible at school too. No one had a clue about how to be by my side and support me when I was suddenly taken out of my adolescence and moved to a space seemingly unknown by all around me. I spent years in this cave and developed the ability to move within its many spaces, and to come out and back in. I like to think that I became a being that could live under and above water and, later, transformed to develop wings. I was able to inhabit my family's and my peers' social environment some of the time but not all the time. The enduring love of my uncle and grandmother felt like a cord that sustained me spiritually and gave me the oxygen my cells needed to continue growing. After all, I was still a child.

As time passed, my family, having always been reluctant participants in the catholic church, left it completely. The church's legacy of political persecution, which the paternal side of the family had endured, stayed with me as a reminder of *the violence* and, centuries before, the holocaust of my indigenous ancestors. Other family members began exploring Protestantism, and my mother later pursued a spiritual path outside of organized religion. Life went on, and though my parents tried their best to bring back our family life, they couldn't. I witnessed a deep sadness in their eyes – a sadness of the soul that couldn't be hidden from me. We bore the pain in silence.

When the time came for me to plan for college, an expected struggle between my father and me came about. My father's parents had grown up in big semi-rural families who struggled to make a living. My grandmother moved to the capital to escape *the violence* and the political persecution that grandfather had suffered. The period in Colombian history called *La Violencia* refers to an undeclared civil war between followers of the two main parties, given impetus by the assassination of Jorge Eliecer Gaitan, a liberal leader (1946 to 1958). My grandmother made a living as a teacher and seamstress. My father, because of his scholastic achievements, was able to attend high school and medical school on scholarships. He was a dedicated son, husband, and professional who had moved solidly to the middle class and wanted his children to stay there. Since there was no wealth or business to inherit, the way for us to continue this accomplishment was through education. However, my plans did not include the medical or science career that my parents wished for me. My interest was in the social sciences and philosophy. This created a burden for my mother, who ended up paying for most of my education as my father refused to do so after my first year in college. From my parents' perspective, choosing a career with such low income prospects would curtail my independence and stability; they thought this would only be a good choice for a wealthy person who did not have to worry about making an income. There is truth in this idea within the context in which I grew up. But I knew I could not betray my heart's desire. I enjoyed the possibility of a choice and prospects for the future resulting from my parents' efforts, work, and class mobility; having dreamed throughout my life about living in another country, I intuited that I would not live in Colombia after college and that I was going to be fine. When I finished college, I migrated to the land that would become my home, although at the time I did not know it.

While high school had been one of the most difficult and painful times of my life, college became a time for opening up, adventure, and blossoming. My times in the darkness of the cave became less frequent. Slowly I emerged, alive and renewed. Looking back, I am aware that I was a misfit in the school I attended because I was not white enough. I was just another girl with black hair and brown eyes; my class origins were dubious, and my last name, "Hernandez," was too common. At the time, I was not aware that many of the experiences I had involved *colorism*. However, as I developed consciousness as a racial being in my social context, I realized the ways in which prejudice relative to skin tone occurred within my own ethnic group. In addition, I was too outspoken, too critical of social issues, and too independent for a young woman. I attended a very established and secular university where, at the time, people of most class backgrounds were welcome. Nevertheless, college offered me environments in which to learn and express myself that were not available at my high school or in my family.

Unbeknownst to anyone in my family, I joined a leftist student group and a women's solidarity group and befriended people who were gay and not necessarily mestizos (like most of us in Colombia). I joined the student march to protest the assassination of Luis Carlos Galan, walking close to the Colombian Palace of Justice Siege in 1985. We could see the smoke and hear the bombs from the university's hills. I walked into downtown Bogotá to see what was happening. I was shocked by the silence of the university and the way in which the media reported the tragedy. For a while, there was little discussion at the school, perhaps due to the collective shock we experienced. The press focused on villainizing the M-19 guerrilla group and highlighting and simplifying the complexity of relationships between the guerrilla's actions and intentions and the Supreme Court. Years later, when I searched for reports on the incidents, I realized the extent of the cover-up by the media. These and many other experiences pushed me into studying and developing practices for peace and social justice while in Colombia and later while studying in the U.S. Having struggled with the ingrained patriarchal practices of Colombian society and having benefited from a middle-class background and elite education, I developed a critical stance toward the cultural environment in which I had grown up. Being a middle-class, heterosexual, cisgender, able-bodied mestiza woman had new meaning in my life. In some way, it set me onto a path that would slowly and steadily build me up like something that resembles the Khejri tree. This is a tree found in extremely arid conditions indicating the presence of a deep water table, known in the Thar Desert of Rajasthan, India, for its medicinal value. As the epigraph in the final section of this essay illustrates, this tree is miraculous in its ability to transform and sustain life.

Bearing Witness: Suffering the Impossibility of Experiencing the Other's Suffering

The social, cultural, and class environment in which I grew up exposed me, close up, to the poverty and economic struggles, sexism and homophobia, and racism that darker-skinned family members suffered. I was an intimate witness to some of my family members' adversities. I learned to discern and respond to their plight not only by speaking truth to it, but also by remaining true to them. For example, my maternal uncle, Fernando, a cisgender, able-bodied gay man, and I had a very special relationship. My Uncle Fernando showed me my wings. He taught me that I could do anything I wanted; I just had to trust myself. In the most simple and magical way, he did this while teaching me to ride a bike when I was around six years old. He helped me overcome my fears, feel my body, and learn to listen and coordinate. He was the same loving being I allowed to hold me during the dark years after my brother passed.

He did not have children and never married; my brothers and I became his surrogate children. We knew of his sexual orientation. When I met his partner, I was elated to see how happy they were. Uncle Fernando was an engineer by training but never found a job in his field and lived a modest life. He loved me unconditionally with a strength that I feel to this day. As I grew up, I realized that he had been hiding a part of his life, including some of his friends and his partner. It pained me to witness how the taboo the family held allowed him to be with us only if he left out a part of himself. He never came out. He knew that I loved him without reservations even though I witnessed in pain how difficult it was for him to be at the receiving end of comments, jokes, and gestures of contempt. When I was old enough to speak up, I challenged those who were blatantly insulting or who delivered microaggressions. Alas, when I was studying in the U.S., Uncle Fernando and his partner were taken away by the AIDS epidemic in Colombia.

I also bore witness to the spanish legacy of racism – deeply intertwined with Colombian culture – which takes interesting forms in a society full of warmth and accommodation. However, as in many other parts of the world, class and color are interconnected. The descendants of the european people who settled in this land, and who took away Indigenous lands in the most violent ways, still own most of it. Truth be told, most of us are mestizos as a result of the systematic rape and enslavement of Indigenous women. I do not know who my Indigenous or spanish ancestors are. I belong to a social class without records and pedigree – yet society maintains those records for the elite. I belong to a dominant group that has appropriated the word "mestizo/a" to identify itself, and we differentiate ourselves from those who claim to be of european descent. My family on both sides is a mosaic of color. The darker ones have had the most trouble making life better for themselves and their families. I am a light brown mestiza, of average height with black hair and brown eyes. I look like any other average Colombian woman, slender and with long hair. My brother is much lighter than me, taller, with black hair and green eyes. My darker-skinned Afro-mestiza cousin and her son have faced discrimination everywhere – at work, in interpersonal relationships, and from her own mother, who cannot accept that she bore a dark-skinned daughter. Our paths not only differed, but were structurally determined; she had less access and opportunity right from the beginning. My relationship with my uncle and cousin taught me about the real-life impact of structural inequity as well as the ways in which solidarity, love, courage, and hope emerge from the margins.

The literature I encountered on transnational feminism, identity, decolonization, and social location in the U.S. made total sense (Mohanty, Russo, & Torres, 1991). My engagement with these ideas is not an intellectual exercise of understanding the other. I have an embodied knowledge of privilege and oppression. I could never be a person, a professor, a systemic thinker, a psychologist, and a therapist who would *not* integrate this awareness and knowledge into my everyday life and work. Identities constructed on the basis of gender, ethnicity, ability, class, and sexual orientation are socially significant, and these context-specific constructs are useful as markers of historical and social location (Martín-Alcoff, Hames-García, Mohanty, & Moya, 2006). These identities intersect in a particular social context, and it is important to identify the structural privileges (i.e. access and opportunity), or lack thereof, that people have simply by virtue of their location (e.g. lesbian, lower-class, fully able-bodied women of color; heterosexual, upper-middle-class, visually impaired women of color).

Bearing Witness to Hope, Joy, and Wonder

My family and my homeland also taught me about hope, joy, wonder, and courage. My grandmothers in particular held a beacon of light for me throughout their lives. They were both hard-working, assertive, smart, and loving women who, as single mothers – due to widowhood or political persecution – had to raise their children at a time in which this task was more daunting than it is today. However, their optimism, hope, and sense of humor were evident when I was with them.

Before I was born, my paternal grandmother, Isabel, almost lost a leg when a young wealthy woman, who was learning to drive without a teacher, lost control of her car and drove onto the sidewalk. After almost losing her life, my grandmother recovered, but one of her legs was severely damaged. She was told that she would have to use a cane the rest of her life. I remember her saying that she never believed this and that she had set out to make her leg work, even if she had to limp. She did it: she limped but never used a cane. She walked everywhere and never dwelled on her injury. She always kept a positive attitude, a sweetness without measure, and the strongest determination I have ever seen. She was certainly like a Khejri tree. An old combatant filled with the wisdom to transform sorrow into joy and find the positive side of life.

The familial, social, political, environmental, and historical contexts in which I was raised created the foundation for my becoming a systemic thinker, a psychologist, and a family therapist. I am grateful for having been born and grown up in a land that nurtured my desire to understand and treat the wounds of interpersonal, social, and historical traumatic stress; to foster resilience; and to develop theoretical underpinnings and applications of feminist and socially equitable therapy models. Some of the memories that stayed with me and which I highlight here involve riding a public bus every morning and afternoon or evening to and from college and passing through a downtown neighborhood where street children lived and where their bodies and labor were sold. I witnessed the pain in their faces every day, while upper-class schoolmates and their families referred to everything they found lacking or reproachable as "Indian" or "indigenous." These people made fun of our ancestors and eagerly identified with everything connected with western Europe or the U.S. Sadly, this is still true. Most importantly, I had a high school social science and philosophy teacher who helped me understand and decode reality through a lens of social justice. At the time, our school was involved in social service with other schools, and the experiences I gained there with his mentoring launched me on a path towards liberation and social justice. I began to get acquainted with the theology of liberation. This later led me to read the works of Paulo Freire and Ignacio Martín-Baró.

My commitment to developing educational and psychotherapeutic approaches to treating the wounds of social trauma and to promoting equity provided the framework for my philosophy of teaching, research, and service as a college professor. I have dedicated a portion of my life to articulating how events taking place at a societal level (the big picture) reverberate in the day-to-day life of the individual and the family (the little picture), and how individuals and families make sense of such events. Likewise, everyday personal experiences tell a narrative about the larger social context. The field of traumatic stress was a natural context for the development of my professional interests. Having grown up in Colombia, with its legacies of decades-long, low-intensity civil war, and, most importantly, the holocaust of Indigenous peoples, I learned firsthand about social and historical wounds, their impact on people's lives, and how people develop adapting and coping strategies. Through my involvement in research projects, as well as educational and human rights activities, I also learned about the crucial role of education, compassion, attunement, and alignment of cognitive and emotional processes in the development of critical consciousness and healing.

Borderland Epistemology

My life in the U.S. expanded my sense of being and opened new horizons in every way. How does a young woman without capital to fund an education in the northern hemisphere get to the U.S.? Through destiny and choice; strong family support in education; a scholastic record of excellence, discipline, and persistence; a dream; and a scholarship. I could not have continued my education in the northern hemisphere without the foreign student scholarship that the University of Massachusetts (UMASS) offered me. I am also indebted to the Puerto Rican educational leaders and administrators who made me a part of the Bilingual Collegiate Program and the Puerto Rican community at UMASS. I carry Puerto Rico in my heart. My parents gathered some of their savings to help me get settled in the U.S.

It was in Amherst and Holyoke, Massachusetts, that I found myself confronted in a very different way with my own class, ability, and heterosexual privilege, as well as racism and sexism. The Counseling Psychology Program was housed in the School of Education, where I met people who had worked extensively with the ideas of Paulo Freire and Martín-Baró and who introduced me to feminist thinking and systemic ideas, social constructionism, and feminism as conceived by women of color and in non-western locations. At the time, the school was an open basket of diverse people and ideas, and I fully immersed myself in it. The works of Martín-Baró have not been fully translated into English. It was my mentors at my alma matter, the University of The Andes, who introduced me to his ideas in addition to contemporary feminist thinking. This helped me launch my initial work with women and human rights in Colombia, and later the beginning of my work on trauma, resilience, and human rights. In the U.S. I learned about second- and third-wave feminism. I am most grateful for the work of Chandra Mohanty and coauthor's (Mohanty, Russo, & Torres, 1991; Mohanty & Alexander, 1996) on third world women and feminism. Their work truly spoke to my heart and helped me clarify my own positions. I also avidly embraced the work of Lillian Comas-Díaz and her colleagues in psychology (Comas-Díaz, 1987; Comas-Díaz & Griffith, 1988; Comas-Díaz and Greene, 1994; Comas-Díaz, Lykes, & Alarcon, 1998).

During those years, the borderlands became very real to me. The stability in my identity that I had experienced prior to coming to the U.S. disappeared, giving way to an open door to expansiveness and more fluidity. That is, my view of gender expanded and I became more critical of rigid binaries; my sense of what class I belonged to changed again; and I became a person of color, a racialized being in this part of the world. Also, my own view and concerns about my body shifted towards expansion and acceptance of broader ways of being in the world. After the demolition of the Berlin Wall in 1989 and the end of the cold war in 1991, I thought a great deal about the meaning of colonization and decolonization in my life and work within the larger context of 500 years of colonization (Mignolo, 1992). Some of my mentors in the UMASS School of Education were working to create awareness on campus. I am grateful for their presence in my life at that time as it was hard to focus on something so painful, even though it was full of possibility (Mignolo, 1992).

The borderlands are the places in-between, where border knowledge and border identities are constructed. Those of us who inhabit these spaces negotiate disparate cultural representations in the attempt to exercise personal and collective agency. By developing self-awareness and by embracing our multiple identities, we can become whole and transcend the barriers that dominant groups have imposed on us. Borderland thinking helps us sort out how to represent ourselves personally and professionally. As people who are habituated to hybridity, we have the right to construct, name, author, coauthor, and implement healing models and methods that apply to the worlds we inhabit. Most importantly, we have the right to dream – with our ancestors and our descendants, and with all nonhuman beings. In developing my own border identity, the writings of Gloria Anzaldúa (1987) gave me support and inspiration.

Borderland thinking does not fit well with dualism, especially the idea that mind and matter involve two ontologically separate categories that cannot be reduced to each other in any way; the mind is equated with a conscious self, and the body belongs to the physical world. How could this make any sense? In structural philosophy, binary opposition is a fundamental organizer of human language and thought. In science, it refers to the dichotomy between "subject" (the observer) and "object" (the observed). As one of the two opposites generally assumes a role of dominance over the other, the categorization of binary oppositions is often value-laden. Though modern science favors a view in which conscious experience is inseparable from the physical brain, the mind and brain being the same, dualism is deeply embedded in the way we conduct our lives in the west. Dualistic thinking, so foundational to western thought, has historically involved power and domination. Since the Enlightenment, european men have sought to completely separate nature from humans and men from women; after the encounter and collisions with other cultures, they also separated savage and civilized, light and dark, etc. Nature became an extension of humans, a passive and reversible object whose parts could be disassembled and categorized and its laws enunciated. In short, nature could be dominated and controlled.

My personal primary frame of reference is that of someone who inhabits the borderlands of bilinguality, binationality, and interculturality. This frame of reference involves an understanding of how knowledge and subjectivity are intertwined with modernity/coloniality and of what the constructing of knowledges of mental health practices in the borderlands can offer us in opening other paths of healing. I insist upon locating our thoughts, pain, vulnerabilities, and joys in the body to speak with an embodied voice. I believe that a decolonizing framework must be anchored in the reality inherent in multiple subjectivity and embodied voice.

I use borderlands thinking in my personal life and in my academic and professional life as a point of departure to situate myself, understand and reach out to others, and travel back and forth in worlds humans and other beings inhabit. According to Anzaldúa (1987, p. 19), the "Borderlands are present wherever two or more cultures edge each other, where people of different races occupy the same territory, where under, lower, middle and upper classes touch, where the space between two individuals shrinks with intimacy." The borderlands are the places in-between, the spaces in which border knowledge and border identities are constructed, the gaps, fissures, and silences of hegemonic narratives; overlapping border spaces and cultural representations that those who inhabit these spaces negotiate to exercise personal and collective agency (Lugones, 2010). For example, when I teach a family life cycle course for master's-level family therapists, a course requirement is that they examine the ways in which social movements in the 20th century and 21st century changed family life. We embark on an analysis of how the environmental movement shapes family life for families in the U.S. as well as the feminist, gay, and civil rights movements. The purpose is to assist in decentering individualistic ideals that overly privilege age, the future, and freedom of choice and to foster a sense of continuity, connectedness, and remembering of other times and other worlds. I bring knowledge and experience back and forth to share, inform, and learn.

From the perspective of scholars in the modernity/coloniality group, borderlands thinking arises from the colonial difference; that is, the wound of coloniality generates the formation of this kind of subjectivity. For Mignolo (2011), border thinking allows us to draw different paths through the recognition of inequality and acceptance of the wound inflicted by the colonial difference, and the enunciation of other knowledges. While teaching at San Diego State University, I supervised students in practice, and usually my classes were a magnet for Spanish speakers from Latin America, Chicanos, Latin@s, and anyone connected to the border. While working with them on examining dimensions of privilege around ethnicity and class in their countries of origin, I included discussions about the history of the unearned privilege we held as a result of the genocide of Indigenous populations since the arrival of Columbus in Abya Yala. Abya Yala is the name that the Kuna people who inhabit northwest Colombia and southeast Panama use to refer to the American continent. I asked them to examine alternatives for taking responsibility for these unearned privileges and to explore implications for their clinical work and development of the self of the therapist.

Like many other scientists (Schmidt & Wolfe, 2009), ecopsychologists (Buzzell & Chalquist, 2009; Roszak, 1995), and systems thinkers (Bateson, 1979), I see no life in a binary way of relating to nature. Venezuelan ecologist Stephan Harding (2006, p. 26) explained that

> science is a dangerous gift unless it can be brought into contact with the wisdom that resides in the sensual, intuitive, and ethical aspects of our natures … . It is only when these other ways of knowing complement our rational approach to the world that we can truly experience the living intelligence of nature.

In his opinion, a new worldview within science and within our culture that integrates conventional scientific reasoning with intuitive knowledge can help us once again experience our planet as animate and filled with wisdom. This view of life and of ourselves on the planet makes us fully aware of our embodied mindfulness, discriminating awareness, and compassion. As a teacher and clinical supervisor, I strive to encourage and actively participate in learning processes that involve critical consciousness, mindfulness, and coexistence with all beings on the planet. I value psychology's contributions to mindfulness, body/mind integration, and experientially centered approaches.

Over time, I have tried to develop conceptual models and empirical research showing how equity and the natural world can be an integral part of healing, to examine the connections between traumatic stress and resilience in historical context, and to expand the ways in which understanding of social location can shape clinical training and supervision. In *A Borderlands View of Latinos, Latin Americans and Decolonization: Rethinking Mental Health* (Hernandez-Wolfe, 2013), I discuss how macrosocietal processes are enacted in the microprocesses of everyday life; I challenge taken-for-granted practices and offer new pathways for therapeutic action. With transparency I crisscross many worlds to situate *nepantla*, the territory for transformation, in the landscape of contemporary academia. My articles in the areas of traumatic stress and resilience, and vicarious resilience examine how social privilege is used in both positive and negative ways. My work on cultural equity in therapy and training, and other works in the field of traumatic stress have been published in Spanish and in English in Spain, México, and the U.S. (Hernandez, 2002a, 2002b; Hernandez & Roberts, 2002; Hernandez and Blanco, 2005; Hernandez et al., 2007; Hernandez et al., 2010; Hernandez-Wolfe, 2011; Almeida, Hernandez-Wolfe, & Tubbs, 2011; Hernandez-Wolfe et al., 2015).

Mestiza Conciousness

I like to use Gloria Anzaldúa's metaphors to describe the part of my journey guided by my Kamentsa teachers, especially Taita Santos Jamioy. The Kamentsa people are only 6,000 plus community survivors of the holocaust wrought by europeans and, later, Colombians. Following their healing traditions, I was able to experience nepantla, Coatlicue, and Coyolxauhqui.

According to Anzaldúa (1987), the process by which mestiza consciousness, or consciousness about hybridity, occurs is a journey whereby we confront multiple ways of knowing, some of which may challenge or coexist with the ones we are familiar with. In this journey, we come to appreciate the wisdom and teachings of all other beings with whom we share the planet (nepantla). We experience a dismantling of the identities we acquired within a colonial mindset that for centuries has driven economic expansion, resulting in the degradation of biophysical systems all over the world. We recover and honor our ancestral knowledge of the medicinal properties of plants, and we appropriate use of the land and healing rituals. Anzaldúa (1987) named this process Coatlicue (she who has dominion over serpents). It refers to the transformative experiences of giving and taking away of life, the contradictions and fusion of opposites, the underground aspects of the spiritual and psychological worlds. It is a challenging space to inhabit, and it invites us to reconstruct our sense of who we are in the context of our natural and human geographies. For me, a key aspect of this process is appreciating how nature shows us the interconnectedness of all life through cycles and chains of food and energy so that the whole system responds to change and at the same time tends to remain balanced and stable. The human mind-brain-body is itself situated within a complex ecological world, interacting with other mind-brain-bodies and with nature and nonhuman beings. These webs of interactions occur at a given moment in time and over evolutionary time. Bateson's idea of the sacred unity (Bateson & Bateson, 1987), the invisible connections that connect living organisms with diverse degrees of complexity, is a mental process and an inherent part of life. Anzaldúa (1987) named this process Coyolxauhqui. After experiencing the challenges of being torn apart in Coatlicue, a process of pulling ourselves together and remembering who we are takes over. This reconstruction of the self is called Coyolxauhqui. The mestiza recognizes the struggles involved in acknowledging the various legacies that she embodies; she cannot claim a single self; she embraces multiplicity as part of her own identity.

In the borderlands, there are translations back and forth; there are continuities and discontinuities. I am connected with my Indigenous ancestors through a way of thinking that places me as a part of a living world, where the use of plants and the flow of the word have a spiritual dimension and are intertwined in the processes of being and learning. However, in Coyolxauhqui, I understand that each of the many perspectives I embrace invoke the power embedded in the colonial process. My writing and speaking about them is an act of resistance that questions epistemic boundaries and elicits the Indigenous hidden legacy into the worlds dominated by those who prefer to forget, or those who view these healing practices as exotic. Anzaldúa's (1987) concept of nepantla describes a path of knowledge and healing. Nepantla connotes the in-between state in which to create alternative spaces in which to live, function, or create. In other words, it is the process of developing political, cultural, or psychological consciousness as a means not only to survive, but to thrive. My multiple-year journey with my Kamentsa teachers, their wisdom and knowledge of plant medicine, helped me through multiple moves and jobs in the U.S., two interracial marriages and two divorces, the choice to not have children, and losses and joys relative to family and friends. They have showed me through ritual, Indigenous plant medicine, and relationship, that I am but a tiny part of life in a grand planet shared with so many other forms of life. Through my mentor and friend Kamentsa Taita Santos Jamioy, I have been able to heal old and newer wounds and have gained the spiritual strength I need to exist in this planet. Being here and now requires solid spiritual strength and connection to stay centered and remember who we are, embrace all beings with compassion, and continue to generate equity with love.

The Borderlands in the U.S. and Colombia, Nepantla, Coatlicue, Coyolxauhqui: Transnational Training

Transnational training experiences may provide future therapists with the opportunity to engage in transformative intercultural learning processes. Lessons in critical consciousness and in how to develop relationships with others through dialogue are possible when we examine global and local issues of equity, history, and social positioning. In 2013 my colleagues Victoria Acevedo, Irene Victoria, and I embarked on an ambitious project: constructing a transnational learning space that would bring together people who wouldn't normally meet, under conditions designed to generate equity in the learning process (Hernandez-Wolfe, Acevedo, Victoria, & Volkmann, 2015). We helped Afro-Colombian women to prepare a setting in which they could enhance their teaching skills and share their rituals with white and mestizo Colombian and foreign audiences, and to think about the future of their own cultural school. The women reflected on (a) their own performance of the new rituals they included to address the welcoming of a new life and the loss of another one; (b) their impact on the students (native and foreign); and (c) their internal decision-making processes and hierarchy. The audience included displaced Afro-Colombian women, family therapy master's trainees from the U.S., Kamentsa ex-governor and psychologist Santos Jamioy, and the three of us. We were hosted by a local, highly ranked university in Colombia. The training consisted of a course, prior to the students' immersion in the city of Cali, that I designed with the following objectives: (a) understanding intercultural learning through collaboration (Falicov, 2012); (b) articulating a practice of family therapy based on principles of collaborative dialogue (Seikkula

& Trimble, 2005); (c) co-constructing a learning space in which trainees examine the notion of dialogue as a responsive and multivocal activity saturated with uncertainty, incompleteness, and multiplicity (Anderson, 2012; Bakhtin, 1990); (d) introducing learning practices consistent with the Latin American Indigenous paradigm of El Buen Vivir (Escobar, 2008; Gudynas, 2011); and (e) examining issues of colonization and decolonization consistent with the views of Latin American authors and social movements (Escobar, 2008; Hernandez-Wolfe, 2013). Detailed information on how this transnational experience was structured and developed can be found in Hernandez-Wolfe et al. (2015). However, I would like to highlight below some key aspects of this learning process.

The students' contact and cooperation with Afro-Colombian women and local professors began as a course prerequisite; it took place prior to their immersion experience in the form of Skype meetings in which they introduced themselves and brainstormed on topics they wanted to pursue with each other. Each group discussed themes that they would like to address in a workshop format during their visit. The Afro-Colombian women met with the anthropology faculty to discuss their needs and plan their workshops for the students. The women suggested gender equity, sexuality, and leadership as themes for workshops. Students selected topics relative to rituals surrounding the birth of a child, loss and grieving, the importance of Afro-Colombian cuisine, and the meaning of community as well as oral traditions involving the recitation and singing of tenths, *coplas*, and other musical forms used in these communities to distinguish the identity of the Afro-Colombian peoples from those of the Pacific Coast.

When the participants came together in person, I asked them to form a circle with an intentional space in the middle in which we could co-create a borderland space. We sat together with our bodies oriented toward each other. A basket placed in the middle served as a metaphor for our collective history, the center of the basket representing community and the outside rim our individual journeys and our connections to the lands we inhabited (Jamioy, personal communication, February 20, 2013). Students participated in rituals to foster appreciation and openness and to help ground themselves and articulate intentionality in their work. The idea was to create integration and balance between "talking about community" and executing actions that demonstrated trust, reliability, camaraderie, solidarity, honesty, and active participation to build community and relational intimacy. Building community helped students expand their engagement in dialogues in which they recognized different horizons and were open to appreciating and experiencing wonder, joy, and play. Guided by some of the traditions of the Kamentsa People (Jamioy, personal communication, January 12, 2013), students learned to become an ecosystem in which each person's consciousness was deliberately oriented to the various elements that constitute the space we occupy and utilize on a daily basis – nature, nonhuman beings, buildings, signs, design, images, classrooms, decorations, and cultural symbols – and to each other. As Bateson (1979) said, just like plants and animals in a tangible ecosystem, relationships and ideas can be the subjects of evolution, extinction, and/or successful flourishing. No ecological system is completely closed; exposure and participation in imagining, producing, and experiencing sound, emotion, discourse, and practices of relating can have a profound influence on ideas already inhabiting our consciousness. While the experience was quite positive for the students, the process was more challenging for the Afro-Colombian women.

Organizational theorists (e.g. Mir & Mir, 2009) have studied knowledge flow in corporations in the context of historical experiences of power differences and economic imbalances that undergird the transnational encounter. Their observations help us not lose sight of the fact that this transnational training experience occurred within the context of two educational organizations with clear mandates to "internationalize education." A big push for the internationalization of U.S. education was launched in the late 1990s for political, economic, academic, and social reasons. The Colombian university offered a long-established institution with high national rankings, rich transnational connections, and myriad social and political projects having various levels of influence in the country.

Following Mir and Mir's (2009) argument, the power differentials between institutions in the U.S. and institutions in "developing countries" like Colombia resulted in a delayed process to get a memorandum of understanding signed and in great differences in the ways in which U.S. faculty were hosted and welcomed in Colombia when they visited and the ways Colombian faculty were hosted and welcomed in the U.S. In my view, this was the result of the oppressive politics and priorities of the institution I worked for; I hypothesize that if the U.S. institution that I am a part of had worked with an educational institution in a country with a similar or more powerful economy, the experience of organizing, contracting, and developing a program may have resulted in a different product relative to the parties' negotiating power. Mir and Mir (2009) contend that this more equal sort of relationship makes for a more governable participant who is less likely to be hostile to the suggestions coming from representatives of the universities – for which access to power and resources is more readily available. While the Afro-Colombian women's participation was carefully planned to involve them actively in a collaborative exchange and decision-making process with the students in the workshops that they were doing for each other, we believe that the influence of the institutions and the country some of us were representing negatively influenced their desire to work with us and to extend themselves to help us with the project. Dr. Victoria consulted with them regularly to discuss their wishes and opinions and to raise critical consciousness relative to their participation in this learning experience. This protected and private space with a liaison they trusted allowed them to develop their own suggestions with less pressure from the other faculty and the students. These consultations were intended to ensure accountability for us and a space of empowerment for them. The women were also paid a fee for their work within the range of what a professional in Colombia would be paid for a three-day workshop. Nevertheless, these measures by no means generated equitable relationships between us.

Mir and Mir (2009) applied Gramsci's concept of hegemony to the process by which power differentials in social groups are maintained by both threats of force and persuasion "to convince subaltern groups in society that the power difference is natural and acceptable" (p. 107). Persuasion seeks the willful acquiescence of subjects to the wishes of the dominant group. Was it possible to avoid manufacturing consent? I believe that this was not entirely possible. The women's status vis-à-vis the Colombian University as an institution was temporarily elevated. Furthermore, unbeknownst to us, and in their desire to offer to us the best of their work, they invited a renowned male community poet who worked full-time as a teacher in a remote town in another state. While none of the women had a stable job with benefits, they paid his expenses in full in addition to a fee for his visit from the funds that we allocated for them. The total cost was very high relative to their earnings from working with us. Professor Victoria, Dr. Acevedo, and I learned about him after the students and faculty arrival in Cali. When Professor Victoria and I debriefed with the women at the end of the student immersion experience, we had a difficult conversation. We needed to problematize less their choice to invite the male poet at such a costly fee. They shared that they wanted to bring the best poet from their community to this audience of foreigners; they assumed that he alone would have something to contribute that they did not have. Thus, not only did they overextend themselves by way of finances, time investment, coordination, negotiation, and giving up of their space with us, but they also underestimated their own gifts and skills in bringing someone that they thought was better. Conversations we'd had with them the previous year on equity and gender emerged again from the point of view of the choices they made and the financial consequences these choices brought about. It was a hard learning experience that brought to the table other issues the group had around decision-making processes and leadership.

Like the Khejri Tree

> Like a true hero, [the Khejri tree] is patient benefactor, generously giving shade from the pitiless heat of the sun, feeding our animals, providing fruits fit for our consumption, releasing nitrogen for our soil, stabilizing dunes, medicating the weak, fueling our fires and supplying the most sophisticated air-pollution filtration system known to man. Over the years this old combatant has seen its surroundings change, as wilderness gives way to rising agriculture, political systems ebb and flow under the weight of oppressive regimes, industrialization, and mechanization.
>
> *Victoria Johnson (2010)*

This miracle tree and the Bishnois community that protected it in AD 1730 in Rajasthan, India, are a source of inspiration for me relative to life, interconnectedness, solidarity, and social and environmental responsibility. As I write this essay, a part of me sits in Bogotá, Colombia, overlooking the beautiful and majestic mountains against the blue sky and behind the home in which I grew up. Another part of me sits in Portland,

Oregon, where I experience home with lush green and creeks that the city offers almost everywhere. The trees there and the trees here, the creeks and rivers there and the creeks and rivers here, the companion animals that I grew up with and the ones I have in my life now, and the loving human friendships I have in both lands sustain a continuity of life that I experience in both of the places that I call home. I view individuals, couples, and families holistically and systemically, and I assist them in tapping into their relational and inner wisdom for healing and transformation. This involves helping them recognize their inner worth, embrace all of who they are, and strengthen their relationships. I integrate experiential/narrative, transgenerational, decolonization perspectives with various modalities of energy psychology and ecopsychology. Like my ancestors, I believe that we are relational beings. Our lives evolve in relationship to ourselves, our partners, our families, communities, and other beings. Relationships are unavoidable. In addition to our human relationships, our companion animals and gardens can also become integral parts of our lives and healing processes.

References

Almeida, R., Hernandez-Wolfe, P., & Tubbs, C. (2011). Cultural equity: Bridging the complexity of social identities with therapeutic practices. *The International Journal of Narrative Therapy and Community Work*, 3, 43–56.

Anderson, H. (2012). Collaborative relationships and dialogic conversations: Ideas for a relationally responsive practice. *Family Process*, 51(1), 8–24.

Anzaldúa, G. (1987). *Borderlands/la frontera: The new Mestiza* (2nd ed.). San Francisco, CA: Aunt Lute Books.

Bakhtin, M. (1990). *Art and answerability*. Austin, TX: University of Texas Press.

Bateson, G. (1979). *Mind and nature: A necessary unit*. New York: Bantam.

Bateson, G., & Bateson, M. C. (1987). *Angels fear: Towards an epistemology of the sacred*. New York: Macmillan Publishing Company.

Buzzell, L., & Chalquist, C. (2009). *Ecotherapy: Healing with nature in mind*. New York: Sierra Club Books.

Comas-Díaz, L. (1987). Feminist therapy with Hispanic/Latina women: Myth or reality? *Women and Therapy*, 6(4), 39–61.

Comas-Díaz, L., & Griffith, E. H. (Eds.). (1988). *Clinical guidelines in cross cultural mental health*. New York: Wiley.

Comas-Díaz, L., & Greene, B. (Eds.). (1994). Women of color: Integrating ethnic and gender identities in psychotherapy. New York: Guilford Press.

Comas-Díaz, L., Lykes, B., & Alarcon, R. (1998). Ethnic conflict and the psychology of liberation in Guatemala, Peru and Puerto Rico. *American Psychologist*, 53(7), 778–792.

Escobar, A. (2008). *Territories of difference: Place, movements, life, redes*. Durham, NC: Duke University Press.

Falicov, C. (2012). Immigrant family processes: A multidimensional framework. In F. Walsh (Ed.), *Normal family processes* (pp. 297–323). New York: Guildford Press.

Gudynas, E. (2011). Buen vivir: Today's tomorrow. *Development*, 54(4), 441–447. doi: 10.1057/dev.2011.86

Harding, S. (2006). *Animate earth: Science, intuition and Gaia*. White River Junction, VT: Chelsea Green.

Hernandez, P. (2002a). Trauma in war and political persecution: Expanding the concept. *American Journal of Orthopsychiatry*, 72(1), 16–25.
Hernandez, P. (2002b). Resilience in families and communities: Latin American contributions from the psychology of liberation. *The Family Journal*, 10(3), 334–343.
Hernandez, P., & Roberts, J. (2002). Resilience and human rights activism in women's life stories. In R. Massey & S. Massey (Eds.), *Comprehensive handbook of psychotherapy: Interpersonal, existential and humanistic approaches* (pp. 413–434). New York: John Wiley and Sons.
Hernandez, P., & Blanco, A. (2005). Violencia política y trauma psico-social. In A. Blanco (Ed.), *11-M: "Atocha Zona Cero"* (pp. 281–310). Madrid: Trocha.
Hernandez, P., Gangsei, D., & Engstrom, D. (2007). Vicarious resilience: A qualitative investigation into a description of a new concept. *Family Process*, 46(2), 229–241.
Hernandez, P., Carranza, M., & Almeida, R. (2010). Mental health professionals' adaptive responses to racial microaggressions: An exploratory study. *Professional Psychology: Research and Practice*, 41(3), 202–209. doi: 10.1037/a0018445.
Hernandez-Wolfe, P. (2011). Decolonization and "mental" health: A mestiza's journey in the borderlands. *Women and Psychology*, 34(3), 293–306.
Hernandez-Wolfe, P. (2013). *A borderlands view of Latinos, Latin Americans and decolonization: Rethinking mental health*. Lanham, MD: Jason Aronson.
Hernandez-Wolfe, P., Acevedo, V., Victoria, I., & Volkmann, T. (2015). Transnational family therapy training: A collaborative learning experience in cultural equity and humility. *Journal of Feminist Family Therapy*, 27(3–4), 134–155. doi: 10.1080/08952833.2015.1092813
Johnson, V. (2010, December 29). Super tree! [Blog post]. Retrieved February 3, 2017, from https://bishnois.wordpress.com/tag/khejri/
Lugones, M. (2010). Toward a decolonial feminism. *Hypatia*, 25(4), 742–759. doi:10.1111/j.1527-2001.2010.01137.x
Martín-Alcoff, L., Hames-García, M., Mohanty, S., & Moya, P. (2006). *Identity politics reconsidered*. New York: Palgrave Macmillan.
Mignolo, W. (1992). The darker side of the Renaissance: Colonization and the discontinuity of the classical tradition. *Renaissance Quarterly*, 45(4), 808–828.
Mignolo, W. (2011). Geopolitics of sensing and knowing: On (de) coloniality, border thinking and epistemic disobedience. *Postcolonial Studies*, 14(3), 273–285.
Mir, R., & Mir, A. (2009). From the colony to the corporation: Studying knowledge transfer across transnational boundaries. *Group and Organization Management*, 34(1), 90–113. doi: 10.1177/1059601108329714
Mohanty, Chandra Talpade, Russo, Anne, & Torres, Lourdes M. (1991). *Third world women and the politics of feminism*. Bloomington, IN: Indiana University Press.
Mohanty, Chandra Talpade, & Alexander, M. J. (1996). *Feminist genealogies, colonial legacies, democratic futures*. New York: Routledge.
Moraga, C. (2011). *A Xicana codex of changing consciousness: Writings, 2000–2010*. Durham, NC: Duke University Press.
Roszak, T. (1995). Where psyche meets Gaia. In T. Roszak, M. Gomes, & A. Kanner (Eds.), *Ecopsychology: Restoring the earth, healing the mind* (pp. 1–17). San Francisco, CA: Sierra Club Books.
Schmidt, G. A., & Wolfe, J. (2009). *Climate change: Picturing the science*. New York: W. W. Norton.
Seikkula, J., & Trimble, D. (2005). Healing elements of therapeutic conversation: Dialogue as an embodiment of love. *Family Process*, 44(4), 461–475.

8

WEAVING IDENTITIES AND THEORETICAL PERSPECTIVES OF CULTURAL COMPETENCY IN *NEPANTLA*

Carrie Castañeda-Sound

> I am an act of kneading, of uniting and joining that not only has produced both a creature of darkness and a creature of light, but also a creature that questions the definitions of light and dark and gives them new meanings.
>
> *Gloria E. Anzaldúa (1999, p. 103)*

Gloria Anzaldúa's quote captures the dynamic act of self-construction and resistance and closely represents my experiences creating my identity and *lugar* (place) as a psychologist, academic, and mother. As a therapist who often utilizes narrative perspectives, I am drawn to dichotomies such as darkness and light because this is where I locate the Borderlands and *nepantla* ("in-between" space) (Anzaldúa, 1999), a phenomenological space where I live as a biracial Chicana. This is a space of resistance to internal and external colonizing forces, and a restructuring of my identity. In this chapter, I will share my *testimonio* to shed light on my evolving perspectives of identity and on clinical and cultural competence as it pertains to work with Latinas in psychotherapy.

Testimonio literature is often situated within social movements resisting oppressive governments or offered as a way to heal from traumatic experiences (Smith, 2010), but, most importantly, a *testimonio* reflects a "part indistinguishable from the whole" (Brabeck, 2003, p. 253) and reveals aspects of a collective experience. Within the field of psychology, *testimonio* is a powerful tool to give voice to the individual experience situated within a communal and historical experience. Engaging in a process of developing one's *testimonio* requires adding a lens of critical consciousness that contextualizes the narrative in sociopolitical and historical contexts, recognizing that authenticity and vulnerability are critical. My *testimonio* will reveal the complexity of my identities and standpoints that are imbued with both privilege and oppression, questions and answers.

Although I personally connect with aspects of the psychological literature about Chicanas and Latinas, my experiences of being biracial are not fully represented in Latino Psychology. I have blended many cultural values from both sides of my family; that is, a White mother and a Mexican American father. An added dimension to my identity is as a fourth-generation U.S. citizen. This identity is often compared to first-generation immigrants and characterized as more acculturated and less physically and mentally healthy than previous generations (American Psychological Association, Presidential Task Force on Immigration, 2012). While research about Latino immigration provides important information about group trends and effects of acculturative stress (American Psychological Association, Presidential Task Force on Immigration, 2012), little is known about the third and fourth generations of Latinos; thus, their rich experiences are overlooked. My *testimonio* will illustrate the nuances of my identities and experience as I relate this *entendimiento* (understanding) to the field of psychology's approach to cultural competence.

My *testimonio* has a foundation in the history of my ancestors. Yet as I've grown, I've delved deeper into the emotional, cognitive, and spiritual forces that helped me embrace these histories to make sense of the present. Since my adolescence, I have struggled with depression, and I often asked, "Why me?" Maestra Grace's quote (in the final section of this chapter) helps me focus on the joy, beauty, and silence in life rather than focusing on the why. I find purpose in de-stigmatizing mental illness, particularly within underserved communities; furthermore, as a psychologist, I am called to practice beneficence (doing good) and revive/restore hope in clients' lives. Once, I was encouraged by a clinical supervisor to share my story of overcoming depression with a client. I remember recoiling at the suggestion not because of the possible clinical implications (this would have been a poor clinical choice), but because of the internalized shame I was holding onto. I was afraid that revealing that aspect of my life would result in rejection from other psychologists and from the field of psychology in general. Six years into my career as a psychologist, I read a *New York Times* article (Carey, 2011) in which Marsha Linehan, the developer of Dialectical Behavior Therapy, shared her experiences with Borderline Personality Disorder. This was awe-inspiring and empowered me to let go of the shame of depression. I realized that if I am going to work to de-stigmatize mental illness and promote wellbeing, I must start with myself. Consequently, I create a space for trainees to explore their preconceived notions about mental health and illness, the impact of context and generational trauma, and the different forms of healing.

¿De dónde eres (Where Are You From)?

My identity cannot be untangled from the Southern California suburb I call home. Located 45 minutes northeast of Los Angeles, Simi Valley is known to be predominantly White, and during the 1980s and 1990s residents proudly embraced the identification as one of the safest cities in the United States (Kelley, 2000). In 1988, it also became the home of the Ronald Reagan Library, and four years later, the location of the trial of the LAPD police officers who beat Rodney King. The verdict of "not guilty" for these police officers was the beginning of the LA uprising. Depending on whom I am talking to, sharing that I grew up in Simi Valley holds multiple layers of meaning and subsequent assumptions about me. With the privilege associated with the opportunities in my small town came an awareness of the demographic differences between my home town and the San Fernando Valley, 14 miles away, where all of my father's family lived. This was my own version of geographical *Borderlands* (Anzaldúa, 1999) and emphasized my biracial identity.

Growing up, the city did not feel as safe to me. For example, I remember being aware at a young age that my gender carried certain risks and that being a girl could involve sexual assault. During my elementary years, I walked home from school and had to pass a house where I learned that a young woman had been raped. Even though I knew little about sex and sexual assault, I felt the trauma and pain from that house and I ran past it as fast as I could each day. I could never put into words the fear and pain I felt, but this deep empathy has translated to an asset in my clinical work. My parents and ancestors passed down a tradition of empathy as a spiritual gift. This spiritual gift, just as many spiritual gifts, can be a double-edged sword – it can be both a blessing and a curse. Because of this, I have to be diligent about maintaining self-care when I do this clinical work and social justice work to avoid secondary traumatic stress (Baird & Kracen, 2006).

¿Eres Uno de los Buenos? *(Are You One of the Good Guys?)*

My great-grandfather was from Chihuahua, Mexico, and immigrated to the United States dressed as a woman to escape his captors during the Mexican Revolution. He opened a small restaurant in Phoenix and was known to ask any stranger who entered "*Eres uno de los buenos*?" He married my great-grandmother Minnie, a young woman from the Tohono O'Odam reservation in southern Arizona, but they divorced soon after having my grandmother. My great-grandfather's survival instincts and focus on knowing a person's heart has been passed on through the generations. Both of my parents were raised in working-class families that held values of resourcefulness and perseverance. These values facilitated my academic career. As a first-generation college student, I experienced feelings of doubt and insecurity (imposter syndrome), consistent with many in that position. I addressed my feelings associated with the imposter syndrome by identifying mentors and empowered colleagues who helped me to connect with my internal power and resilience. Resilience, power from within, and a deeply felt worthiness are the resources that I continue to pass down as my legacy to my students.

Revealing Dichotomies in the Family History

My grandparents resided all their lives in Canoga Park, California. Filomeno (Fil) and Maria both worked picking oranges in the fields when they were young, but as adults, Fil worked at Water & Power and Maria worked as a custodian at a local elementary school. Maria passed on a love of education and learning to me. I remember my cousin and I going with her while she finished cleaning the classrooms. We loved pretending to be teachers while our *abuela* (grandmother) worked. She loved her work and was proud of the contribution she made. She was fearless and waged private battles against the school district's proposals to rezone the schools. She explained to me that the rezoning would have meant substandard resources and education for her children, so she organized the other mothers and they flooded the school board meetings and made their voices heard. This theme of protest and civil rights can be traced to Maria and then to my father. If I complained about injustices to my father, his immediate response was that I should organize a protest. He "walked the walk" and was a leader of his labor union at his place of employment. He also ingrained in me a duty to give back to the community that has given me so much.

My mother's side of the family has a long history in Kansas and Oklahoma as ranchers and farmers. Her ancestors were European American with a strong English and German influence. My grandmother on that side, Avesta, was unique for her time in that she married and divorced three times and, for many years, was a single mother supporting her three daughters. She held many jobs such as waitress and grocery cashier, and she was one of the "Rosie the Riveters" during World War II. She is another example of a strong woman who influenced me to be resilient and push through the hard times.

As I explored by mother's ancestry, I found stories of shame and oppression. For example, I have learned that my mother's great-grandfather was a member of the Ku Klux Klan. No one wants to talk about this history, but it helps me understand how the ideology of white supremacy is passed down through generations, both overtly and covertly. Additionally, my mother's great-great-grandfather (maternal side) was Jewish but stopped practicing his religion due to the anti-Semitism in the United States in the late 1800s. This ancestry helps me understand the context and history contributing to my upbringing and reminds me how pride, shame, and oppression can be passed through the generations (Hardy & Laszloffy, 1995).

When my mother married my Mexican American father in 1970, both of their families were shocked. My mother was a divorceé with two small boys, and my father was six years her junior and had just completed his enlistment in the Marines during the Vietnam War. With time, my maternal grandparents embraced my father. Being very acculturated, he was adept at straddling the two cultures, and the only time I heard him speak Spanish was with his parents, extended family, or close friends. I noticed that whenever he went "over the hill" from Simi Valley to San Fernando Valley, his identity shifted. As a result, I learned how to live in the Borderlands by watching him.

I asked many questions about my ethnicity, but my mom had no understanding of ethnic-racial socialization. For instance, at 5 years old, I entered a Halloween costume contest and the announcer introduced me as a Spanish princess. As I walked across the stage, I was confused and angry, because I just saw myself as a princess. My mom laughed it off, but the experience happened again in first grade when friends told me I couldn't play the role of Cinderella in their game because I had brown hair and eyes. I felt hurt and alienated, but more than anything I felt different. These experiences were pieces in the puzzle of my identity development. I equated difference with confusion and exclusion. It was then that I realized I am neither White enough nor Mexican enough.

At times, I was deluded into thinking I fit in, and then I would be reminded of my difference. For instance, the first time I was the recipient of a racial slur was in high school. I was walking down the street and when a car drove by, the kids all yelled in unison, "Beaner!" As I looked around to see if there was someone else they were yelling at, the realization that they knew I was Mexican American shocked me more than being called a racial slur. Even my maternal grandmother saw me through the lens of whiteness and was surprised when people saw me as Latina. When I was in my twenties, a stranger asked me a question in Spanish, and while we were having a conversation in Spanish, my grandmother asked my mother how this stranger knew I spoke Spanish. My mother then had to explain that I look Mexican American. This experience revealed to my grandmother the way the world sees me: in that moment, my grandmother restructured my identity, expanding it to include how she saw me and how the world saw me.

Critical Consciousness of my Different Identities

I have heard different terms to explain my identity – biracial, biethnic, *mestiza*, and mixed, but my chosen identification since my mid-twenties has been Chicana. Hurtado (2003) eloquently describes this label as "a political move to highlight its 'in-between' position in the interstices of multiple social, economic, and cultural systems" (p. 24). I experienced a *cultural awaking* in my undergraduate years when I took my first Chicano studies class. My Chicano studies courses inspired and empowered me to learn the full history of my ancestors. My *critical consciousness* further developed during my graduate training at the University of Utah, where I embraced the identity of a Chicana Feminist. As a first-generation college student, pursuing a doctorate in counseling psychology was terrifying, but moving from California to Utah was an even greater shock to my microsystem. It was outside the (dis)comforts of California that I truly connected with the intersectionality of my identity. I ventured out of the field of psychology to critical studies in the field of education, and I found that the works of Gloria Anzaldúa, Patricia Hill Collins, bell hooks, and Kimberlé Crenshaw give meaning to the lives of my clients as well as my own. Rather than solely naming the multiple identities, these authors gave the full picture of people's lives, which included the historical role of social inequities, the debilitating impact of being at the wrong end of power, and the spiritual movement of speaking truth to power. My exposure to these scholars was the reason that I added a year on to my studies. I worked as a teaching assistant in the Chicana/o Studies program so I could delve deeper into critical studies within Latinx communities. That year validated my work and selfhood and is a time when I witnessed the power of syncretism and theoretical pluralism (Comas-Díaz, 2014) as it applied to my clinical work.

Decentering Whiteness

With little ethnic-racial socialization from my parents, my emerging young adulthood was spent seeking sources of knowledge and experience to understand and give words to my biracial experiences. As I decentered whiteness and explored my Mexican ancestry, others accused me of "rejecting my White side" or "pretending to be someone else." Although that is how others perceived it, I was on a journey of liberation in my exploration, and in many regards, I was "giving birth to [myself]" (Comas-Díaz, 2016, p. 164). This journey involved cultural socialization. Typically parents are the source of cultural socialization, which involves overtly and covertly transmitting to their child a sense of pride and knowledge about the history, traditions, and beliefs of their ethno-cultural group (Araujo Dawson & Quiros, 2014; Douglass & Umaña-Taylor, 2016; Hughes et al., 2006; Hughes, 2003). Furthermore, strong ethnic identity in Latino parents predicts cultural socialization of children and preparation for dealing with bias (Knight, Bernal, Garza et al., 1993). As my parents managed a blended family with my two older European American brothers (from my mother's first marriage), our family de-emphasized Mexican American cultural socialization, which led to the promotion of color-blindness and egalitarianism, but little discussion of race (Hughes et al., 2006). This context left little room for racial socialization.

Racial socialization involves instilling racial pride and group identity, and it prepares the child for race-related bias and discrimination by providing coping skills and perspectives for understanding race relations (Hughes et al., 2006; Rollins & Hunter, 2013). The Latinx community involves a variety of racial identities, and with my lighter skin color, I have benefitted from skin color privilege. It wasn't until I became a mother of darker-skinned children that I revisited exploring the gaps in my racial socialization. As a mother of multiracial children, I work hard to model critical consciousness, but an important area of growth was my awareness of my need for racial reparenting (Malsbary, 2016). Consequently, I sought outside sources to help me fill the gaps in my racial socialization. These close friends, mentors, *curanderas*, and extended family were my "psychospiritual *rebozo* (shawl)" (Comas-Díaz, 2016, p. 164) that embraced, enlightened, and protected me during this developmental period.

In line with the psychological research, my children initiated dialogue about their racial identity in preschool; their questions never came from a place of distress, but rather from innocent curiosity (Bernal, Knight, Garza, Ocampo, & Cota, 1990). Some of my daughter's questions were: Will my skin be light like yours? Will my children have skin color like me? After my daughter watched a video about the civil rights movement that showed how the police hit African American protestors with water cannons, her response surprised me. She said, "That was really mean (pause); I'm Black and that could have been me!" I was taken aback because I realized that she saw herself in those videos. As a child, I was always an outsider looking in when seeing these videos, while she felt a sense of kinship. This elicited a dialogue about the differences between dark skin and African American heritage; we then had a long discussion about her ethnic heritage and her ancestors' challenges with oppression and their successes. We also discussed racial discrimination and prejudice, and my daughter expressed a developing understanding of oppression. In addition to her sense of kinship and empathy, she embodies a quiet healing presence. In these moments, I can help and guide her, but I realize she is teaching me more than can ever teach her.

Language and Collective Identity

My critical consciousness deepened when I committed to learning the Spanish language while in Mexico. Beyond affectionate words like *mi'jita* (my little daughter), my father did not speak to me in Spanish. When my father was a child, he was hit on the hands with a ruler if he and his friends spoke the language at school, sending a loud and clear message that Spanish was devalued in public spaces. He spoke Spanish with his parents and siblings in my presence, and they often switched into Spanish when they didn't want me to know what they were saying. I felt like an outsider to their "secret" language, and these instances illuminated my whiteness and my outsider status in my own family. As a result, when I had the chance to study Spanish in middle school, I embraced it wholeheartedly. I saw Spanish as a connection between my grandparents and myself – a way to finally feel more Mexican.

After studying abroad in Mexico, I realized that being bilingual in the United States was a form of social capital within Latinx communities. Someone's ability to understand and speak Spanish was used as a way of testing one's "Mexicanness." Gloria Anzaldúa (1990) called this the ethnic test; it includes making assumptions about how "real" a person is as a Chicana or Mexicana based on Spanish fluency. Other dimensions of identity (e.g. social class, geographical location, country of origin, generational status since immigration, etc.) add to the degree of legitimacy when being assessed as a "real Chicana." In my last year of graduate school, another Chicana student said to me, "Well, you're not *really* Chicana, because you're also White." I was angry and felt betrayed, but I am inspired by the validation of Anzaldúa (2000), who shared in an interview that

"The experiences of biracial and multiracial people are very important and we need to hear about them. For a lot of these people it's like juggling all these cultures and none of the cultures want them" (p. 186).

Only when someone feels like an outsider do they constantly work to fit in. Rather than deconstruct the internalized discrimination in this practice, I worked to find a way to fit in by shifting between Spanish, English, and Spanglish. Language switching as well as shifting between my ethnic identities took an emotional toll, especially knowing I was complicit with the bifurcation of my identities in my silence when people assumed both my parents were either White or Mexican. My silence was fueled by a fear of rejection from people that were "really" Mexican or White. As my knowledge and critical consciousness heightened in *nepantla*, they were compounded by a spiritual *conocimiento* (awareness and consciousness) grounded in my indigenous heritage, which informs my clinical work.

Application to Clinical Work

Re(visioning) Multicultural Competence

Cultural competency in the practice of psychology has been a focus of scholarship, application, and debate for the last 40 years. Competency benchmarks are relevant in the training of future psychologists and impact the curriculum of training programs. As a Chicana who completed her training in Counseling Psychology between 1997 and 2005, I recall a concerted effort by multicultural scholars to define and promote an understanding of multicultural competency. As a student, I remember thinking that competency was the "holy grail" and a destination for my focused study, while simultaneously thinking that so much was missing from our understanding of working with Latinas and Latinx communities. Now, 12 years after my doctoral training, the majority of that time having been devoted to the scholarship and training of future therapists, particularly within the Latinx community, I have developed a more nuanced understanding and approach to cultural competency that is grounded in the concept of cultural humility.

Cultural humility is a term coined by Tervalon and Murray-García (1998) to further the field of multiculturalism within primary care settings. They conceptualized cultural humility as encompassing critical self-reflection, lifelong learning, and institutional accountability. While early multicultural theories in psychology embraced the importance of knowledge, skills, and attitudes (D. W. Sue, Arredondo, & McDavis, 1992), at the time of my training, less attention and guidance was placed on institutional accountability and lifelong learning. As a result, my misunderstanding that multicultural competency has an endpoint has been challenged and reformulated to include a multitude of factors such as process-oriented models (López, 1997) and multidimensional models that include scientific mindedness, dynamic sizing, and culture-specific resources (S. Sue,

1998). I have come to envision a woven mat as a symbol for understanding the process, dimensions, and texture of cultural attunement in a clinical setting. Traditional woven mats are made by hand and are common across many different cultures worldwide (e.g. the Philippines, Tonga, Samoa, South Africa, First Nations). When examined closely, these woven mats use different materials, such as straw, cedar bark, bamboo, reeds, or the leaves of a variety of plants native to the local environment. The materials may be coarse or fine to the touch, and they serve different functions, for instance as wall dividers, as clothing, as a place to sit or sleep, for the floor of canoes, or for use in burial (Smithsonian Institution, n.d.). The materials are critical, but more important is the skill required in the weaving. The knowledge needed for weaving is often passed down across generations. This offers a metaphor that fits with psychotherapy and cultural attunement. The different materials that comprise these mats remind me of the variety of cultural stories (e.g. values, acculturative stress, oppression) and problems (e.g. trauma, depression, and anxiety) that vary in complexity, degree, and intensity during a clinical encounter. When working with Latinas, I consider the "materials" that comprise our interaction to include my stimulus value, the problem that brought them to counseling, but also their cultural values and beliefs, ancestral history, stories of pride and shame as well as their connectedness/disconnectedness to collective identities.

Just as mats serve a variety of functions, I consider the most appropriate and functional theories and techniques for my clients. I work from an integrationist perspective, but primarily draw from feminist and liberatory paradigms, and I use techniques from narrative and schema-based cognitive psychotherapy. As I develop a relationship with the client, the theories and techniques serve a function that is congruent with the client's worldview. Although not a psychological theory, Anzaldúa's (1990) conceptualization of *nepantla*, the space "in-between," helps me conceptualize clinical work when my Latina clients are growing in psychospiritual awareness and critical consciousness. For example, *nepantla* is a culturally relevant conceptualization of the phenomenological experience of acculturative stress, ethnic identity issues, and/or navigating oppressive systems. *Conocimiento* is a different dimension and embodies an awareness and resistance of the social hierarchy and power and privilege individuals encounter and may have internalized. Finally, similar to psychotherapists in training, the skills required to design and create woven mats take many years and practice. Once the basic skills are acquired, the artistry and the natural inclination of the weaver can emerge. Some weavers stand out with exceptional ability, but what is impressive to me is the continued practice and commitment to improve their craft. This informs my approach to supervision and training; I encourage my students to learn the basics of counseling and then develop their natural inclination as a psychotherapist. I often begin by asking what they love to do outside of school, what helps them to feel connected and at peace, and what gives them inspiration and energy. This is a great way for students to disconnect from their academic persona and bring to the surface their whole person. For example, one of my students is an accomplished musician and singer, and in her clinical practicum she works with incarcerated youth. One of her more difficult clients writes rap songs, and in one of their sessions he shared the lyrics of one of his songs. She created a "hook" between two of the lines, and the client responded with surprise and appreciation. She shared that the therapeutic exchange shifted the quality of their therapeutic relationship. She connected to an aspect of his identity that was important to him. I encourage students to expand their notions of healing to include culturally centered interventions, such as artistic expression (drumming, dance and *danza*, art, spoken word, etc.). As a result, I firmly believe that growing towards cultural competence requires humility, continued effort and growth, and an appreciation for the different textures and materials that make up clients' lives.

Resistencia y Autocompasión *(Resistance and Self-Compassion)*

> If it weren't for the stones in its path the river wouldn't sing ...
>
> *Grace Alvarez Sesma, (Kumiai/Yaqui/Chicana),* Curanderismo, *the Healing Art of Mexico*

As I approach a mid-career milestone, my professional interests have shifted from solely research and teaching to a need to be more involved in clinical practice and supervision of students. My goal is not just to teach about multicultural psychology and Latinx psychology, but also to model this for my students in our university's clinic. I also am shaping my identity as a leader, and I look to the wisdom of my ancestors and mentors as I venture in this direction. When I dream of the legacy of my professional life, I imagine continuing to teach, supervise, and collaborate with community members to provide services for women, youth, and families that are empowering and informative about holistic, culturally congruent wellbeing. In the words of my great-grandfather, I want to be "*uno de los buenos*" (one of the good guys).

References

American Psychological Association, Presidential Task Force on Immigration. (2012). Crossroads: The psychology of immigration in the new century. Retrieved from www.apa.org/topics/immigration/report.aspx

Anzaldúa, G. (1990). *Making face, making soul: Haciendo caras: Creative and critical perspectives by feminists of color.* San Francisco, CA: Aunt Lute Books.

Anzaldúa, G. (1999). *Borderlands/La Frontera: The new mestiza* (2nd ed.). San Francisco, CA: Aunt Lute Books.

Anzaldúa, G. E. (2000). *Interviews/Entrevistas.* Ed. A. Keating. New York: Routledge.

Araujo Dawson, B., & Quiros, L. (2014). The effects of racial socialization on the racial and ethnic identity development of Latinas. *Journal of Latina/o Psychology*, 2(4), 200–213. doi: 10.1037/lat0000024

Baird, K., & Kracen, A. C. (2006). Vicarious traumatization and secondary traumatic stress: A research synthesis. *Counselling Psychology Quarterly*, 19(2), 181–188.

Bernal, M., Knight, G., Garza, C., Ocampo, K., & Cota, M. (1990). The development of ethnic identity in Mexican American children. *Hispanic Journal of Behavioral Sciences*, 12(1), 3–24.

Brabeck, K. (2003). *Testimonio*: A strategy for collective resistance, cultural survival and building solidarity. *Feminism & Psychology*, 13(2), 252–258.

Carey, B. (2011, June 23). Expert on mental illness reveals her own fight. *The New York Times*, p. A1.

Comas-Díaz, L. (2014). Multicultural psychotherapy. In F. L. Leong, L. Comas-Díaz, G. C. Nagayama Hall, V. C. McLoyd, & J. E. Trimble (Eds.), *APA handbook of multicultural psychology. Vol. 2: Applications and training* (pp. 419–441). Washington, DC: American Psychological Association.

Comas-Díaz, L. (2016). Mujerista psychospirituality. In T. Bryant-Davis, L. Comas-Díaz, T. Bryant-Davis, & L. Comas-Díaz (Eds.), *Womanist and mujerista psychologies: Voices of fire, acts of courage* (pp. 149–169). Washington, DC: American Psychological Association.

Douglass, S., & Umaña-Taylor, A. J. (2016). Time-varying effects of family ethnic socialization on ethnic-racial identity development among Latino adolescents. *Developmental Psychology*, 52(11), 1904–1912. doi: 10.1037/dev0000141

Hardy, K., & Laszloffy, T. (1995). The cultural genogram: Key to training culturally competent family therapists. *Journal of Marital and Family Therapy*, 21(3), 227–237.

Hughes, D. (2003). Correlates of African American and Latino parents' messages to children about ethnicity and race: A comparative study of racial socialization. *American Journal of Community Psychology*, 31(1–2), 15–33. doi: 10.1023/A:1023066418688

Hughes, D., Rodriguez, J., Smith, E. P., Johnson, D. J., Stevenson, H. C., & Spicer, P. (2006). Parents' ethnic-racial socialization practices: A review of research and directions for future study. *Developmental Psychology*, 42(5), 747–770. doi: 10.1037/0012-1649.42.5.747

Hurtado, A. (2003). *Voicing Chicana feminisms: Young women speak out on sexuality and identity*. New York: New York University Press.

Kelley, D. (2000, May 9). Simi Valley retains place as safest city in the U.S. *L.A. Times*. Retrieved from http://articles.latimes.com/2000/may/09/local/me-28198

Knight, G. P., Bernal, M. E., Garza, C. A., Cota, M. K., & Ocampo, K. A. (1993). Family socialization and the ethnic identity of Mexican-American children. *Journal of Cross-Cultural Psychology*, 24(1), 99–114. doi: 10.1177/0022022193241007

López, S. R. (1997). Cultural competence in psychotherapy: A guide for clinicians and their supervisors. In C. J. Watkins (Ed.), *Handbook of psychotherapy supervision* (pp. 570–588). Hoboken, NJ: John Wiley & Sons Inc.

Malsbary, C. (2016, June 13). Racial re-parenting [Blog post]. Retrieved from https://cultureraceimmigration.com/2016/06/13/racial-re-parenting/

Rollins, A., & Hunter, A. G. (2013). Racial socialization of biracial youth: Maternal messages and approaches to address discrimination. *Family Relations: An Interdisciplinary Journal of Applied Family Studies*, 62(1), 140–153. doi: 10.1111/j.1741-3729.2012.00748.x

Smith, K. M. (2010). Female voice and feminist test: Testimonio as a form of resistance in Latin America. *Florida Atlantic Comparative Studies Journal*, 12, 21–37.

Smithsonian Institution. (n.d.). Sharing native cultures: Grass mat. Retrieved from http://alaska.si.edu/record.asp?id=264

Sue, D. W., Arredondo, P., & McDavis, R. (1992). Multicultural counseling competencies and standards: A call to the profession. *Journal of Counseling and Development*, 70(4), 477–486.

Sue, S. (1998). In search of cultural competence in psychotherapy and counseling. *American Psychologist*, 53(4), 440–448. doi: 10.1037/0003-066X.53.4.440

Tervalon, M., & Murray-García, J. (1998). Cultural humility versus cultural competence: A critical distinction in defining physician training outcomes in multicultural education. *Journal of Health Care for the Poor and Underserved*, 9(2), 117–125.

9

TRANSFORMING DEVELOPMENT THROUGH JUST COMMUNITIES

A Lifelong Journey of Inquiry

Ester R. Shapiro (aka Ester Rebeca Shapiro Rok)

> The struggle is inner: Chicano, indio, American Indian, mojado, mexicano, immigrant Latino, Anglo in power, working class Anglo, Black, Asian—our psyches resemble the bordertowns and are populated by the same people. The struggle has always been inner, and is played out in outer terrains. Awareness of our situation must come before inner changes, which in turn come before changes in society. Nothing happens in the "real" world unless it first happens in the images in our heads.
>
> *Gloria E. Anzaldúa (1987, p. 87)*

Family Storytelling as Cultural and Intergenerational "Time Travel" across Borderlands

There are many ways to share my stories of the living, evolving, contested history of my Cuban Jewish Eastern European American family continuously shaping my life and work as a Latinx Psychologist, educator, and healer. Here and now, I want to explore Anzaldúa's central insights, opening the chapter, about how crossing Borderlands/overcoming blockades, imposed and internalized, commences through an arduous, continual, and rewarding journey of personal inquiry and discovery. I became a culturally centered, developmental-systems-oriented psychologist first as a strategy for personal survival in decoding complexities of my Latinx immigrant family experiences. I came to understand why a bookish, perceptive girl had to be harshly disciplined to know, desire, and embrace her "place" in preserving a particular vision of the family's future. Enduringly, I have dedicated my life's work to articulating how all families, including my own, mobilize meaningful cultural/spiritual resources to overcome hardships, especially in contexts of inequality, and how to develop purposeful awareness permitting us to evaluate and transform these experiences. Informed and challenged by dialogues across differences, I join with others cultivating Gloria Anzaldúa's Borderlands "*conocimiento*" on an arduous path towards critical consciousness inspiring collective action. As Anzaldúa underlines in the opening epigraph, we internalize our sociopolitical worlds as lived experiences, and emancipation begins with our inner re-visioning of these choreographies. Similarly Maria Lugones (2004) describes tools needed for transformation requiring first the clarity of challenging anger in confronting relations of unequal power and only then pursuing empathic "world traveling" towards the goal of establishing hard-won coalitional consciousness and solidarity in a shared struggle for social change.

Inspired by these writers/guides, and by my family storytellers who helped me time-travel to the Russian/Polish border in the early 1900s or to rural Cuba in the 1930s, I would add that our personal past is a shared, complex experience, contingent/responsive to contexts of both time and space, especially to the catalytic moment in time when we connect with the courageous writer, beloved friend, cherished teacher, mentor, or healer who recognizes a dimension of self, necessary but societally devalued, by which we wish to live. We share a wellspring of provisional sociopolitically informed stories we tell ourselves and others to creatively mobilize cultural resources and solve real, material, current problems of shared intergenerational development Entre Mundos/Between Worlds, especially under conditions of inequality (Shapiro, 1996, 2013, 2014; Shapiro and Alcantara, 2016). Our culturally informed stories/counter-stories are themselves creative resources, offering continuity in the face of disruption, honoring family members' heroism in facing everyday and catastrophic hardships on behalf of our survival, reweaving the fabric of heritage too often violently, deliberately torn to enforce intersecting inequalities. With these *respaldos*/this backing, we can transfigure/transform our lives, more deliberatively choosing what we wish to live by. I learned to collect, cultivate, and cherish as well as question, reimagine, and revise our multi-voiced, evolving intergenerational family stories, from my Havana childhood in a bilingual Spanish/Yiddish household through a Spanish/English adolescence in South Florida, college and graduate studies in Massachusetts, working as a clinical psychologist and educator in Boston, and now as an elder with aging, ailing parents.

I want to share what I have learned about our impactful role as teachers, mentors, and healers, inspired by Paulo Freire's "pedagogy of love" (Darder, 2015) and mobilizing what Bluck, Alea, and Ali (2014) call reminiscence as growth-promoting "time travel," in guiding meaningful dialogues supporting transformational learning. Accompanied by Anzaldúa (1987, 2015), I appreciate that those of us questioning an unjust world are handed a story of our deviance and required conformity by an oppressive society and its enforcers, often including our families. Lovingly, loyally, we find ways to live by these constraints, turning ourselves against ourselves until the time and place when we can choose, instead, to live by what we truly love and see most clearly, our path illuminated by the clarity of our yearning for justice and righteous anger. When first defying unjust demands, we experience what feels like a lonely transformative process of death and rebirth. We may begin with what appears to others like an *arrebato/* crazy rebellion, yet we are moving towards clarity and wholeness, from darkness to light. We identify kindred spirits and are comforted by companions in "*la lucha*"/the struggle, within just communities we join and help create. Now aged 65 and a cancer survivor, with responsibilities to past and future generations, I appreciate how even pasts shadowed by sorrow or violence remain rich renewable resources on behalf of joyous, arduous present lives and hoped for futures when we preserve capacities to see clearly, love open-heartedly, protest injustice, and act on purpose-full visions.

Where I Write from: Searching for Cuba as Necessary and Forbidden

For nearly 30 years, I have taught, learned, and practiced at the University of Massachusetts, Boston, a unique urban public university with a mission deeply grounded in Paulo Freire's participatory education and co-creation of knowledge through community partnerships that strives to educate students and generate knowledge contributing to local and global inclusion and equity. I teach diverse undergraduate students in Psychology and Latinx Studies, and graduate students in a culturally oriented Clinical Psychology PhD program as well as in a new multiethnic studies program in Transnational, Cultural and Community Studies. I work with colleagues at the Mauricio Gaston Institute for Latino Public Policy, named after a Cuban American activist who was a beloved, inspiring faculty member until his untimely death, founded and directed by his widow, my friend and colleague Miren Uriarte. Thanks to this community, I have focused my work on "wellness as fairness" (Prilleltensky, 2012), requiring material, procedural, and interpersonal justice as foundational to our human dignity and thriving. My extended family has called me *loca/arrebatada/*crazy and *podrida/*rotten for my love of books, traitorous for choosing others over family, pitiable for my lack of children, poor marital choices, and limited wealth. With compassion, respect for ethics in telling stories not exclusively my own, and, when needed, righteous anger, I travel back in time to retrieve my multifaceted lived experiences, "finding what was lost in plain view" (Shapiro, 1994b).

I was eight when my family left Cuba, as their early support for the values of Cuba's revolution vanished once the new government turned towards socialism. Yet I experienced and cherished Cuba's distinctive, curious, and open-hearted approach to cultural encounters, captured by Cuban anthropologist Fernando Ortiz's concept of transculturation as a process of mutual transformation, even as Africans and Europeans met under conditions of power inequalities (Bernal and Shapiro, 2005; Ortiz et al., 2014). Sadly my family's grief-stricken response to displacement and loss of their beloved Cuban life was to disavow Cuba and reaffirm our commitments to Jewish family continuity and material success. Required to speak Spanish at home and to socialize exclusively within our extended family, we were forbidden to have non-Jewish friends, locating our Cuban identities narrowly within politically conservative Miami Cuban Jewish communities. Like all children, attuned to my family's grief and vulnerabilities, I worked hard to refashion myself in loyalty to the new story of our lives, in which our temporary sojourn in Cuba led us to the United States, the true Promised Land. I appeared rebellious in my early adulthood life choices: instead of allowing my father to choose college, career, and husband for me, I insisted on attending college and remaining in Massachusetts, choosing Clinical Psychology graduate school instead of Medicine or Law. My ailing 88-year-old father recently said to my sister, "I wonder, if I hadn't allowed Ester Rebeca to move away to college, if all of you would have stayed here." In my mid-twenties, when my cousins were joining family businesses and launching highly traditional gendered families, I married an older (Jewish) graduate student who had custody of his 8-year-old son. Looking back, I now see my choices as secretly honoring family expectations while preserving my professional path.

Yet I obeyed what had become internalized prohibitions against contact with Cuba, while slowly exploring my "Latinidad" through friendships and professional experiences with Latino/a communities in Amherst and Boston, unaware of the price paid for severing those worlds. I remember at a party celebrating my successful dissertation defense on adult development during transition to parenthood, my faculty advisor, feminist sociologist Alice Rossi, exclaimed: "Ester, you look like a different person when you speak Spanish, so animated!" Guillermo Bernal, a Cuban American fellow student in the University of Massachusetts, Amherst, PhD program, became my first guide back to my "Cubanidad" as politically informed and grounded in both my family lived experiences and my culturally informed professional identity. But as he and other Massachusetts friends returned to Cuba via the Cuban American Antonio Maceo Brigades of the late 1970s, I was not ready to confront these powerful, internalized blockades. When I moved to Boston and my two sisters followed, becoming social workers focused on Latino/a communities, we established roots and extended family who shared our values. We befriended Latina professionals, among them Cuban Americans and immigrants from across Latin America and the Caribbean, who shared our political commitments to social justice service. Through these friendships, I launched a search for my specific Cubanidad, one that defied imposed, conservative narratives and appreciated the values of Cuba's socialism.

My first marriage dissolved in my thirties when my stepson left for college; among our many conflicts were my husband's refusal to have more children, jealous intolerance of my family, social life, and yearning for Spanish/Latinidad/Cubanidad, from which he felt excluded, and his inability to support my strivings for an academic career. Reflecting at the time, with sisters, friends and in psychotherapy, I was shocked that my seemingly rebellious choices and insistence on independence and gender equality surreptitiously reproduced familiar choreographies of my loving but shy, submissive mother's marriage to my domineering, tyrannical father. Seeking to rebuild my life on a more secure foundation, I reconnected to these disavowed Cuban experiences and commitments/*compromisos*, visiting Cuba for the first time in 1989 and joining a community of Cuban Americans of my generation seeking these connections who created *Bridges to Cuba* (Behar, 1995). I met Cuban Jewish cousins, having been unaware they existed because they had remained to build the revolution and had been excommunicated. I was introduced to my second husband within this community, a Boston-based Cuban American journalist, scholar, and activist focused on Cuban, Caribbean, and Latin American history through the voices of its creative artists. Falling in love, we discovered similar enraged disavowals and enforced silences in our childhoods within outwardly angry, secretly grieving Cuban exile families. Together, both scholars and educators, we have built a home dedicated to knowledge for a just world, in which transculturation of Cuban, African, Jewish, and Socialist Democratic cultural, religious/spiritual, and political traditions inform/transform one another. These rediscoveries have shaped my evolving trans-national/cultural/disciplinary education and family storytelling.

Borderlands Travel as Journey of Inquiry

Everything I know, teach, and continue learning about our culturally and socio-politically grounded family lives, our opportunities to collectively learn from lived experiences and transform our worlds, has emerged from a journey of inquiry (Shapiro, 2005, 2014) that began in studying my family's responses to challenges of survival at the crossroads of everyday family life in collision with politics and history. The challenges were as true for my twice-immigrant family – survival depending on their documentation status, fearing the destitution of poverty – as for my immigrant students and their families today. They live with the burdens of poverty, often in the shadows, fearing they or their loved ones, hard at work supporting local and transnational families, could yet face a cruel, disruptive, and life-threatening incarceration and deportation for the civil violation of lacking the right paperwork for U.S. sojourn. From family, from colleagues and community collaborators, from patients and students, I learned that in this often arduous, at times indifferent or deliberately cruel, and always blessed world, opportunities for surviving and thriving are not created equal. Yet as I learned first from family, the audacious and determined could overcome and triumph, creatively identifying resources where at first it seemed nothing could flourish, preserving our past and protecting our futures in defiance of destructive forces. Creatively, through the alchemy of love, drawing on cultural and spiritual resources expressed through routines and rituals of everyday life, we discover ways to turn scarcity into abundance.

Seeking to understand how gender equity was both constructed and subverted within the rhythms of family life as these intersected with societal inequalities, I became a student of the many avenues through which we mobilize multifaceted resources supporting shared development, through major transitions like reproductive decision-making, childbirth and parenting, adolescence/coming of age, illness, dying, and death, recognizing that our best responses require justice in our opportunities to meet daily life demands, what Latinx/Latin American feminists call "*lo cotidiano*"/the everyday (Shapiro, 2005, 2014). Initially trained in clinical developmental psychology, family therapy, and life-course sociology, and learning public health and critical health psychology through my work with transnational Latin American and U.S. Latinx women's health and social movements (Shapiro, 2000, 2005, 2014), I appreciated the *encaje*/interweaving of personal and societal processes with our families – biological and chosen kin – as the crucible supporting equitable, shared development throughout the family life course (Shapiro, 2013). I call myself "A Clinical Psychologist in Recovery" and a "Born-Again Health Promotion Researcher," because my training for licensure in biomedically based, diagnostic clinical psychology has been transformed by my life-course-grounded, transdisciplinary journey of inquiry. Many of my students are intimidated or alienated by the term "research" until introduced to transdisciplinary and participatory action research (Baum, MacDougall, & Smith, 2006; Leavy, 2011), supported by cultural theorist Appadurai's vision of research as a human right:

> Research is a specialized name for a generalized capacity, the capacity to make disciplined inquiries into those things we need to know, but do not know yet. All human beings are, in this sense, researchers, since all human beings make decisions that require them to make systematic forays beyond their current knowledge horizons.
>
> *(2006, p. 167)*

My research is informed by my own interpretation of my Cuban Jewish American identities and values; it is increasingly conducted with students as partners, actualizing these values together with them within communities that have cultural heritage formed from many historical strands. Education mobilizing inquiry for social change becomes a mutually empowering and healing practice connecting personal struggles on behalf of families and communities with solidarity for change.

Writing Grief as a Family Process

Studying family life-course transitions as opportunities for growth promotion, I transitioned from the culturally and politically informed environment of my Amherst PhD program to McLean Hospital for internship, at a time when Freudian psychoanalysis ruled Boston practice and DSM II was still in use. I was diagnosed as "borderline" due to my interest in working with faculty applying relational and developmental approaches. I next did child and family postdoctoral studies at Judge Baker Children's Center, where I joined like-minded colleagues.

I was especially fortunate to work at The Family Support Center with a new transdisciplinary, multiracial team rooted in Community Mental Health and Civil Rights movements and focused on cultural and social resource understandings of family experiences after a loved one's death. Grounded in our own lived experiences with bereavement while also listening closely to our patients, we challenged dominant Freudian theories requiring "decathexis," or letting go of internalized/imagined relationships with the deceased, especially for children experiencing a parent's death – a deeply destructive belief contradicted by emerging evidence. I had listened to my paternal grandmother, Abuela Berta, speak of the devastating sudden death of her father and brother due to a bridge collapse – "accidental," though bridges to Polish Jewish communities were typically not maintained. I knew that my Abuela Berta, her two younger sisters, and her mother, suddenly a family of women with limited means of support in a dangerous war-torn region, had moved forward with courage to create successful lives. They were resilient even if also shadowed by these impactful losses. My Abuela Berta named all three of her children with variations of her father's name: Nachemie/Consolation. As a working team at Judge Baker Children's Center, instead of using imposed diagnostic categories to patient's presenting problems, we began by exploring our own life struggles with death and loss in diverse community contexts. Together we asked: what existing and new resources helped us, our loved ones, and the African American, Puerto Rican, Salvadoran, Lebanese, and other immigrant families we met move forward with lives diminished but not extinguished by loss? As our patients became co-investigators, their lived experiences of grief and growth joining with our evolving knowledge, tested in the crucible of their own lives, we were able to see challenges like poverty or incarceration and cultivate cultural resources like family bonds and spirituality, that were invisible under ideological biomedicalization. Having theorized family life-course transitions using emerging developmental systems theories and qualitative methods, I brought that contextual perspective to writing on grief and shared development, highlighting cultural/spiritual family resources including transformed, continuing bonds with the deceased as resources nurturing positive developmental outcomes, what an emerging literature termed "resilience" (Shapiro, 1994). Recognizing these possibilities for growth even in contexts of inequality and adversity, working from transdisciplinary perspectives mobilizing critical consciousness and social resources, we could relieve suffering while supporting new meaningful relationships and reasons for living in response to a loved one's death.

Learning and Teaching in the House of Memory: Discovering Resources for Flourishing

Exploring the developmental uses of memory within the interdisciplinary field of applied cognitive psychology as it informs our knowledge of adult development and aging, Bluck, Alea, and Ali (2014) describe the personal past as offering opportunities for "time travel," return to reminiscences that can help us face unfolding challenges of adult development and aging by exploring new insights and dimensions of relationships in ways that allow us to face new, evolving demands. The authors – three of the four from Trinidad, a rarity in our field – review the work of important cross-disciplinary adult development theorists and researchers, including psychoanalysts Erik Erikson and Carl Jung, sociologist Beatrice Neugarten, gerontologists Robert Butler and James Birren, feminist philosopher Simone De Beauvoir, as enduringly useful historical antecedents. On my syllabus for an APA required course in the Clinical Psychology PhD program, Social and Cultural Bases of Behavior, I use Bluck et al.'s paper to bridge different historical eras in understanding positive developmental contexts for emergence of symptoms in adult life. My own graduate education took place in a different era, heavy on theory-based, sociopolitically decontextualized "schools of psychotherapy" and light on accountability gained through systematic inquiry, including our own sources of subjectivity. Our APA-approved program in Clinical Psychology strives to balance cultural accountability and critical reflexivity with demands of training in diagnosis and in research-supported/evidence-based practice. I engage students in personal, family-centered cultural reflection narratives and clinical practice observations in response to readings, exploring contexts of adult and family development supported by cultural resources and burdened by inequality. As teacher and mentor, I help students explore a menu of readings, set like an abundant table, so each can choose what most inspires curiosity and best answers urgent questions, sharing our journey of inquiry. Together, we assess dynamic societal contexts responsible for facilitating or impeding positive coping and growth, environments within which all of us respond as best we can to daily demands and challenging transitions, even as opportunities for thriving or exposure to suffering are structured unequally. What does research offer when, instead of focusing on diagnosis, we first ask: How do we best use culturally grounded relationships and spiritual resources, loving compassion, righteous anger and collective action to respond to life's burdens and remake contexts of our own/shared development towards self-determined, desired goals?

Continuously learning from my own life experiences, formed in contexts of political upheavals over ideologies contesting who had the right to live well and flourish and who must be dominated, abandoned, exploited, or destroyed, I bring my life-course developmental systems training into conversations with Paulo Freire's critical pedagogy as well as critical race and feminist women of color perspectives on how societal oppression and abuses of power "get inside" us to enforce oppression and how Psychology as a discipline colludes with these processes (Fine and Cross, 2016). Freire's pedagogy was deeply informed by the humanist, "Neo-Freudian" feminist and Marxist psychoanalysts, like Erikson, Fromm, and Horney, as well as by moral philosopher Martin Buber's emphasis on the ethics of dialogue in which we are responsible for appreciating the subjectivity of others (I/Thou) rather than their objectification (I/it), viewed as a sacred trust. In *Pedagogy of the Oppressed*, Freire's (1970) emphasis on the importance of critical consciousness also drew from Martinican psychiatrist Frantz Fanon, especially *Black Skins, White Masks* (1952). Fanon's revolutionary work, emerging in French colonial Algeria from his innovations in culturally meaningful, egalitarian treatment, believed that to challenge internalized, racialized colonialism as it operates within us required real-world decolonization. Students from my research team presented applications of Fanon's work to practice-based research with University of Massachusetts Boston women students in recovery from psychiatric hospitalization in contexts of gender-based violence, with Palestinian refugee communities, and in responding to an unjust firing of Latinx staff at a local community health center through organized protests. All conducted social-justice-oriented dissertations, with careers actualizing these ideals.

An Unexpected Opportunity for a University Career

First in my family to graduate from college, I grew up in a Cuban Jewish family whose multiple migrations had taught them to focus on financial achievement and to mistrust education as nurturing critique rather than family loyalty. In love with books, I knew absolutely nothing about planning the life of a scholar I had always dreamed of. Unable to get a faculty position in Boston and unwilling to displace my family to move for a job, I chose instead to contribute to collaborative educational and practice settings challenging the status quo, at a turning point in clinical practice, helping create interdisciplinary psychoanalytic institutes (Meisels and Shapiro, 1989) and supervising community practice on multicultural teams. I was fortunate to get the opportunity to teach at the University of Massachusetts, Boston, when my Amherst PhD program mentor, Castellano Turner, became the inaugural Clinical Program Director for a new PhD program focused on cultural, developmental, and social justice training. The University of Massachusetts Boston is an urban public university for commuting working students, a majority of whom identify as non-White, are from immigrant and working-class backgrounds, and are first in their families to attend college. We offer one of the critical engines of educational opportunity in a state with the highest indexes for quality of life for the wealthy and educated and intersecting inequalities for the poor, particularly our Latinx immigrant and Black communities. Due in part to successful opposition from powerful private institutions in Boston and our Amherst flagship state campus, University of Massachusetts, Boston, was initially mandated to develop only undergraduate, and later graduate, programs that would not compete directly with these more powerful institutions. I joined the faculty in 1989 to coordinate Practicum Training for the University's new culturally and developmentally oriented Clinical Psychology PhD program, with my teacher Cass Turner as the founding director and Joan Liem as the visionary guide who made the case for founding a program with what remains a unique training approach. I discovered that across the campus my colleagues and future collaborators included the newly formed Mauricio Gaston Institute for Latino Public Policy and Community Development and other community-partnered research institutes working for social justice. Many of our faculty were guided by Paulo Freire's writings, as his translator and co-author Donaldo Macedo taught critical pedagogy in Applied Linguistics. I approached clinical practicum training from a whole-student developmental perspective, seeing students' community-based clinical experience, along with their research interests and guiding sense of purpose, as steps that could help achieve professional goals while also positioning them to have maximum impact as agents of change.

In 1990, my first year teaching Clinical Psychology students a course in Child Developmental Psychopathology emphasizing realistic contexts of distress and positive growth-promoting resources (I refused to teach a course focused primarily on child diagnosis and DSM III), an African American student saw me struggling to describe my Cuban Jewish racial/cultural identity. She suggested I read James Baldwin's 1984 essay, "On Being White … and Other Lies." Baldwin eloquently argues that Southern and Eastern European immigrants considered "non-White" were invited to "become White" in the United States as long as they agreed to Black/White definitions of racism. He asserted that given our historically recent experiences with German extermination, Jewish immigrants choosing "Whiteness" were the worst offenders. This insight into my own racialized political history has helped me teach students of all backgrounds how to understand their "place" in webs of intersecting inequalities imposed by our families, societies, and ourselves in unwitting collusion. By opening my mind/heart to my Cuban Jewish experience of transculturation, supported by my return to Cuba and my second marriage, I began to cultivate the Afro-Cuban spiritual traditions that have become part of my own heritage, pedagogies, and healing practices. Returning to Cuba often, I have found much to admire in the socialist revolution's commitment to universal, high-quality, integrative, family-centered health and mental health care available in neighborhoods while also providing specialized care sensitive to psychological needs (Shapiro and Bernal, 2013). I traveled to Israel only once, in 1990, visiting my Abuela Berta's youngest sister, my great-aunt, Yochebed and the family she established in Palestine in 1936 when she took charge of her ailing mother who refused to immigrate to pagan Cuba. I found the open expressions of racism towards Arab and Palestinian communities and justification of violently imposed occupation intolerable, and I have been unable to return.

I was fortunate to have allies for my culturally oriented, practice-based theoretical writing within Psychology and across campus, as my tenure in 1996 was contested though eventually approved by the department, then denied by the College Personnel Committee (CPC), accompanied by a vicious letter of justification that was deliberately designed to destroy any confidence I had in the value of my own work. In my letter of rebuttal, I successfully argued that within a new practice-based PhD program in a historically undergraduate institution, my work in applied, culturally informed clinical scholarship and my role in designing and supervising community-based practicum training was consistent with our institutional values and definitions of scholarship. In the midst of this fraught process (I had my fifth miscarriage shortly after receiving the negative CPC letter) I had a dream: our campus is located on a peninsula surrounded by Boston Harbor, and I dreamed that I and a male colleague in Psychology whose tenure had been approved were together on a small motorboat approaching the university library. He was allowed to disembark, but I was not. This image echoed the 1939 voyage to Havana of the *St. Louis*, a ship filled with German Jewish immigrants who due to increased immigration restrictions were not permitted entry in Cuba or the United States and were forced to return. Having fought for my place in this institution, as if my life depended on it, I now share my strategies for preparing a successful tenure case with colleagues, and my story is instructive for faculty whose work defies disciplinary categories. But institutional violence in educational settings leaves its mark, resonating with histories of violence, and I have not (yet) applied for evaluation required for promotion to full professor.

Writing Family Histories for Public View: Ethical Challenges

In my forties, I joined Latinx and other feminist colleagues in Gender and Cultural Studies writing politically informed *testimonios*/personal narratives, beginning with how I overcame both political and family prohibitions to return to Cuba (Shapiro, 1996), initiating a transformation as I challenged the official story of our Cuban American exile. I found that sharing critical, contested transitions across generations in my Cuban Eastern European Jewish family helped me reflect on an arduous past to illuminate the path ahead. With my beloved paternal Aunt Consuelo's consultation and permission, I wrote my first family story, "From Belorus to Bolondron: A Daughter's Dangerous Passage" (Shapiro, 1999), about the coming of age of Nachame/Consolation/Consuelo in 1936, en route from an early childhood in the strictly controlled ghetto life in the dangerous Bloodlands of the Russian/Polish border to the open society of their small town in rural Matanzas province, Cuba. Consuelo's voluptuous body, her exuberant personality, and her blond-haired, green-eyed exotic beauty initiated a flurry of unacceptable courtships from important men in Bolondron. My grandparents charged her two younger brothers with her surveillance so my grandfather could deliver beatings, though these did not succeed in stopping her unacceptable non-Jewish romances. By the time Consuelo was 17, she was twice married through arrangements in the Havana Jewish community. Teaching Adolescent Psychology as "Coming of Age in the Context of Culture" and encouraging undergraduate students to become co-investigators of their own lives, I often told her story, framing it as a cautionary tale for my own coming of age between cultures, a battle I won though struggling with my own experiences of violently enforced gender roles. In that story at that time, both my Tia Consuelo and her mother, my Abuela Berta, still living, I noted that my *abuela* had always favored her two sons – my father Nachemie/Jaime, the youngest and best-liked, and his older brother, the taciturn, responsible Neiach/Noel – and shut out my Tia Consuelo, insisting she belonged to her husband's family now. I reflected that after the untimely deaths of her father and older brother and the many struggles of their all-women family, her own life had contradicted the gender traditionalism that she then enacted and enforced. Together, her sons joined her in caring for my chronically ill Abuelo Lazaro while, at the same time, lifting their family business to impressive success, first in Cuba and then in South Florida.

After publishing a series of these family stories, from the feminist standpoint that I had the right to speak from my silenced voice, I came to appreciate that these were not only mine to tell. Additionally, my understanding of these stories and the purpose for telling them evolved with time as our shared lives unfolded. For many years, I kept writing but stopped publishing these family stories, concerned that I had not fully considered impacts of family storytelling on the many others involved. Writing about cooking for my sister's wedding or about using Santeria as a supportive resource when my husband and I briefly separated, I placed details in print that would remain fixed and public. Although I showed those most directly involved the manuscripts in draft, I began to feel uneasy about sharing intimate details of others' lives without more careful consideration of methods and ethics. I have come to identify this work as "autoethnography," which goes beyond personal narrative or testimony to conduct systematic inquiry on how our lives reflect sociocultural processes (Chang, 2016). Tolich (2010) argues that individuals discussed in our autoethnographies deserve anticipatory consent regarding issues that may emerge now and in the future and require "process consent" as the project evolves through stages of discovery and disclosure, and he acknowledges the coercive possibilities when seeking consent only after a manuscript is completed. He notes "internal confidentiality" as a central concern since family members may learn things about each other that were shared in confidence. Although Tia Consuelo assured me that she didn't care what anyone thought of her, I found myself flinching when reading what others had cruelly relayed about her unacceptable behavior and the violent discipline they believed she deserved. Her great-grandchildren have asked me to share these family stories, an aspect of our intergenerational family lives that now reach past a century of living memory, recognizing I am now their sole guardian. I take these responsibilities to heart and am seeking responsible ways to do so. I have continued to draw on family stories as sources for shared learning in my teaching, now much more aware of the ethical implications of sharing these family stories. Teaching community-engaged research ethics as part of training in qualitative, creative-arts-based methods and participatory research across courses, we explore how our lived experiences are both a unique source of knowledge and grounded in our unique subjectivities. Still sensitive to the need to protect the privacy and vulnerability of past, present, and future family members, and to the provisional nature of these stories – invocations of ancestral stories on behalf of a specific time, place, need, and conversation – I am ready to write family stories for public view again.

Revisiting Family Stories: Balancing Tradition, Innovation, and Equity

On the Cultural and Intergenerational Borderlands

When I wrote the first sentences of this chapter, I started here: Looking back in intergenerational time and space for this narrative, I see how I was fortunate to grow up in my close-knit, polyglot, Polish/Byelorussian Jewish extended family in Havana, later transplanted to South Florida, lovingly cherished by my two intrepid, determined, though domineering grandmothers, who survived wars and revolutions across continents encompassing most of the 20th century and the dawn of the 21st. Their living examples spoke more enduringly to me than their silent collusion in often violent family enforcement of strict patriarchal roles and materialistic values, particularly those restricting my educational aspirations, viewed as encouraging my disobedience and endangering my marriage prospects and future as a wife and mother, prohibitions I fiercely fought. How it comes to be that women in our families, with their many strengths, collaborate as enforcers of family-centered gender inequality has been central to my life's work. I appreciate, with Anzaldúa, that while we must work to transform our inner worlds, we also have to act in the world of real politics and policies or we slide into complicity. Fine and Cross (2016) challenge Psychology for its colluding with inequality when only fighting oppression by cataloging individual deficits/damages. Observing my world in light of past experiences, I continue to learn from the evolving Cuban revolution and from global/transnational gender equity, civil rights, and human rights movements, which remain works in progress in these dark times. I appreciate that maintaining power inequalities requires careful social policing and strict mind control, and liberation requires first recognizing painful experiences of internalized oppression and social targeting through which the ideologies of intersecting gender, race, and class inequalities are imposed and maintained. I have also come to appreciate the centrality of culturally grounded, gender equitable family roles in easing burdens of an unjust society and creatively protecting our capacities to survive when necessary and flourish when possible.

Both my *abuelas*, each born on a different war-torn border of Poland, steered their families through dangerous times at critical crossroads of politics and history as these fateful forces collided with the specific timing of births, bar mitzvah ceremonies (in my generation, for boys only), coming of age, courtships and weddings, illness and deaths punctuating the flow of our multiply transplanted, continually evolving family lives. Respected as the guiding elders of our twice-refugee extended family, in their vigorous forties in 1952 when I was born, both *abuelas* compellingly contradicted the rigid gender roles adopted by our extended family in Cuba and strictly enforced during our immigration and resettlement in South Florida in 1960. Both lived long lives allowing them to know their great-grandchildren within often transplanted, at times struggling, yet ultimately thriving families. *Mis abuelas*/my grandmothers differed in many ways – my maternal Abuela Adela, the youngest in her family, arrived in Cuba as an adventurous, sociable adolescent and responded open-heartedly to the openness of a multiracial Cuban culture, in ways exemplified by her exuberant Cuban Jewish cooking and hospitable open-door policy. Introduced to her husband, my reticent Abuelo Salomon, through an island-wide network identifying elegible Jewish bachelors, she spoke to us in a mix of accented Spanish with some Yiddish, reflecting her Cuban transculturation. My paternal grandmother, Abuela Berta, became the responsible oldest and co-parent after the accidental deaths of her father and oldest brother coincided with the start of World War I. She fell in love with my handsome, pampered, frail Abuelo Lazaro and formed her young family on the Russian Polish border. This included her eldest, my exuberant Aunt Consuelo, lovingly remembered; her middle son, my taciturn Uncle Noel; and my father, Jaime, her youngest and favorite child – their lives always on the edge of famine or catastrophe until their just-in-time immigration to rural Cuba in 1936. Abuela Berta was far more guarded with outsiders: speaking to us in Yiddish mixed with Polish and Russian, she sternly warned that friends could always betray and only family could be trusted. Her desiccated, Polish-style holiday brisket was untouched by Cuban influences, food consumed for survival only; her bereaved family survived during World War I when their home was seized for a military hospital thanks to her mother's ingenious recipe for potato peel soup made from commissary discards.

First in Cuba, then later in Cuban Jewish enclaves in South Florida, both *abuelas* honored rules and roles of Cuban Jewish patriarchy while, at the same time, clearly subverting them: they ran successful family businesses through multiple migrations, while elevating their husbands and sons into positions of business and family authority and marrying off their daughters as required by tradition. Both adored me as a bookish, observant, and curious girl, entrusting me with cherished family stories of struggle and survival. Yet they also unquestioningly accepted my father's often violent enforcement of his patriarchal authority over his wife and three daughters. As in many other periods of history, women may be called on to take the mens' role during times of crisis, but patriarchy like all forms of power protects its privileges, and societies return to traditional gender roles for continuity and security. In our family, traditional gender roles became even more entrenched as our transplanted multigenerational family achieved economic success. When, unexpectedly, the nationalist Cuban revolution became allied with communism, my initially supportive family made plans to become refugees in the United States, rejecting dreams of a just and equal society and turning to family loyalty and material security as the most enduring values. There, our extended family became part of a Cuban American migration that vociferously attacked Cuba's revolution, accepted the many associated privileges of their cold war visas and enduring political power and economic supports, while refusing those opportunities to other immigrant communities.

Closing Reflections: Psychology of Shared Development and Social Justice

While both *abuelas* shared stories of remembered lives in now vanished villages, kin and neighbors murdered, cemeteries desecrated, and of the enduring losses that punctuated their life stories, they did so as lessons for living, surviving, and thriving in unpredictable times and unfamiliar places. Listening closely to my *abuelas*, I became a witness to lost lives in far-away geographies, appreciating my own family life in the larger flow of historical time. Recognizing my obligation to honor their sacrifices I have also critically interpreted these values, informed by my own understanding of Jewish ideals, my childhood appreciation of Cuba's distinctive cultural values and socialist revolution, and my adult exploration of Latinidad/Cubanidad. Pursuing my own transculturation, I have embraced a far more inclusive concept of the communities within which I wish to be accountable to those values, in ways that many in my family find suspect. I find it intolerable that in my name as a Jew, Israel continues an illegal and inhuman occupation of Palestinian lands. I visit Cuba often and have friends and collaborators there though, alas, no remaining family. I have insisted on my own interpretation of family loyalty, one in which I reject family values of material prosperity and unquestioned togetherness, choosing instead to live by values highlighting educational opportunity as an ethical obligation and sacred trust. Accused of family disloyalty, I argue that even though I sometimes defied my parents as an adolescent, chose my own education and career far from home, selected my own unsuitable husbands and live and work in Boston away from extended family, I am actually the most loyal. Unfaithful to family unity and material success, I remain faithful to our Cuban Jewish transculturation, both transforming and maintaining our deeply held Jewish values viewing *Tikkun Olam*, healing of the world through a striving for social justice, as a sacred trust.

My life as a woman whose love of education took me far from my family remains a mystery to most of the extended family in South Florida. Unable to bear my own children, I have sought and found ways to transform the weight of this enduring sorrow into other forms of generativity. I do so as a devoted *tia/* auntie and as a dedicated teacher and mentor to students and colleagues in both university and community settings. Yet, facing curiosity, cruel recrimination, or pity for my choices, inevitably resonating with my own regrets, I choose socially conscious love combined, when needed, with a clarifying dose of righteous anger. My politics have taught me powerful tools for promoting wholeness through knowledge, allowing me to lovingly, respectfully, with disobedience and confrontational resistance when necessary, act in ways that transform our own contexts towards greater justice. I look back on our often courageous, at times meanly competitive, and always forward-looking family with admiration and compassion, with righteous anger when necessary to my survival, and with determination to live by my values. With these family stories, I affirm that even within our most arduous experiences we can continue to discover rich insights, renewable resources, and supportive communities. These discoveries assist us in moving forward, guided by a sense of purpose in achieving meaningful goals.

Only by insisting on my rights to interpret my life story and act upon it on my own terms can I live by the principles of politically critical, spiritually and ethically informed revolutionary love animating my life choices. As I face the end of my parents' lives and uncertainty of my own health, I once again feel fortunate for this opportunity to reminisce. I can afford to exercise the power of compassionate listening because I have learned to do so without turning against myself. With health and travel restrictions due to sequelae from my cancer treatment, I visit my elderly, ailing parents as often as I am able. I attend family celebrations, where I affectionately/ethnographically observe the transplantation of a form of close-knit, Spanish-speaking, Polish shtetl life surviving anachronistically in contemporary South Florida. The contradictions between family values and actions, the complex, contingent family stories that were told uniquely by each family member while they claimed to subscribe to a harmonious whole, intrigued me. More importantly, they offered me a foundation for understanding shared, intergenerational development, particularly during family life-course transitions, and a path towards my own independent interpretation of our shared lives, and the knowledge and values I chose to live by. They taught me the great value of the optimistic preferred story, one in which loss galvanizes purpose. Yet I also watched closely as our family relationships often contradicted these official stories. I too chose my preferred story, one in which loving compassion and appreciation of life experiences resulting in such divergent views helped me understand, protect myself, and forge my own independent path. I learned to discern enduring strains of sorrow that often underly harsh angers, translating my understanding into a more complex, multifaceted, and inclusive story.

My life within my twice-uprooted, refugee immigrant family has offered me an open door to the rich experiences and challenging puzzles of human development as our intergenerational lives in time and place abruptly and forever changed. Continuously, consistently time-traveling to the past on behalf of an arduous present and hoped for future, my look back in time is not merely through my own memories of events, but with recognition that lived experiences are far more complex than we can capture with words in any language, even more challenging when lived in translation. I share our collective memories, reassured that transplanted roots also grow deep. I learn from and with my students, appreciating their own arduous journeys towards wholeness through the redemptive power of education, offering my mentorship as they select a professional path permitting them to give back to their communities. Antonia Darder, scholar of emancipatory education, writes:

> Understanding *love as a political force* is essential to understanding Freire's revolutionary vision of consciousness and transformation … love constitutes an intentional spiritual act of consciousness that emerges and matures through our social and material practices, as we work to live, learn, and labor together.
>
> *(2015, p. 49)*

Darder, like Freire, insists that a politics of love is foundational to our work as we face oppression and seek within our daily realities the seeds of possibility for transformation.

I write now at a time in U.S. history where the desecration of Jewish cemeteries has resurfaced in climates of increased impunity among White supremacists and anti-Semites. They remind us that we can renew our sense of purpose and dedication to justice by remembering our past while connecting this knowledge to the coalitional/collaborative fight for justice across communities. Although I may fight my discipline of Psychology for its unexamined collusions with biomedicine or its overly narrow, decontextualized research methods and practices protecting societal inequalities, I could not have asked for a better disciplinary home for my journey of inquiry and the meaningful work I do today.

References

Anzaldúa, G. (1987). *Borderlands/La Frontera: The New Mestiza*. San Francisco: Aunt Lute.

Anzaldúa, G. (2015). *Light in the Dark/Luz en lo Oscuro: Rewriting Identity, Spirituality, Reality* (Ed. A. Keating). Durham, NC: Duke University Press.

Appadurai, A. (2006). The right to research. *Globalisation, Societies and Education*, 4(2), 167–177.

Baldwin, J. (1984). On being white … and other lies. *Essence*, 14(12), 90–92.

Baum, F., MacDougall, D., & Smith, D. (2006). Participatory action research. *Journal of Epidemiology and Community Health*, 60(10), 854–857.

Behar, R. (1995). *Bridges to Cuba/Puentes a Cuba*. Ann Arbor, MI: University of Michigan Press.

Bernal, G., & Shapiro, E. (2005). Cuban families. In M. McGoldrick, J. Giordano, & N. Garcia-Preto (Eds.), *Ethnicity and Family Therapy* (3rd ed.; pp. 202–215). New York: Guilford Press.

Bluck, S., Alea, N., & Ali, S. (2014). Remembering the historical roots of remembering the personal past. *Applied Cognitive Psychology*, 28(3), 290–300.

Chang, H. (2016). *Autoethnography as Method*. Abingdon, UK: Routledge.

Darder, A. (2015). *Freire and Education*. New York: Routledge.

Fanon, F. (1952). *Black Skins, White Masks*. New York: Grove Press.

Fine, M., & Cross, W. E., Jr. (2016). Critical race, psychology, and social policy: Refusing damage, cataloging oppression, and documenting desire. In A. N. Alvarez, C. T. Liang, & H. A. Neville (Eds.), *The Cost of Racism for People of Color: Contextualizing Experiences of Discrimination*. Washington, DC: American Psychological Association.

Freire, P. (1970). *Pedagogy of the Oppressed.* New York: Continuum.
Leavy, P. (2011). *Essentials of Transdisciplinary Research: Using Problem-Centered Methodologies.* Walnut Creek, CA: Left Coast Press.
Lugones, M. (2004). *Pilgrimages/Pregrinajes: Theorizing Coalitions Against Multiple Oppressions.* New York: Rowman & Littlefield.
Meisels, M., & Shapiro, E. (1989). *Tradition and Innovation in Psychoanalytic Education.* Washington, DC: American Psychological Association, Division 39.
Ortiz, F., Gonçalves, J. F., & Morton, G. D. (2014). The human factors of Cubanidad. *HAU: Journal of Ethnographic Theory*, 4(3), 445–480.
Prilleltensky, I. (2012). Wellness as fairness. *American Journal of Community Psychology*, 49(1–2), 1–21.
Shapiro, E. (1994a). *Grief as a Family Process: A Developmental Approach to Clinical Practice.* New York: Guilford Press.
Shapiro, E. (1994b). On finding what had been lost in plain view. *Michigan Quarterly Review*, 33(3), 579–590.
Shapiro, E. (1996). Exile and professional identity: on going back to Cuba. *Cultural Diversity and Mental Health*, 2(1), 21–33.
Shapiro, E. (1999). From Belorus to Bolondron: A daughter's dangerous passage. In M. Agosin (Ed.), *The House of Memory: Stories by Jewish Women Writers of Latin America* (pp. 230–240). New York: Feminist Press.
Shapiro, E. (Ed.). (2000). *Nuestros Cuerpos, Nuestras Vidas* [Our Bodies, Our Lives]. New York: Seven Stories Press.
Shapiro, E. (2005). Because words are not enough: Transnational collaborations and Latina revisionings of health promotion for gender justice and social change. *NASW Journal*, 17(1), 141–172.
Shapiro, E. (2013). Family resilience and chronic illness. In D. Becvar (Ed.), *Handbook of Family Resilience* (pp. 385–408). New York: Springer Press.
Shapiro, E. (2014). Translating Latin American/US Latina frameworks and methods in gender and health equity: Linking women's health education and participatory social change. *International Quarterly of Community Health Education*, 34(1), 19–36.
Shapiro, E., & Alcantara, D. (2016). Mujerista creativity: Latin@ sacred arts as life-course developmental resources. In T. Bryant & L. Comas-Díaz (Eds.), *Womanist and Mujerista Psychologies* (pp. 195–216). Washington, DC: American Psychological Association.
Shapiro, E., & Bernal, I. L. (2014). Integrated mental health systems: The Cuban experience. In S. Okpaku (Ed.), *Essentials of Global Mental Health* (pp. 152–161). Cambridge: Cambridge University Press.
Tolich, M. (2010). A critique of current practice: Ten foundational guidelines for autoethnographers. *Qualitative Health Research*, 20(12), 1599–1610.

PART V

Mentorship and Leadership

10

MAPS OF MEMORY

Oliva M. Espín

> Maps are useful guides, but they are site-specific ideological constructions and are quickly dated by the earthquakes of history.
>
> *Juana María Rodríguez (2003, p. 39)*

All memory is memory of place, space, or location even when that "place" may not be a concrete or physical space. However, in my case, concrete spaces are deeply intertwined with my place in life and with the specific places in which I have found myself. Those places and spaces and the memory of them have made me who I am. Moreover, personal memories and narratives based on those memories evolve in the context of relationships – to other persons, to stated and unstated expectations of particularly important groups of people in our lives, to collective memories valued and shared in the context of specific cultures, even to entities that may be interpreted as fiction by others, such as what we understand as God or the Divinity. And, in turn, those memories developed in relationships become "the story of the self" (Freeman, 2007).

Indeed, all "lives are lived at the intersection of individual and social dynamics; life stories are correspondingly structured by multiple narrative logics and frames" (Maynes & Pierce, 2008, p. 43). But it seems to me that this is especially true for my life and personal story. The particular historical and social circumstances of Cuba followed by years lived in different countries, each with its own cultural, social, and historical context, before finally coming to reside in the United States have shaped my life narrative and sense of self in ways that are not typical. It is a given, that all "personal narratives are contextualized by, reflect on, and explore the individual's place in collective events and historical time" (p. 43) and that "personal narratives both specify and are contextualized by particular historical moments" and "emerge in historically specific cultural and institutional settings"

(p. 45). Yet, because "individuals are shaped by their contexts, but never reducible to them" (p. 67), I know that my memories and life narrative are my own and, as such, different from others who may have similar experiences of immigration and exile in a variety of contexts.

Thus, even though I share with others some of the particular historical, cultural, and social circumstances of those places that are central to my memories, there are ways in which the accumulation of multiple contradictory experiences, of memories and places, creates for me a rather jumbled picture that requires a peculiar effort at making sense of it all. This jumble is the uniqueness of my story. I know I could have become a different person if only a few junctures and contingencies might have been different or not have happened at all, if I had lived in places other than the ones where I found myself at different points in my life. As I have written before, "I do not know and will never know the person I could have been had I not left my country. The only me I know is the one that incorporates the consequences of migration" (Espín, 1999, p. 1).

I am made of intersections, memories, and maps of places where I have learned and grown to be who I am, some of which do not even exist anymore. My "mattering map" (Kaschak, 2011) and the maps of my memories forever moving and transforming themselves as they shift, taking center stage or fading into the background as events and circumstances call on them to come to the fore or recede, as happens for everyone else. The change characteristic and sense of instability of the first three decades of my life may have exerted a pressure on me that created memories and altered some expected patterns of identity.

In a sense, there is nothing unique about that. All human beings experience shifting conditions in their life priorities and their understanding of the meaning of their memories. But, I think that because of the multiplicity of concrete geographical spaces and historical contexts in which I have lived, my life has had so many shifts that the maps of my memories of places and spaces, emotional as well as physical and concrete, have been and continue to be more unstable and shifting than those of many others.

Through the years, I have shared autobiographical details in my professional writing to illustrate some points or to respond to requests to provide accounts of my life for a variety of purposes. I have presented accounts of my life as a psychologist, a feminist, a feminist therapist, an immigrant, a lesbian psychologist; descriptions of my spirituality, my intersecting identities, and other variations (e.g. Espín, 1991b, 1993, 2005, 2008b, 2014a, 2014b, 2015b, 2017; Kawahara, 2017). I have also been writing a memoir about my childhood and adolescence in Cuba that is nearing completion (Espín, in preparation). Therefore, when I received the request from the editors of this volume to write about my experiences as a Latina psychologist, I began to wonder what I could say that I had not said already, how many distinct versions of my life I could have to narrate. The proverbial nine lives of cats, obviously, do not apply to me. Regardless of the multiplicity of cultural, historical, and geographical contexts in which I have lived, I am just me.

Am I being repetitive when I narrate my autobiographical memories? I hope that because "autobiographical memory is always selective" and "the ways that particular emotional experiences will be expressed will be a function of the specific context in which one is sharing one's life story" (Fivush, 2004, p. 81), the stories I am about to tell sound sufficiently fresh and descriptive of what my life experiences and, specifically, my life as a Latina psychologist have been.

And so I have decided to go back in my mind to the many places where I have lived and let the geography of my memories be the guiding thread of this writing, which means it must start in Cuba.

Map of an Island Home: Fear, Love, and Loss

Cuba has always been foremost in my mind. I have never, unlike other immigrants, wanted to forget where I came from. In fact, I went back to Cuba less than three months ago, this time with a group in which most participants were mental health professionals or students in the field. The trip included visits and conversations with Cuban psychologists, which of course, evoked my memories of being a university student there. The trip also included repeated travel on the street where I lived for ten years during my childhood, a street that is full of memories of financial deprivation and physical constraint.

My father had a small elementary school and an adult commercial academy in a rented top-floor flat on that street. We lived in two rooms in the back of that flat. The bustling street of my childhood is still there; it is still one of the main thoroughfares in the center of Havana. The heavy traffic then and now makes this street feel like a forbidden and dangerous space. There was no playing in the street or with neighborhood kids. And more than ever, the street reeks of poverty, intensified by the decay of Havana buildings after six decades of disrepair. On that street, in the back rooms of that flat, I read voraciously, fantasied, imagining other possible lives and places, and played at being Joan of Arc over desks and chairs when the students were not around.

Most children grow up among family members at home, playmates, classmates, and teachers at school. I had all that. I attended a Catholic school ran by nuns for middle-class girls – on a scholarship as we could not have afforded it otherwise. But also, at home, I met my father's students. Not so much the girls and boys of the day elementary school, but rather the women and men evening students and their teachers, all of whom were working adults who studied or taught after their day jobs. They talked about all sorts of things I would not have had contact with were it not for the peculiar circumstances of sharing living space with that adult evening school. Among my father's adult students and their teachers, surrounded at an early age by different stories and contradictory opinions, I started wondering about what makes human beings "tick." I guess the curiosity awakened by those overheard conversations started opening the door to my interest in psychology.

Then, when I was fifteen, the high school curriculum included a Psychology course. I suppose the fact that my favorite teacher taught it contributed to my interest in the subject. But aside from the teacher, I thought the content of the course was captivating. The emotions, the unconscious, dreams, and other topics were intriguing. What William James, Sigmund Freud, or Carl Jung had written about this or that topic was fascinating. The course followed a model that compartmentalized in separate chapters each one of those topics as well as intelligence, the will, the brain, temperament, character, personality, and so on. Needless to say, none of the authors discussed were women, nor was there any mention of any woman or anyone who was not European or North American contributing to knowledge in the field. Despite its limitations, that high school course made me decide I wanted to be a psychologist. And although several decades, countries, and political dramas interfered with that early dream, I never abandoned it.

Perhaps I should say I grew up in a Cuba where middle-class professional women were very present. The nuns in my school were highly educated women with doctoral degrees in Physics, Literature, Mathematics, as did the lay teachers, who were also women. The 1940 Cuban Constitution guaranteed equal rights in voting, property, and education for women. And even though, as in any country, laws don't necessarily provide equal access to opportunities for everyone, the remnants of the strong Cuban women's movement of the 1920s and 1930s (Stoner, 1991) were still manifest in the lives of my teachers in the 1940s and early 1950s since they had lived through that movement in their youth. Perhaps this is also the moment to say that although pre-revolutionary Cuba is routinely depicted as a corrupt place owned by the United States and the mafia, this is not what my memory tells me or what the historical record reveals. The Cuba I grew up in, despite political and economic problems caused by the unequal distribution of resources, was a place full of poetry and music as well as pride in our history of struggle against domination by both Spain and the United States. This writing is not the place to engage in political diatribe. But I do need to say that even though I grew up under constricting poverty in a society where race and gender inequality were evident, I grew up feeling great pride in being Cuban, surrounded by smart women whose example led me to believe that I, too, could achieve what I wanted. Men like my father and his brother, who was my godfather, encouraged my intellect and made me feel capable of much, regardless of whatever forces might have militated against my ambitions.

Concretely, Batista, who had made himself "President" when I was in my early adolescence, closed all public universities when Fidel Castro and his comrades disembarked in Oriente province in November 1956. I had started university a few weeks before, after graduating from high school in June of that year. I had also started working, tutoring children, to help support my family. I spent hours in buses going to children's homes. And since the closure of the University of Havana had interrupted my opportunity of formal studying, I used those times to read. Among other books, I read all of Karen Horney's works in Spanish translation while riding on Havana's buses.

After the fall of Batista, the revolutionary government reopened the universities, but at the beginning of the Revolution, psychology was not a priority. Psychology was seen as a "bourgeois" discipline, useful only to rich people. Eventually, psychological services were incorporated into the national health services. But by then I had left the country, after a year studying Psychology with a scholarship at the private Catholic University of Santo Tomás de Villanueva located in the outskirts of Havana.

In between, before entering Villanueva, I had experienced a serious crisis. I suffered from nearly constant panic attacks that almost incapacitated me. On multiple occasions, I was certain I was about to suffocate because no air seemed to reach my lungs no matter how deeply I inhaled. At other times, I became certain that I had been stricken with some strange and deadly disease that was creeping into my bones and destroying me from within. As the episodes succeeded one another, they were compounded by my constant fear of the fear. I was either experiencing a panic attack or terrified that I would begin experiencing one shortly.

The director of an organization of Catholic college women I belonged to, who was a psychologist, offered me free therapy for over a year. She helped me explore my life history and the causes of my panic attacks from different angles. After eighteen months of therapy, the frequency, intensity, and duration of the episodes subsided. Eventually they disappeared. I have never again experienced panic attacks. Having a vivid proof of the effectiveness of psychotherapy, I became ever more convinced of the value of psychology.

As I write about these emotionally charged memories of childhood and adolescence, I am aware that like all autobiographical memory, mine probably contains distortions. The events of my early life are complicated by their entanglement in Cuban history, which creates varied reactions and opinions from those around me about what my life must have been like. However, I know that some of my memories of childhood and adolescence are etched in stone. I have encountered those memories in full force every time I returned to Cuba. Despite all the limitations of human memory, now that I have lived most of my life, I know those memoires are basically true and they unquestionably reveal the building blocks of my life. I also know that the historical events I have lived through shaped my interest in understanding how "the personal is political" and how the political becomes transformed into the personal. That interest has persisted throughout my life.

No Maps for this Road: Uprootedness and Aching to Belong

I left Cuba in 1961 shortly after the failed Bay of Pigs invasion, thus joining the ranks of the millions of displaced people of the world who are "condemned to the limbo of not belonging" (McDowell, 1999, p. 2). As I have written before, having immigrated to another country, no matter how long ago, means you are always from somewhere else. You are always betwixt and between, neither here nor there. Many important events of your life have occurred in another place. Who you are is influenced by absence; the absence of people and places that shaped those events. Distance from your original place necessitates understanding yourself from a different geographical and cultural setting than the one in which many of your memories were encoded. You have to organize your memories in a certain way to make them intelligible in your new context; you have to explain details that would otherwise have been taken for granted. Sometimes I feel as if I have to explain myself constantly in order to be understood by those who matter to me in this new life and place (Espín, 2015b, p. 35).

After leaving Cuba, I lived in Spain and Panama for a few years, and I worked for a few months in Miami as a teacher aid. In March 1964, I moved to Costa Rica. There, in 1969, I finished a B.A. in Psychology at the Universidad de Costa Rica while also working full-time as a teacher of psychology, religion, and literature in a girls' high school and administering a residence for women students near the same university. This last was a volunteer job I performed as a member of the Catholic college women's organization I had belonged to in Cuba since my late adolescence. During those years of repeated moving, Costa Rica was my most permanent place, the one closest to being a second home. And yet I learned there another lesson about the plight of those who live away from their home country, which eventually I incorporated in my work with and about immigrant women: there are lots of cultural variations even among those who share a heritage. The sense of being "different" was not as vivid there as it later became in the United States. But despite similarities in language, customs, and values, I always had a sense of not fully belonging. There was the sound of popular folk music that was familiar to everyone but me. And there was my memory of another popular folk music that only I knew. There was the unfamiliar taste of food that was a daily staple for the others. And there were tastes that I longed for which were unknown or inaccessible in that country. I learned to enjoy Costa Rican food and love Costa Rican music. My friends, co-workers, and classmates forgot to include me in their list of foreigners. And yet, occasionally, the subject of my nationality would come up when someone was angry with me or when I could not remember events in Costa Rican history. To this day, those years in Costa Rica are very close to my heart, and my Costa Rican friends continue to be central in my life. But they know, as I know, that I am not really Costa Rican (Espín, 1991b, p. 155).

It helped that it was a politically stable place, in contrast to neighboring Panama where, before moving to Costa Rica, I had been living in early 1964 during a serious confrontation between Panamanian students and Canal Zone inhabitants. Days of violence and destruction that resulted in the deaths of more than twenty Panamanians and four U.S. soldiers, and eventually forced the development of new Canal treaties between the two countries, evoked my fears of past political violence. Political instability continues to scare me because I have witnessed too much of it. But being in Panama during those dramatic days made me realize that the world is not easily divided in two dimensions of good-bad or right-wrong. Comments I heard describing the events in Panama as a "communist plot" contrasted sharply with the love of country and resistance to foreign domination that I knew motivated my Panamanian friends who had participated in the turmoil. Simple explanations of human behavior were, again, not fitting. I had seen the holes of the gunshots on walls and columns; they were proof that the U.S. "Zonian" forces had not been shooting in the air but at the "assailants" who had tried to raise a Panamanian flag in the Canal Zone, which was legally Panamanian territory. The crisis made evident multiple variations and nuances in human motivations and sociopolitical forces that could not be explained in a dichotomous way. Despite the relatively brief time I lived in Panama, I learned important lessons about ambiguity at that historical juncture. More important for my understanding of psychology, I also learned that human emotions and behaviors do not only have a psychic origin or explanation. I reaffirmed then what I had started to realize years earlier in Cuba – sociocultural, political, and historical contexts are essential components of individual psychology and identity. This has been a central tenet of all my work in psychology.

From Costa Rica, I had gone to Belgium with a fellowship to do a doctorate in Psychology, which was cut short by an ill-fated marriage and divorce. Being a married woman in a country where I could not get money out of my own savings account without my husband's permission was a shock to my sense of self after having lived an independent working life for more than a decade. This marriage also taught me other things that have proven useful for me as a therapist and in helping students understand the plight of women who suffer domestic abuse … because I was at the verge of becoming one of those women and I experienced how hard it is to extricate oneself from that confusing mixture of love and fear. I know it was a miracle that I was able to get out of that situation. I learned then, as I am relearning now that I am married to a woman, that while the institution of marriage is protective and legitimizing, it is also restrictive and limiting even in the best of circumstances.

Shifting Maps of Identity

I had married a man in my early thirties partly because I was afraid to be a *solterona* – an "old maid" – partly because it had never occurred to me that there were other alternatives to fulfill my emotional needs. But I soon fell in love with a woman and went through a coming out process. Coming out as a lesbian before 1973 created anxieties about my professional life: Could I be a psychologist if I was "sick"? Never mind that I did not feel sick at all but, in fact, felt more alive and complete than ever. Luckily, in a few years the sick label disappeared and I found colleagues who shared my identity and professional interest concerning sexual orientation.

After that failed marriage in Belgium, I came to the United States to finish my doctorate and immediately moved to Montreal to teach at McGill University, supervising francophone students. It was after that time in Canada that I moved to the United States. In other words, I did not have a stable home for more than a decade, plus I lived my life split between Spanish, English, and French during those years, which added language homelessness to the mixture, as I will discuss later.

Although I had previously lived in Florida for several months at a time and had finished my doctorate there, my "real" introduction to the United States happened in Boston, where I began an academic position at Boston University. Almost immediately after arriving in Boston in 1975, even though my primary job was as a professor educating therapists-in-training, I became part of Womanspace, a Feminist Therapy Collective. I slowly developed a small private practice. My clients were women from diverse cultural backgrounds. Working with them, I developed and applied my understanding of feminist psychology and feminist therapy (Espín, 1994a). My appreciation of feminist therapy – and of the importance of social justice perspectives in the practice of psychotherapy and in the training of psychotherapists – developed and grew. The effervescence of feminist thought that surrounded me in Boston was a determining factor in my life and career. I know the feminist movement was strong in other places at that time, but my location in Boston had specific characteristics that had to do with the predominant theoretical perspectives in Boston's clinical environment and its preeminent role in the development of feminist psychology theory. Feminist psychology theories were being developed prominently in Boston at the time. I was lucky then to be in group supervision with Jean Baker Miller (1976).

My training in Costa Rica had included a strong psychodynamic component, particularly of the Cultural Psychoanalysis of Horney, Fromm, Sullivan, and Fromm-Reichman. But in Boston, where psychoanalytic theories flourish, I deepened my understanding of it and, specifically, of Object Relations and Self-Psychology. I found that I could mix them with the theoretical perspectives prevalent in my doctoral training, which had been mostly Person-Centered Rogerian, and with my feminist understanding of the social world. In the personal construction of my own theory of psychotherapy practice, I incorporated relevant concepts of established theories to the insights I had developed about cultural, political, and historical forces and my commitment to social justice and feminism.

While discussions about the integration of social justice and clinical services are now more common (e.g. Aldarondo, 2007), this was not a prevalent conception in the 1970s and 1980s. Feminist therapy was one of the few exceptions. Despite individual and theoretical variations, feminist therapists share a basic consensus that "feminist therapy [… is a …] transformation of the way in which therapy is understood and practiced" (Hill & Ballou, 1998, p. 5). A short, mostly unknown book entitled *Psychology and Social Change* (Pizer & Travers, 1975), published when I was at the beginning of my career, also offered me a rare confirmation of psychology's potential to effect social change. I remember reading this little book while waiting for the train in an underground station in Boston – again, the memory of places that bring to life defining moments in my understanding of who I was and wanted to be as a Latina psychologist. I don't think it is a coincidence that in my itinerant life I have done a lot of reading on buses, trains, and planes.

The belief that societal oppression can be the cause of psychological distress, held by feminist therapists and other like-minded psychologists in the northern hemisphere, was shared by Latin American psychologists. I had started reading several of them in Spanish in my search for integration of my Euro-American graduate training and my Latin American experience. Psychologists such as Ignacio Martin-Baró (1994), Elizabeth Lira, and others like Lira & Piper (1997) had made me ever more aware in the late 1970s that "the practice of psychology is intrinsically political and intrinsically ideological and all our professional work is equally political and ideological" (Lira & Piper, 1997, p. 126). From the perspective of these Latin American psychologists – reluctant witnesses to the psychological impact of political/social violence on individuals – "incorporating the social context to the study of subjectivity has allowed us the understanding of how intrapsychic suffering is directly related to experiences lived in the social and political realms" (p. 109). Regardless of differences in theoretical background and practice as well as geographical and sociocultural contexts, there is a consensus among these practitioners that psychotherapy *is a political act.* I have made mine and sought to transmit this understanding to my students in my decades of training psychotherapists (Espín, 2006b, 2014b, 2015a).

Mapping a Promising Home: Women, Migration, Sexuality, and Language

In 1990, I came to California as a professor in the oldest Department of Women's Studies in the country, at San Diego State University, to which I later added part-time work teaching doctoral students at the California School of Professional Psychology. Paradoxically, being in Women's Studies allowed me to grow and develop as a psychologist by incorporating some important insights and currents of thought shared by other disciplines that are mostly ignored within psychology. While, before, the issues I wanted to explore professionally were deemed less than deserving because they focused on women who belonged to non-dominant social groups, such as Latinas or immigrants and refugees, and, moreover, I was exploring those issues using non-conventional methods, I now found myself in an environment that encouraged the scholarly exploration of experience as a source of knowledge (Espín, 1997a). In my new academic context, my long-term interest in cultural and ethnic issues in psychology (Espín, 1991a, 1994a, 2006b;

Espín & Gawelek, 1992; Kawahara & Espín, 2007, 2012) and exploratory methods of psychological inquiry (Espín, 1988, 1994b, 1996a, 1999) came to fruition.

Also, although I had written about immigration and gender before coming to California, almost immediately upon beginning my position in Women's Studies I started actively publishing about this topic and produced several books and articles in rapid succession. It is my work on the life experiences and narratives of immigrant and refugee women, particularly as it concerns issues of sexuality, that has constituted the bulk of my work and is closest to my heart and life experience (e.g. Cole, Espín, & Rothblum, 1992; Espín, 1987b, 1992, 1994b, 1995, 1996b, 1997b, 1999, 2006b, 2010; Espín & Dottolo, 2015). Specifically, issues of sexuality and identity for Latina women, both lesbian and heterosexual, had been the focus of some of my writing (Espín, 1984, 1987a, 2012a). I extended my focus and developed major research projects on life narratives of women immigrants from across the world. Women of various sexual orientations and identities were centrally included (Espín, 1996a, 1996b, 1997b, 1999, 2000).

This work reaffirmed my belief that human motivations cannot be attributed only to psychological causes or just measured and captured in simple variables. Although there is important learning to be gathered from laboratory and experimental methods, statistical data are not the only valuable source of information – there is more to human beings than what can be measured or counted.

In my work with and about women immigrants, issues of language were always present. Observing how clients and participants switched languages in a therapy session or any time in research interviews when "touchy" topics such as sexuality came up, it progressively became obvious to me that the connection between language, identity, and memory was paramount (Espín, 1993, 1999, 2006a, 2013, 2015b).

As I said earlier, being an immigrant in different countries and cultural spaces made it

> clear to me that there were many valid ways of being human and that human development had many different healthy courses. Most importantly, experiencing myself in different countries and different languages taught me things about who I am that I would have never had access to had I not experienced myself in these cultural and linguistic contexts.
>
> *(Espín, 1993, p. 410)*

The experience of living my life in the context of different languages has been significant in the development of the maps of my memory – an experience that is shared by many immigrants. In my early migrations, I encountered dialectical variations within Spanish, but I still felt as if I was at home in language. There were things I shared with my friends in Spain, Panama, and Costa Rica, however, that became difficult to share with my close friends in Canada and the United States. I felt that no matter how fluent I was in English, my innermost feelings continued to be in Spanish. The deepest part of myself remained hidden from people who were extremely important to me, no matter how hard we all tried (Espín, 1991b, 1992). My sense of not being "quite there" when expressing emotion or remembering details from my past while speaking in English is corroborated by research on the topic of multilingualism and memory (e.g. Javier, Barroso, & Muñoz, 1993; Kazanas & Atarriba, 2014; Schrauf, 2003; Schrauf, Pavlenko, & Dewaele, 2003; Schrauf & Rubin, 2003). In other words, language itself and the place where a language is spoken creates a deep connection to the memories evoked or "forgotten." As Schrauf and Rubin (2003) put it, for me, as for other multilingual immigrants, my "mother tongue is tied to innumerable concatenations of vividly remembered, half-remembered, and nearly forgotten contexts in which [I] came to communicative and cultural competence, learning where and when and how to be unconsciously 'native'" (p. 134).

Maps of the Spirit (... and Home?)

Lastly, I do not want to finish this "journey" through my life without mentioning the role and importance of spirituality in influencing who I am. As a child, I wanted to be a saint more than anything else. I wanted to be Joan of Arc, Rose of Lima, or any of the other women saints whose lives I read about or saw depicted in films. I played at being a hermit, a martyr, or a saintly heroine – behind my bedroom door, in the garden of my grandmother's house, or anywhere I was free to fantasize. And I endured some mocking from my sister and classmates as a consequence. My aunts and grandmother thought it very funny that when asked what I wanted to be when I grew up, I always said I wanted to be "a nun or an actress." I never became either, but I can say with a smile that I have been a bit of both most of my life.

However, all was not solitary prayer or fantasy. In 1958, when I was nineteen, I won a small fortune on Cuban TV answering questions about religion and went to Europe by myself for three months with my winnings. And when I came to Women's Studies at San Diego State, I started recovering the stories of the saints of my childhood using feminist and psychological perspectives and insights and started teaching courses, presenting, and publishing on these proto-feminist women's lives and my personal spiritual connections to them (e.g. Espín, 2004, 2008a, 2008b, 2011a, 2011b, 2012b, 2014a).

Ironically, San Diego has been more permanent for me than I could have ever imagined. I have lived here longer than anywhere else, and although I continue to travel and live temporarily in other places, I have come back here for almost thirty years. And here I continue to wonder what would my life have been if I had not been an immigrant and lived in different contexts and languages; if I had not pursued the topics and used the methodological approaches I have. Without overestimating my own foresight – which, in fact, was not there – I know I went against the grain and took risks that could and did endanger my possibilities of career advancement. But taking those risks ended up making it possible for me to contribute to the field and, hopefully, to a better understanding of the psychology of women immigrants and Latinas. For the obedient little girl wanting to become a saint that I was, being rebellious against established disciplinary norms was somewhat appalling and contradictory. And yet I know that following my inner compass has ended up being the fulcrum on which my professional life has become what it is.

Because I have lived in so many different places and because my life has taken so many turns, my memories are linked to specific spaces – countries, cities, places where I have worked and played and lived. Each one of them has had a specific impact on who I am as a psychologist and a Latina. And perhaps because the search for a stable home has been elusive for most of my life, I hold on to those memories and to symbolic tokens of home. One of them is my quaint collection of mini model houses from all over the world, that I have acquired on my multiple travels. If I can't feel I am at home anywhere, at least I can have all these beautiful little houses. I don't think it is a coincidence that according to Aztec astrology, I was born on the sign of The House. The House sign is characterized by the search for strong foundations and a need to settle down that might never be achieved. People born under The House sign tend to be "givers" and listeners, as psychologists are supposed to be. According to Aztec astrology, The House is linked to a true respect for the secret aspects of one's self that, no matter how much we try, are always shrouded in mystery. I won't pretend to know what every thing and every turn in my life means. But if I could have talked to my younger self, I would have told her that despite the instability and disruptive uncertainty, a map was getting built in my kaleidoscopic soul that now feels like home.

References

Aldarondo, E. (Ed.). (2007). *Advancing social justice through clinical practice*. Mahwah, NJ: Lawrence Erlbaum.

Cole, E., Espín, O.M. & Rothblum, E.D. (Eds.). (1992). *Refugee women and their mental health: Shattered societies, shattered lives*. New York: Haworth.

Espín, O.M. (1984). Cultural and historical influences on sexuality in Hispanic/Latin women: Implications for psychotherapy. In C. Vance (Ed.), *Pleasure and danger: Exploring female sexuality* (pp. 149–164). London: Routledge and Kegan Paul.

Espín, O.M. (1987a). Issues of identity in the psychology of Latina lesbian women. In *Lesbian psychologies* (pp. 35–55). Urbana, IL: University of Illinois Press.

Espín, O.M. (1987b). Psychological impact of migration on Latinas: Implications for psychotherapeutic practice. *Psychology of Women Quarterly*, 11(4), 489–503.

Espín, O.M. (1988). Spiritual power and the mundane world: Hispanic female healers in urban U.S. communities. *Women Studies Quarterly*, 16(3/4), 33–47.

Espín, O.M. (1991a). *Ethnicity, race, class, and the future of feminist psychology*. San Francisco, CA: American Psychological Association.

Espín, O.M. (1991b). Roots uprooted: Autobiographical reflections on the psychological experience of migration. In F. Alegría & J. Ruffinelli (Eds.), *Paradise lost or gained: The literature of Hispanic exile* (pp. 151–163). Houston, TX: Arte Público Press.

Espín, O.M. (1992). Roots uprooted: The psychological effect of historical dislocation on the lives of refugee women. *Women and Therapy*, 13(3/4), 19–32.

Espín, O.M. (1993). Giving voice to silence: The psychologist as witness. *American Psychologist*, 48(4), 408–414.

Espín, O.M. (1994a). Feminist approaches [to therapy with women of color]. In L. Comas-Díaz & B. Greene (Eds.), *Women of color and mental health* (pp. 265–286). New York: Guilford Press.

Espín, O.M. (1994b). Traumatic socio-historical conditions and adolescent development: Letters from V. In C.E. Franz & A.J. Stewart (Eds.), *Women creating lives: Identities resilience, and resistance* (pp. 187–198). Boulder, CO: Westview Press.

Espín, O.M. (1995). "Race," racism, and sexuality in the life narratives of immigrant women. *Feminism and Psychology*, 5(2), 287–302.

Espín, O.M. (1996a). *Latina healers: Lives of power and tradition.* Encino, CA: Floricanto Press.

Espín, O.M. (1996b). Immigrant and refugee lesbians. In E.D. Rothblum & L.A. Bond (Eds.), *Preventing heterosexism and homophobia* (pp. 174–183). Thousand Oaks, CA: Sage.

Espín, O.M. (1997a). *Latina realities: Essays on healing, migration and sexuality.* Boulder, CO: Westview Press.

Espín, O.M. (1997b). Crossing borders and boundaries: The life narratives of immigrant lesbians. In B. Greene (Ed.), *Ethnic and cultural diversity among lesbians and gay men* (pp. 191–215). Thousand Oaks, CA: Sage.

Espín, O.M. (1999). *Women crossing boundaries: A psychology of immigration and the transformations of sexuality.* New York: Routledge.

Espín, O.M. (2000). Crossing borders and boundaries: Gender and sexuality in the life narratives of immigrant women. In E. Olstein & G. Horenczyk (Eds.), *Language, identity, and immigration* (pp. 123–140). Jerusalem, Israel: Magnes Press.

Espín, O.M. (2004). How Joan of Arc saved my life. *Psychotherapy Networker*, 28(3), 95–96.

Espín, O.M. (2005). The age of the cookie cutter has passed: Contradictions in identity at the core of therapeutic intervention. Presentation at National Multicultural Conference and Summit, APA, Los Angeles, CA.

Espín, O.M. (2006a). Gender, sexuality, language and migration. In R. Mahalingam (Ed.), *Cultural psychology of immigrants* (pp. 241–258). Mahwah, NJ: Lawrence Erlbaum.

Espín, O.M. (2006b). A feminist look at the kaleidoscope of identity. Presentation, Association for Women in Psychology, Ann Arbor, MI.

Espín, O.M. (2008a). "The destiny of this people is my own": Edith Stein's paradoxical sainthood. *Cross Currents*, 58(1), 117–148.

Espín, O.M. (2008b). My "friendship" with women saints as a source of spirituality. In C. Rayburn & L. Comas-Díaz (Eds.), *WomanSoul: The inner life of women's spirituality* (pp. 71–84). Westport, CT: Praeger.

Espín, O.M. (2010). A psychology of immigrant and refugee women. Presentation at University of Klagenfurt, Austria.

Espín, O.M. (2011a). The enduring popularity of Rosa de Lima, first saint of the Americas: Women, bodies, sainthood, and national identity. *Cross Currents*, 61(1), 6–27.

Espín, O.M. (2011b). Female saints: Submissive or rebellious? Feminists in disguise? In D. Eibl, M. Jarosch, U.A. Schneider, & A. Steinsiek (Eds.), *Innsbrucker gender lectures I* (pp. 135–164). Innsbruck, Austria: Innsbruck University Press.

Espín, O.M. (2012a). "An illness we catch from American women"? The Multiple Identities of Latina Lesbians. *Women & Therapy*, 35(1/2), 45–56.

Espín, O.M. (2012b). The interplay of criollo identity, colonial politics, and gender in the enduring popular appeal of Rose of Lima. In P. Golinelli (Ed.), *Agiografia e culture popolari /Hagiography and popular culture* (pp. 355–366). Verona, Italy: Universita degli Studi di Verona.

Espín, O.M. (2013). "Making love in English": Language in psychotherapy with immigrant women. *Women and Therapy*, 36(3/4), 198–218.

Espín, O.M. (2014a). Saints in the Cuban heat. In E. Facio & I. Lara (Eds.), *Fleshing the spirit: Spirituality and activism in Chicana, Latina and indigenous women's lives* (pp. 102–112). Tucson, AZ: University of Arizona Press.

Espín, O.M. (2014b). *Reflections on weaving the personal, theoretical, and professional in psychology*. Presentation at The Legacies of Professor Oliva Espín, American Psychological Association, Washington, DC.

Espín, O.M. (2015a). Psychotherapy as a tool of restorative justice. Presentaion at Feminist interventions and restorative justice: Research, reflexivity, therapy and performance, Association for Women in Psychology, San Francisco, CA.

Espín, O.M. (2015b). A geography of memory – A psychology of place. In O.M. Espín & A.L. Dottolo (Eds.), *Gendered journeys: Women, migration and feminist psychology* (pp. 29–51). Basingstoke, UK: Palgrave Macmillan.

Espín, O.M. (2017). "Caminante no hay camino": The road is built as you walk. In M. Kopala & M. Keitel (Eds.), *Handbook of counseling women* (pp. 34–40). Los Angeles, CA: Sage.

Espín, O.M. (in preparation). *My native land is memory: Stories of a Cuban childhood.*

Espín, O.M. & Dottolo, A.L. (Eds.). (2015). *Gendered journeys: Women, migration and feminist psychology*. Basingstoke, UK: Palgrave Macmillan.

Espín, O.M. & Gawelek, M.A. (1992). Women's diversity: Ethnicity, race, class and gender in theories of feminist psychology. In L.S. Brown & M. Ballou (Eds.), *Personality and psychopathology: Feminist reappraisals* (pp. 88–107). New York: Guilford Press.

Fivush, R. (2004). The silenced self: Constructing self from memories spoken and unspoken. In D.R. Beike, J.M. Lampinen, & D.A. Behrend (Eds.), *The self and memory* (pp. 75–93). New York: Psychology Press.

Freeman, M. (2007). Narrative and relation: The place of the other in the story of the self. In R. Josselson, A. Lieblich, & D.P. McAdams (Eds.), *The meaning of others: Narrative studies of relationships* (pp. 11–19). Washington, DC: American Psychological Association.

Hill, M. & Ballou, M. (1998). Making therapy feminist: A practice survey. In M. Hill (Ed.), *Feminist therapy as a political act* (pp. 1–16). New York: Haworth Press.

Javier, R., Barroso, F. & Muñoz, M. (1993). Autobiographical memory in bilinguals. *Journal of Psycholinguistic Research*, 22(3), 319–338.

Kaschak, E. (2011). The mattering map: Multiplicity, metaphor and morphing in contextual theory and practice. *Women and Therapy*, 34(1/2), 6–18. doi: 10.1080/02703149.2010.532688

Kawahara, D.M. (2017). The amazing life and times of Oliva Espín. *Women and Therapy*, 40(3/4), 323–333. doi: 10.1080/02703149.2017.1241571

Kawahara, D. & Espín, O.M. (Eds.). (2007). *Feminist reflections on growth and transformations: Asian-American women in therapy*. New York: Haworth Press.

Kawahara, D. & Espín, O.M. (Eds.). (2012). *Feminist therapy with Latina women: Personal and social voices*. New York: Routledge.

Kazanas, S.A. & Atarriba, J. (2014). Multilingualism and memory. In C.A. Chapelle (Ed.), *The encyclopedia of applied linguistics* (pp. 1–7). New York: Wiley.

Lira, E. & Piper, I. (Eds.). (1997). *Subjetividad y política: Diálogos en América Latina*. Santiago, Chile: Instituto Latinoamericano de Salud Mental y Derechos Humanos.

Martín-Baró, I. (1994). *Writings for a liberation psychology*. Ed. A. Aron & S. Corne. Trans. A. Aron. Cambridge, MA: Harvard University Press.

Maynes, M.J. & Pierce, J.L. (2008). *Telling stories: The use of personal narratives in the social sciences and history*. Ithaca, NY: Cornell University Press.

McDowell, L. (1999). *Gender, identity and place: Understanding feminist geographies*. Minneapolis, MN: University of Minnesota Press.

Miller, J.B. (1976). *Toward a new psychology of women*. Boston, MA: Beacon Press.

Pizer, S.A. & Travers, J.R. (1975). *Psychology and social change*. New York: McGraw-Hill.

Rodríguez, J.M. (2003). *Queer Latinidad: Identity practices, discursive spaces*. New York: New York University Press.

Schrauf, R.W. (2003). A protocol analysis of retrieval in bilingual autobiographical memory. *The International Journal of Bilingualism*, 7(3), 235–256.

Schrauf, R.W., Pavlenko, A. & Dewaele, J.-M. (2003). Bilingual episodic memory. *The International Journal of Bilingualism*, 7(3), 221–233.

Schrauf, R. & Rubin, D. (2003). On the bilingual's two sets of memories. In R. Fivush & C.A. Haden (Eds.), *Autobiographical memory and the construction of a narrative self: Developmental and cultural perspectives* (pp. 121–145). Mahwah, NJ: Lawrence Erlbaum.

Stoner, K.L. (1991). *From the house to the streets: the Cuban woman's movement for legal reform, 1898–1940*. Durham, NC: Duke University Press.

11

ENTRE FRONTERAS

Thriving with Optimism, Purpose, and Connectivity

Patricia M. Arredondo

To survive the Borderlands you must live sin fronteras / be a crossroads.
Gloria Anzaldúa (1987, pp. 194–195)

In 2001, I was president of the Society for the Psychological Study of Ethnic Minority Issues (Division 45), an honor and a responsibility. At our annual ceremonies held during the APA conference in San Francisco, I was charged with giving a presidential address. I had heard others speak in the previous years and wondered how esoteric I wanted to be, how scientific a presentation to make, or what other foci that would be relevant to the mission of Division 45. Since then and in subsequent keynotes, I have chosen to be more self-revealing such that the motivation and meaning of my life's work comes through more than in other conference talks. "Mujeres Latinas: Santas y Marquesas" (Arredondo, 2002), based on that presidential talk, was the first time I really spoke about my origins and their relationship to my scholarship, social justice endeavors, and passion for women's leadership. Thus, the invitation to contribute to this text in the company of other Latinas I hold in high regard seems like a moment of arrival, one of those unexpected events I would not have considered in my lifetime. What is a little different in this narrative and also present in more recent speaking engagements is my willingness to talk about disappointments, experiences of marginalization and racism, and other incidents that caused me to redirect my purpose. My voice has changed and allowed me to bring attention to incidents I am certain other Latinas have suffered too. I am grateful to be at a place in my life where I can be candid and proud. Sharing reflections of oneself is humbling, but I hope that this narrative will provide both inspiration and a sense of identification with my uneven pathway and how I have managed during times of challenge. I will try to end each section with a *consejo*, a statement of encouragement and affirmation.

Framing the Narrative

There is a broader context for meaning-making of my sense of thriving and optimism *entre fronteras*, of navigating the personal and professional simultaneously. A construct I learned from reading Erik Erikson (1975) many years ago is that of "history-taking and history-making," and I believe this describes how I am framing and relating this narrative.

As I will share, my endeavors as an academic, organizational consultant, and institutional administrator have always been culture-centered. My curiosity is like that of an anthropologist, beginning in formative childhood years and continuing to this day as I advocate for multicultural competency development and social justice principles. I believe my zeal for learning about people's cultural personas is not so different from that of some well-known anthropologists. The studies of anthropologists (Ruth Benedict, Clyde Kluckhohn, Elaine Strockbeck, Margaret Mead, and others) who lived among communities different primarily because of their "non-mainstream" lives illuminated as well as patronized the lives of thriving indigenous groups in Australia, Hawaii, New Zealand, and so forth.

Place, or geographical location, was at the forefront of their inquiries, as they tried to understand people in place. I too believe this is an important springboard for self-understanding. Place informs socio-historical, sociocultural, political, and economic forces that shape one's worldview. In my life, place and places have been formative, and although many of us describe our lives in terms of generation or major life events, I will integrate themes that address origins of place as well as subsequent situations that deepened my multicultural competency development, personal evolution, approaches to psychotherapy, and of course my mentorship.

Consejo: Reflect on your origins and landmarks in your life, consider how these have informed your sense of Latina identity and personal empowerment.

La Filosofía

I have chosen to speak about thriving and optimism because I have always held a worldview of positivity, of human assets rather than shortcomings or deficits, and of empowerment. The metaphor of the "borderlands" is one I have borrowed repeatedly from Gloria Anzaldúa's remarkable feminist reader, *Borderlands/La Frontera* (1987). Additionally, I frequently invoke Julia de Burgos' poem "*Yo misma fui mi ruta*" (1953) because it affirms the self-determination that has often taken me down uncharted pathways. I hope to reveal in this chapter how I have lived these metaphors as, I believe, so many other Latinas have, and to inspire our younger generations to claim the *frontera* as a source of identity development and strength.

Like my water sign, I have always been adaptable, moving toward the social inequities I could not walk away from and endeavoring to lead changes that would reduce or eliminate injustices. As I have advanced career- and age-wise, I have framed my career to promote knowledge, cultural competence, and mentorship to benefit others. My philosophy is one of giving back, being an example, and leaving a legacy, the legacy of a proud Latina, a psychologist who continues to persevere so that others will thrive and give back in turn.

My life's work is culturally and contextually informed and gender-centric, empowered by a feminist father and a traditional mother, a yin and yang. Cultural socialization has taught me the art of nurturance and instilled in me a desire to inspire and motivate others – this is my worldview. I see myself as a mentor of stepchildren, family members, students and colleagues, men and women alike. I have also taken to heart the identity tasks put forth by Erik Erikson's (1968) life tasks of generativity rather than stagnation and integrity in place of despair.

Consejo: Regardless of your age, consider the legacies you want to leave behind.

Siempre hay Comienzos/There Are Always Beginnings

I am a Moon Child, a Cancer, born in mid-July at the early hour of 5:38 a.m. This astrological water sign signaling adaptability and movement has been a conscious and unconscious force for me. My worldview has always been that the glass is half-full rather than half-empty; that having faith in possibilities means being able to be purposeful in pursuits that may benefit others; and that it is through the practice of connectivity that what seems daunting to pursue alone becomes more feasible and fun along the way, because of connections with others. This I learned from my family as we practiced *familismo, respeto*, and *tener orgullo* as a unit of nine and with extended *familia.*

My identity as a Mexican woman, daughter of low-income, achievement-oriented, and supportive immigrants, is immutable and a source of pride. Running through my veins is the spirit and determination of a proud, risk-taking Oaxacan *abuela* who lived with a *Sí se puede* attitude through her entrepreneurship, nurturance, and encouragement of her grandchildren, and a strong faith in God and the Virgen de Guadalupe. Doña María Estefana Zaldívar Morelos modeled caring but not selflessness, pragmatism, and a sense of self-determination that inspires me to this day.

Perhaps it was Mamá's risk-taking behaviors that encouraged decisions I made. Initially unconscious of her example, upon reflection I notice choices I made that took me to new and unique places. Illiterate, Mamá ran away from home at age 13 to avoid marriage to an older man. She migrated *al norte* through Texas, Kansas, Illinois (where my mother was born), and eventually Lorain, Ohio (where I was born). She raised four daughters and later some of my cousins, outlived my grandfather, who died of alcoholism at the age of 44, and died of cancer at 88. The death of my grandfather meant a new chapter in her life and set in motion many actions not typical of women of her station in life. She is a true icon for me.

Mamá took a job at the steel factory doing women's menial work – sweeping floors. All along she was planning, and she used her income to buy her first home; later she purchased a second home. Her spirit of entrepreneurship also stood out; each house became a source of income as she rented rooms to immigrant men who worked in local factories. When I have pondered a difficult personal situation over the years, including a new home, a move, or ending a relationship, I think of her common-sense approach to managing life, her calmness, and the generosity that resulted from her risk-taking. She only grew impatient when others did not do their part, but her patience and compassion were enormous.

Growing up with my unique Mexican American identity in Lorain, Ohio, I was readily cognizant of my assumed "difference" from others, who were of European American and Mexican and Puerto Rican heritage. My early ethnic identity images were based on comparison of myself with others, primarily in terms of ethnicity, socioeconomic status, nationality, and color. I grew up working class but did not appreciate this fact until I studied sociology as an undergraduate. Just about everyone in South Lorain had immigrant heritage or was African American.

I attended a Catholic school comprised primarily of Slovenian children, as did my siblings. Here I developed my sense of academic competency as I endeavored to be the best student and received support from the nuns. However, I always questioned my academic successes, because I was in an unfamiliar world. My parents always said homework first, but I never turned to them for help with homework. The truth was that I felt the sense of difference based on ethnicity and color that persisted for many years. This was the initial borderland experience for me. Perhaps it had to do with being the "different" one in the room, the only non-White person at the table, or, later, leading others early in my career. Thankfully, I have integrated these aspects of identity confusion.

Consejo: A sense of being different should in no way diminish your appreciation for your "Latina-ness." As an individual, you are unique and different; *ten orgullo*. We are different and can be proud of this.

Latina-Specific Cultural Values as Influences

Gender roles were clearly articulated in terms of roles, rules, and responsibilities. The Catholic Church, very rules-oriented, specified behaviors for women that aligned with my socialization as a Latina girl and teenager. Being raised in a traditional home, with my mother as the homemaker and my father as the external breadwinner, meant I took on many helping roles. In a family of seven children and as the second-oldest girl, I had a lot of responsibilities. In many ways, these activities benefitted me over the years, and I like to remind other Latinas of the competencies we acquired. Among these are multitasking, alternative ways of thinking, perspective-taking because we were always having to take on roles on behalf of others, empathy, caring, problem-solving, and initiative. I hope this does not sound too idealistic, but I have found over the years as an administrator, supervisor, and psychologist that these skills served me well.

Now, I would be less than honest if I did not also call out how roles, rules, and responsibilities also silenced Latina girls and women, gave us messages about being subservient and powerless, and placed undue burdens on us based on gender identity. *The Maria Paradox* (Gil & Vázquez, 1997) illuminated the ten rules of marianismo communicated both subliminally and overtly to most Latinas. Admittedly, I learned about putting others' needs first and not asking for help. I heard my mother say we did not discuss personal matters out of the house and that she had to be the consummate homemaker – making drapes and slip covers, baking three days a week, and following routines that modeled an ideal household. I guess perfectionism and control, especially of household and care-taking tasks, were modeled for me. Mind you, I never heard my father criticize my mother; however, she had her own tapes (internalized messages about what is right and wrong) that drove her need to do it all.

After I read *Isabella: The Warrior Queen* (Downey, 2014), I reflected on her complex and powerful life story and recognized how her worldview as a woman was so strongly shaped by religion. No matter that she was gifted and more capable than her husband Ferdinand and her brothers, she also treaded carefully in negotiations with them, empowering them through her wit because otherwise they would surely flounder. Outside of my home, I witnessed enabling of men by women and ways that men could be the victims that women had to nurse. This was not a reflection of my parents; in fact, it was quite the opposite. Their relationship was built on respect, sharing of responsibilities, and equity. I have always said that my father was a feminist before I knew the term. Thus, it was the nurturance and modeling of my parents and my maternal grandmother that instilled in me an orientation to servant leadership and a loyalty that persists.

Consejo: Most role models for Latinas were in our home, our *familias*. Always remember the lessons they taught you.

Intersectionality Informing my Life Work

In the world of academia, my identity was always salient – at least to me. As a student, I was generally the only Mexican American in a class, and later in my career, I was the only Latina faculty or administrator – generally the first too. I was the "twofer" – filling two Affirmative Action categories – that of a woman and a person of color. At first, I was surprised by the term, but since it was not within my control, I continued with my long-standing motivation: *to do everything twice as good as everyone else.*

I am a multidimensional person informed by my given identity factors – being Mexican American, being a woman, being heterosexual, and my age; these are priorities as well as visible attributes for how I express myself. I also have secondary identity factors that have changed in their level of importance for me over time. Currently, these secondary dimensions are relationship status, health, geographical location, and employment. My primary identity factors are more visible than the secondary factors, and they are ones that I was born with, unlike the secondary factors that are based more on opportunity and choice. These dimensions of identity come from a model I developed to show the wholistic identity of immigrants and how the immigration event sets in motion many life changes. The Dimensions of Personal Identity model (Arredondo et al., 1996) describes me and other Latinas as the sum of many parts rather than just those articulated through simplistic stereotypes.

The primary identity factors of ethnicity and gender always informed my sense of intersectionality even though others wanted to pigeonhole me as "Mexican." To distinguish myself and to deal with internalized racism as a Mexican meant taking on the belief that I had to be twice as good as everyone else. This belief motivated my educational performance. Grades 1–8 with the Sisters of Notre Dame were reinforcing of my goals to excel and to do so independently of color, gender, socioeconomic status, and ethnicity. Through many years, I struggled with the issue of color and how I felt it made me stand out, but in a less than affirming way.

As an undergraduate Spanish major, I became more informed and conscious about my mixed racial heritage. Growing up, I sometimes said I was Spanish as though this would minimize the prejudice I often felt because of my Mexican heritage. Times have changed. In all presentations or class lectures, I inform participants that being born Mexican American means I am a mestiza – and I am proud of this identity. From Mamá, I have Oaxacan and Zapotec indigenous heritage. Of course, I also have "Spanish" heritage, principally from my father's family. In fact, there is a town in northern Spain named Arredondo. I do find it limiting to check census boxes that give you only choices of Black Hispanic and White Hispanic. I believe I skipped this the last time and wrote in Mexican American.

Fortunately, we now have literature by Latinas/os on the topic of colorism and how we must own what this represents to our sense of shared historical identities (Adames & Chávez-Dueñas, 2016). I am surprised when family from Mexico or colleagues in the U.S. do not see me as a "person of color." The fact that this is verbalized by the latter always provides an opportunity to impart a brief history lesson about *mestizaje* and my mestiza identity.

Consejo: As Latinas, we are all born as multicultural and multiracial beings; be proud.

Placing my Whole Self into my Work as a Psychologist

Without a doubt, this lifelong recognition of the salience of my gender and ethnicity and socioeconomic status identity has influenced my orientation in counseling and psychology. My years in private practice gave me the opportunity to work primarily with women professionals and college women from different ethnic heritages. The majority were not Latinas or other women of color. Still, my intersecting identities were the framework that I applied when counseling with these women. All had an ethnic heritage, conflicts because of their lessons of marianismo, and power dynamics to navigate in their male-dominated workplaces. The glass ceiling is one example of the anti-woman workplace climate.

My early work with the Boston Psychological Center for Women informed my teaching as a junior professor at Boston University. I worked with professional women from different backgrounds, and I always seemed to consider how alike we were in terms of our gender socialization and, for many of them, experiences of limiting messages about being a woman or, for some, encountering workplace inequities based simply on gender identity. Although we were different in terms of ethnic heritage, I always found my Latina woman identity to be a valuable lens for assessing these women's orientation to self-empowerment, family relationships, and self-efficacy. I was curious about how much color, gender, and occupation informed their worldview and generally introduced these topics for their consideration and also to "normalize" what could not readily be explained about their sense of marginalization.

Perhaps it is obvious that my conscious awareness of my ethnic heritage, color, and appearance and my indigenous roots have allowed me to empower women clients and students across the spectrum.

Embracing my Immigrant Family Heritage

Immigrant identity development, adaptation, and mental health stressors have been a strong force in my professional work. Admittedly, I use the lens of immigration and its effects on individuals and families to examine other types of life changes that individuals experience (Arredondo et al., 2014). For example, moving from home to a college campus, moving to a new geographic location for employment, or going through a life change like divorce or an illness begets examination of one's identity and who one "is." I have been inspired by my family's acculturation processes and their ability to navigate in a society hostile to Mexicans and to working-class men and women who spoke minimal English, like my grandmother, or who spoke with a marked "Mexican" accent, like my father. They taught me how to demonstrate strength and not to apologize. They never made excuses about barriers of racism and sexism. In fact, my father was a leader among White bowlers. He was skilled at the sport and was also elected to the presidency of one of the three leagues with which he bowled. He was a great example of leadership for me and my siblings.

My grandmother engaged in what I would call missionary work from her home. Perhaps this is behavior she learned growing up in a small collectivistic village in Santa Ana, Oaxaca. She made friends with young neighborhood children when her grandchildren were gone or grown-up. These children were her helpers around the kitchen, running errands for her, picking veggies in her garden, and being friends to her dogs. Of course, they earned a little money and she always sent them home with some food for their parents and siblings. This model of giving and gifting continues to inspire my behavior. I readily contribute to charities, but ones that are for causes like farmworkers, American Indian schoolchildren, and domestic shelters. I like to think that Mamá's example to me and these children were ones that they too emulated as adults.

Consejo: Remember to honor your elders. In our *familias* is where the learning begins with examples for leading and caring.

Claiming my Bicultural, Mestiza Identity

Early on, I was aware of what I have called my bicultural identity and was affirmed by reading Anzaldúa's *Borderlands/La Frontera* (1987). She captured my lived experience, though different from hers, by using the borderlands concept. Further, she raised the idea of marginalization because of her intersecting dimensions of identity – a Mexican American on the Texas-Mexico border, an artist, and a lesbian. I have always picked up on how women, in particular, experience marginalization and how this affects their sense of wholeness, self-worth, and empowerment in the midst of the value of their bicultural experiences. This concept has come readily into my clinical work, my teaching, and my consulting. I have always sought to promote inclusionary thinking and practices, and I have attempted to guide others to consider how they may be more inclusive without judgment, starting with themselves. In the academy, I have worked with many students of color and always sensed how important it was for them to hear that they were OK and competent for the program. I try to normalize their discomfort or lack of confidence that increases in their doctoral program by talking about stereotype threat, the Eurocentric norms of the profession and most training programs, and, of course, the fact that they see no one who looks like them among faculty.

My zeal for inclusive environments and the importance of empowering individuals historically lacking power in the workplace led me to develop a Bilingual Bicultural Counselor training program at Boston University and, later, my consulting company, Empowerment Workshops (1985–2001). I put my values and preparation as a psychologist to work.

Consejo: We are *mujeres* with multiple talents; always aspire broadly and with purpose; our communities and *familias* will benefit.

Resilience in a Racist, Sexist Society and Organizations

As a woman of color in the U.S., it is easy to be the recipient of many "isms." Regardless of education, awards, and career achievement, discrimination and prejudice have been a part of my life. Noteworthy experiences have always been work-related, although I am certain they occurred in other public settings as well. With my career so salient, I took these situations more personally at first, but then had to accept them and move on. However, this in no way minimizes the fact that these occurrences were ones of discrimination and racism.

Experience #1 was being passed over for a leadership role as director of a high school guidance department in favor of a White woman with fewer credentials. There was no logical explanation, but I could surmise from the superintendent's explanation that he felt that "wealthy" professional parents would feel more comfortable with her. I felt a sense of both betrayal and loss. My early school dreads of being different and not being good enough flooded me as I tried to get beyond this disappointment. Fortunately, I ran into one of my doctoral advisors that day. Dr. Maria Brisk, a bilingual education advocate, a female Don Quijote, consoled me and told me to move on. "There is more that will come your way," she said affirmatively. She was correct. I like to share this example because of the imprint the experience could have had on me, having longer negative outcomes. When we suffer a disappointment, I advise sharing with a trusted colleague or friend who will say the right thing.

Example #2 is about feeling prejudice and exclusion not that long ago. I was hired for a senior academic position and came to realize that the provost was not happy to have me there. She saw me as the president's hire and friend. My initial portfolio was based on experiences with another university and it also put me in the spotlight. She did not like this and was not willing to give me more responsibilities. Colleagues know that my work ethic is excessive, and I felt underutilized. Her idea was that I go out and about and get to know the Latino community. I had already set these activities in motion through other colleagues so I did not need her permission to do this. It was her condescending tone accompanying her recommendation that irked me; I know when I am being patronized. In this instance, feeling insulted, I wanted to push back and prove her wrong. I then questioned myself and wondered if I was in the right place because, looking around, I knew I was the only Latina in a high-ranking administrative role. Fortunately, I shared the experience with a couple of friends at the university, allowing me to let go of my need to prove her wrong.

I mention xenophobia, fear of foreigners, because as Latinas or another competent women of color, we create unease for other women. So often I have sensed the low expectations, competition, and envy, particularly from White women. I am an accomplished, confident, and highly regarded woman of color, and for some women, this is a threat. Although the academy tends to marginalize women, some, I have learned, marginalize other women in turn. Sadly, women with the queen bee syndrome are the ones who more often act out (Arredondo, 2011).

Example #3 came at an advanced career position, much to my surprise but perhaps a further test of my fortitude and affirmation of my purpose. A reorganization took place at my institution, displacing me from the senior position I had assumed less than three years previous. Moreover, as most of us often do, I stepped into a second major role for a year, working around the clock and traveling across the country. I believed in the importance of the educational mission until I began to see the termination of positions held by other senior persons of color. These behaviors showed me the lack of genuine care for institutional diversity statements and a regression to the norm – all-White leadership. I could hardly believe I was at square one with no true empathy from the person who had hired me. My talents and visibility as a senior Latina in a city in need of Latina/o leadership was readily dismissed. I was not happy.

With a firm decision in place, I had to plan my leave within 60 days. This meant many good-byes, assessing my next steps, and supporting those whom I had hired and was now leaving behind. My decision was to engage my *dignidad*, to demonstrate that I was stronger than ever in spite of this act of indignity. My supervisor had asked me to resign, and I refused. After all, it was her decision, not mine. Thus, I told my direct reports that I was not choosing to leave; I wanted them to hear truth from me.

In my departing talk, I addressed the challenges of facing adversity with dignity and how to move on with grace. To this end, I created a paradigm for thriving that includes the following "P" motivators: planning, preparedness, passion, pragmatism, persistence, patience, and pride. These are words I live by and that guided my next chapter. I once again heard the words of Julia de Burgos' "*Yo misma fui mi ruta.*"

Consejo: We all grow from adverse and positive experiences as we walk the borderlands. In fact, it is the adverse experiences that in retrospect I have found to be the most valuable, the ones that have led me to persevere, strengthen my belief in myself, and thrive.

Mothering and Mentoring

Mothering or parenting is something I have practiced for many years; it is the sense of generativity or contribution to other generations. It began as an older sister of five younger siblings, and to this day I find there is some of this behavior occurring with my siblings, though more from a sense of support. I have six stepchildren, who I am very close to. When they were teens or younger, I can say with certainty that I played an active mothering role with at least four of them. It seemed natural to step in and make sure DH graduated from high school, that CV got money for an emergency dental procedure, and that I could be with LA upon the birth of her first child. This 35-year long-term relationship now extends to their children. High school and college graduations, family visits to Hawaii and California, and annual summer gatherings on Cape Cod have strengthened our family relationship.

Mentorship is what I exercise with students and clients or employees; I am very aware of boundaries and do not attempt to "take care of them." I am the founding president of the National Latina/o Psychological Association (NLPA), an organization that fills me with pride for how others now lead. I see my nurturing role in professional settings from NLPA to the workplace more as one of mentorship, coaching and empowering.

Consejo: In the process of being a mentor, one also learns and grows.

Empowerment – My Approach to Psychotherapy

I was trained as a psychodynamic psychotherapist and followed a Rogerian style of counseling practice initially. However, even in training, I found the counseling rituals to be very sterile and not sufficient to engage with high school students who were focused on the here and now. These young people were going through enormous change –navigating a new culture, learning English, and feeling a sense of responsibility to their parents. This led me to engage in what we call narrative therapy. I wanted to hear their stories and invited them to describe how they had arrived in the U.S. and how life was treating them. In Spanish, we call this *la plática*, or small talk (Arredondo et al., 2014). This mode of exchange is highly relational and empowering and comes from both Latina-centric and womanist principles of valuing the relationship. Erikson's (1975) psychohistorical framework was about understanding another through their stories, not just in the here and now, but from their past lived experiences. Thus, I used psycho-educational interventions with the immigrant adolescents so that their voices could be shared.

I have always been pragmatic and Reality Therapy with high school immigrant students seemed more welcoming as they addressed issues of fitting in, academic challenges, and changing relationships with their parents. I could hear their stories of loss of friends and other family members as well as their struggles to be accepted in a new, culturally different environment where now they were the visible minority. These are experiences I could readily relate to from my own background, and it gave me the opportunity to affirm their identity conflicts and multiple change processes.

With my women clients, I knew I needed to look beyond the limiting texts that tended to pathologize women, rendering them depressed and helpless. My own life experiences also provided me with varying frames of reference as I have already discussed. To expand my knowledge about women, I indulged myself with readings including Simone de Beauvoir's *The Second Sex* (1949/1972), Jean Baker Miller's *Toward a New Psychology of Women* (1976), and writings about historical Mexican icons such as Sor Juana de la Cruz and La Malinche. I was inspired by these women, who I considered change-makers, pioneers, and borderland navigators. I needed alternatives to the limited male-developed counseling theories.

In the actual counseling encounters with women clients, individual and group, I began to apply CBT practices and engage some psychodynamic and culture-centered frameworks to get at old issues that were interfering with the women's relationships and careers. *Feeling Good* by David Burns (1981) was especially useful to help clients reframe their thinking. I assigned women homework so that together we could impact negative thoughts that impeded their sense of power and control. In the psycho-educational workshops, the women prepared cultural genograms and read articles about women and power, women's self-esteem, and other affirmative self-help literature. At the time, the concept of codependence was very prominent, often blaming women for holding on and not individuating. To this end, I saw it as my responsibility with women and Latinas/os to affirm that interdependence is a positive quality. This is the culture-centered approach. I would say that I thought about the women's and the immigrant students' situations through the lens of cultural socialization and how this shaping impacted how they saw themselves and the value of their relational orientation.

Consejo: Never be afraid to step out of counseling paradigms that are sexist or lacking in culture-centeredness. Interdependence needs to be affirmed.

Engaging and Learning from International Encounters

My curiosity about cultural differences inspired my deep interest in traveling outside of the U.S. and then doing work internationally. I was fortunate that my first husband also enjoyed international travel that led us to Mexico, Egypt, the Soviet Union, Turkey, and other countries I had never dreamt I would visit. In these pre-1985 encounters, I traveled with deep observation skills. I was curious about how people dressed, moved, communicated, laughed, and rode public transportation. I wanted to learn about the country's culture, and this occurred through visits to spiritual sites, museums, and, once again, just through watching how people were. Of course, this was very cursory learning, but it still gave me some place-specific insights about cultural differences. I was always curious about the women in these countries. What roles did they play? In these countries, the women were not hidden. They were in plain view as merchants, consumers, mothers, and grandmothers. I noticed their collectivistic style when with families and their direct eye contact when selling products. Some stereotypes about women as invisible beings outside of the U.S. were readily dissuaded for me.

For the past 20 years, I have engaged in considerable travel that was career related. This has included presentations at international conferences in the Netherlands, China, the Dominican Republic, South Africa, and Mongolia, among others. The diversity among these countries continues to fuel my appreciation for multicultural competency development and how I must continue to learn about the deep history, values, and tradition of other cultures.

Guatemala is a country I have visited almost annually since 2002. I have been an instructor and consultant to new programs in clinical psychology and counseling at Universidad del Valle in Guatemala City. In one of my first visits, I was asked to teach Multicultural Counseling, and Counseling with Women. Yes, I have taught both courses in the U.S.; but Guatemala? I knew that my curriculum needed considerable adjustment so that I could teach with relevance.

I visited bookstores in Antigua to find books that would inform me about history and cultural differences within the county. For example, I could not overlook the 30-year civil war that intentionally annihilated Indian people, nor the fact that the majority spoke indigenous languages such as Quechua. This was the multicultural context in Guatemala that I had to bring to the classroom and which, I learned, was ignored by many of the women from primarily European heritage. The class turned out to be somewhat of an awakening for these graduate students in terms of their multicultural identity, their gender socialization, and their power because of color and family.

The Counseling Women class turned out to be provocative. As had happened with my women clients, when you begin to examine differential opportunities and treatment in society toward women, awareness gets heightened. It was not my intention that the women become anti-men, but all began to question the family and institutional inequities. In this regard, as they prepared to be counselors and psychologists, I emphasized that this personal awareness-building would enable them to consider the worldview of their clients and the barriers they may face as women.

My travels to different countries and cultures underscore that women are powerful and driven to make a difference everywhere. They rarely receive the visible recognition they deserve, but this still does not prevent them from advancing causes and being leaders. For me, the good fortune is to have these lived encounters that continue to deepen my understanding about how women express themselves and demonstrate their sense of empowerment. Because most of my experiences have been with women from working-class and service as opposed to affluent backgrounds, from male-dominated countries, and with little opportunity for social mobility, I have gained knowledge of how they make progress in spite of adversities. I could never acquire this knowledge from a textbook, and in turn I can describe these rich lived experiences to my students and to readers.

Local Experiences Become Global

Throughout my life, I have intentionally found myself engaged in different cultural experiences, the majority involving women or led by women. These engagements have demonstrated to me the power of women and their deep caring for their families and others – like my *abuela.*

One of my favorite examples occurred in Tempe, Arizona. I was invited by a Muslim woman leader to join her and other women for dinner. They wanted to honor me after I spoke about social justice at a community event. I was in awe of the beauty of their dresses, their headscarves, and the lavish foods they brought. We sat in a circle of about 20, and so began the evening with introductions. Fortunately, the convener went first, followed by the other women; I went last. Every single woman introduced herself in relationship to her family – her spouse and his occupation, her children, and her volunteerism. I know some were professional women, but this was not a part of their presentation. Quickly, I adapted my introduction to specify my six stepchildren, though with no mention of their father. I did brag about them and how much we were united by making time to be together.

In her autobiography, *My Beloved World*, Justice Sonia Sotomayor mentions her relationship with new colleagues: "we'd found much more than work to talk about, having discovered our background had plenty in common" (2013, p. 291). Being with the Muslim women was an important lesson for me about the bonds women can have cross-culturally.

Crossing Domestic *Fronteras*/Boundaries

It has always been easy for me to move about in communities that are new to me to learn about the people who settled there by choice or who arrived there through different circumstances. I am referring particularly to immigrants and their families and to American Indians, peoples it should be well-understood are part of my life story.

One of many enriching experiences with immigrants began for me in 2004 and continues today. I was introduced to South Ranch, a Habitat for Humanity community in South Phoenix. Home to 120 families, primarily Mexican immigrants, South Ranch is a hidden story about immigrants' goal orientation, self-efficacy, and resilience. I engaged a team of graduate students from 2004 to 2005 to participate in the lives of these families and prepare a thesis. They clearly benefitted from this community research project. I have returned to South Ranch to continue to write the narrative of why this has remained a sustainable community after 20 years. These are the narratives about immigrant resilience I want to document and promote.

Consejo: Always look for assets among people who are often minimized and underappreciated.

The Blessings of Being a Latina Psychologist

It's hard to say when I decided on a career in counseling, but I had many pushes over the years. First, there was my concern and caring for my older sister and her long-term mental illness. I recognize my compassion for her as a preadolescent. Unlike our family doctor, I knew she was not going to "outgrow" her condition. As an adolescent, I volunteered at La Capilla, the mission for newly arrived Puerto Rican families. This was my first helping experience, alongside the missionary nuns dressed in their dark brown robes. I helped to register families and learned about where they came from and what they needed. In the process, I also began to recognize cultural differences between people of Mexican and Puerto Rican heritage. These island people were away from the familiar warmth of San Juan and other locations in Puerto Rico. They ate different foods than Mexicans, and their Spanish sounded a little different. I wanted to learn as much as possible, and being a volunteer with people who shared my language and similar heritage was enriching.

Reflecting on these early experiences further clarifies why I chose to become a counselor and psychologist. Though an introvert, I like people. Over the years, I took advantage of my work positions to engage in community outreach in Boston and other locations. I played the traditional role of faculty activist, business owner, and civic leader, giving myself permission to shake off my discomforts about being different or the only Latina in the room. I learned to claim my competencies as a change agent, multicultural consultant, and astute Latina professional.

Consejo: Professional networking and engagement have multiple benefits for us as Latinas. First, we can expose ourselves and our professional prowess to others who have doubts about us, and second, we give ourselves the opportunities to practice our competence and to affirm our Latina womanhood at the same time.

Avocations and Interests, Always Culture-Centered

My professional and personal identity is informed by my education as well as relationships and personal interests. I attempt to engage in multiple interests that I have had for many years. Among these are the arts – broadly speaking. I enjoy visiting museums where I live and travel, particularly ethnic-centered museums like the Heard (American Indian) Museum in Phoenix and the National Museum of Mexican Art in Chicago. Reading has also been a source of great enjoyment for me since I first got my library card at age six. I enjoy fiction and nonfiction alike, especially murder mysteries and biographies. The mysteries help me escape and do some crime solving, while the biographies are stories of inspiration. More recently, I have begun to read Spanish-language novels with women as the protagonists. With *Arráncame la Vida* (Mastretta, 1990), set in the earlier part of the 20th century, I became totally captivated by the determination of a woman to transcend the limits of her position as wife of a state governor. She believed in equity for women and always challenged the status quo; this was sometimes to no avail, but she tried – as have many women. Though her lover was killed, she never stopped seeking true love, much to her older husband's distress. I cheered when she finally became her own person after his death. I have recently been given murder mysteries in Spanish. This is another opportunity to improve my vocabulary and to escape.

Collecting and admiring art has been a long-term passion; my first husband and I shared this interest, and in 1975 I began to collect art, especially Mexican art, that decorates the high walls in my home today. Signed lithographs by Siquieros surround me. Another focus of my art purchases is paintings of women, especially indigenous women and women of color. For the last few years, I have purchased art by local artists, a way to have my money stay in local communities. My art with brown and black women fills my home with vibrant colors. This makes me smile.

As for music, I am a strong aficionada of classical, particularly Mozart, Beethoven, Bach, and Vivaldi. Thanks to my mother, we were introduced to the waltzes of Straus, opera, and the big band sound. Perhaps it goes without saying that I enjoy Mexican classics sung by both older and contemporary artists. I am enthralled by Placido Domingo, Natalia Lafoucarde, Juan Gabriel, and Los Tigres del Norte and other groups. Once again it is the Spanish language and the emotions in the music and songs that stir me.

A final outlet, probably one that seems less culturally congruent for a Latina psychologist, is my love for golf. Although I always saw golf as an "awkward" sport played by White men, once I took lessons, I was enthralled. I think it had to do with the focus and discipline that is required and the idea that one is competing with oneself. I can play golf alone and have done so many times. It is a sport I would like to play as long as possible – whether I hit the ball well or not!

Latina Self-Care

I do some form of physical exercise every day and have done these activities for many, many years. It is part of my lifestyle. Currently, I walk a little more than a mile three to four times a week and do yoga-like exercises daily. I want to keep my legs strong because as my father told me, your legs are key to health; he lived to be age 93. Self-care also means eating well and keeping up with health appointments. These may sound like routine procedures, but if we do not adhere to multiple forms of self-care, like healthy eating and regular health screenings, we may put ourselves at risk.

Consejo: Taking care of the mind, body, and spirit is essential to a Latina's wellbeing.

Spirituality

I am not a regular churchgoer, but I do believe in higher powers. I have faith that guides my optimism and hopefulness about humankind; I rely on faith especially now in the midst of horrible assaults on people's humanity, such as separating families and children with the immigration terror.

In counseling, I have always inquired about individuals' religious upbringing or spiritual practices. I want to know how beliefs may be anchors or barriers for some. For me, there is an intricate relationship between culture, religion, and gender socialization, but I cannot make assumptions; I always ask.

Being Grateful

In rereading some highlights of my story, I hope they do not come across as self-serving but, rather, as examples of how to face adversity, affirm our cultural identity, and look at our lives as exemplars for others. Last year, colleagues Ed Delgado-Romero and Angela Romero-Shih engaged in a history-taking project with me. I am grateful for their example in "Patricia Arredondo: Creating a Pathway for Cultural Empowerment" (2016) because they capture my voice in an authentic way. I hope I have done similarly in this piece on thriving with optimism, purpose, and connectivity *entre fronteras*. My career has been nonlinear but constantly evolving, as has my Latina-empowered identity. I have been purposeful in promoting culture-centered knowledge and experiences to advance cultural competence and mentorship – and this is my continuing commitment.

The word *dignidad* has always been part of my moral compass. As Latinas, we are exemplars, scrutinized and admired, complex and inspiring. *Dignidad* is how we can model our self-respect, *orgullo* in our Latina *identidad*, and our character. And I hope my legacy will be one of affirming Latinas to own their eclectic selves, to carry themselves with *dignidad*, and to never apologize for their beautiful ethnic identity.

References

Adames, H. Y., & Chavez-Dueñas, N. Y. (2016). *Cultural foundations and interventions in Latino/a mental health: History, theory and within group differences*. Abingdon, U.K.: Routledge.

Anzaldúa, G. (1987). *Borderlands: la Frontera: The new mestizo*. San Francisco, CA: Aunt Lute.

Arredondo, P. (2002). Mujeres Latinas-santas y marquesas. *Cultural Diversity and Ethnic Minority Psychology*, 8(4), 1–12.

Arredondo, P. (2011). The "borderlands" experience for women of color as higher education leaders. In J. L. Martin (Ed.), *Women as leaders in education: Succeeding despite inequity, discrimination, and other challenges* (pp. 275–298). Westport, CT: Praeger Press.

Arredondo, P., Gallardo-Cooper, M., Delgado-Romero, E. A., & Zapata, A. L. (2014). *Culturally responsive situational counseling with Latinos*. Alexandria, VA: American Counseling Association.

Arredondo, P., Toporek, R., Pack Brown, S., Jones, J., Locke, D. C., Sanchez, J., & Stadler, H. (1996). Operationalization of the multicultural counseling competencies. *Journal of Multicultural Counseling and Development*, 24(1), 42–78.

de Beauvoir, S. (1972/1949). *The second sex*. Ed. and trans. H. M. Parshley. Harmondsworth: Penguin.

Burns, D. D. (1981). *Feeling good*. New York: Signet.

de Burgos, J. (1953). Yo misma fui mi ruta. Retrieved from http://upr01.upr.clu.edu/español/Julia_de_Burgos

Delgado-Romero, E. A., & Romero-Shih, A. I. (2016). Patricia Arredondo: Creating a pathway for cultural empowerment. *The Counseling Psychologist*, 44(8), 1212–1235.

Downey, K. (2014). *Isabella*. New York: Doubleday.

Erikson, E. H. (1968). *Identity and the life cycle*. New York: W. W. Norton & Company.

Erikson, E. H. (1975). *Life history and the historical moment*. New York: W. W. Norton & Company.

Gil, R. M., & Vazquez, C. I. (1997). *The Maria paradox: How Latinas can merge old world traditions with new world self-esteem*. New York: Perigee.

Mastretta, A. (1990). *Arráncame la vida*. Mexico, DF: Editorial Planeta Mexicana.

Miller, J. B. (1976). *Toward a new psychology of women*. Boston, MA: Beacon Press.

Sotomayor, S. (2013). *My beloved world*. New York: Vintage Books.

12

GRACIAS A LA VIDA!

The Empowering Journey of a Latina Psychologist

Melba J. T. Vasquez

Gracias a la vida (Thanks to the life).

Poem by Violeta Parra

As I sit to write this, my mother is in intensive care at the Dell Seton Medical Center in Austin, Texas, 30 miles north of her home time in San Marcos. She is on her seventh hospital visit in as many months, and this time, the transient ischemic attacks (TIAs) have led to a couple of more severe strokes. She cannot swallow or speak well, her left side is paralyzed, and when she does speak, this fully bilingual woman is insisting that all speak only Spanish. My mother will soon be 85 years old; she is only 18 years older than I am. I am the oldest of seven children. My mother has been my role model, my mentor, my guide during critical times. She attended the American Psychological Association convention with me twice; she encouraged and supported me in so many ways.

At the same time, my spouse of 37 years is challenged with a diagnosis of Parkinson's and frontotemporal degeneration. He was diagnosed with Parkinson's in January of 2016, and his neurologist believes that the general anesthesia of a knee replacement surgery in March of that year uncovered an underlying neurological degeneration, or dementia. He is still mostly my loving, kind, generous husband, but the frontal lobe seems affected, and he can no longer engage in sequencing; his ability to engage in activities that require following several steps has dissipated. This is the man who was a teacher, a school principal, and who then, after early retirement, obtained a second master's degree in social work and was in independent practice with me for over 20 years. He is also the person who took over all financial and household responsibilities when I ran for and served as president of the American Psychological Association. He was my primary consultant for complex and challenging political and organizational issues during that period. He can no longer track the complexity of the issues involved in those dynamics.

My two personal and professional supporters are now significantly debilitated. I have cried more in the last year than in the previous ten! This is a very painful, humbling, and grief-filled period and phase of my life. I am learning a significant amount during this traumatic period. I share these personal events because I wish to be as "present" and genuine in this *testimonio* as possible. I will also share my career development and significant experiences, including key developmental events as I view them now.

I have had a unique combination of challenging experiences throughout my life, as have most Latinas willing to take risks. Yet when I step back from this painful period of my life, I know that I have also been very fortunate and experienced many wonderful opportunities. But as Mercedes Sosa sings, "*cambia, todo cambia!*" (everything changes). She also sang, "*gracias a la vida.*" So, I am aware that I am experiencing a very significant set of changes in my life. I am also feeling very grateful and appreciative for the life I have had to date.

Influential Experiences – Family and Community Support

The oldest of seven children, I grew up surrounded by the unconditional love of a large Latino/a family in central Texas. I believe that we were clear about our identities as Mexican American, and although we experienced discrimination, I believe that this supportive environment developed by my immediate and extended family and community created a strong foundation to face the world and to build my career as a Latina counseling psychologist. I also grew up at a time when Mexican Americans and African Americans were socially segregated from White populations. In my view and experience, this created a bond between these identity groups as well as with a few European American allies.

Despite having only elementary education and being working class, both my parents were politically involved at the grassroots level and engaged in civil rights activities. They articulated a strong belief in and support for education. They, in fact, influenced all of their seven children to obtain at least associate's degrees, and all my siblings are contributing members of society. I am proud of all my siblings and of my hard-working parents. My mother obtained a GED, and a bachelor's degree (while I was in graduate school); she was the first Latina to serve on the local school board and eventually became director of a Community Action Program, part of President L. B. Johnson's War on Poverty. My mother continued to be very active in her community, and initiated and cofounded Centro Cultural Hispano de San Marcos (see www.sanmarcoscentro.org/home.html), which just celebrated its seventh anniversary in 2017 with a gala fundraiser. The event, with keynote speaker John Quinones, was sold out with a waiting list to attend. My mother was unfortunately not able to attend due to the severity and recency of her strokes, and I and one of my sisters make comments in her stead. Our mother always emphasized by word and by action the importance of education, the values of a strong work ethic, and of giving back to the community. She believed passionately that it is *critically important* to help others to have opportunities to actualize their strengths and potential.

Mentors in Graduate School and in Early Career

I feel fortunate to have been encouraged to enter a doctoral program in counseling psychology, because that particular specialty has developed values of diversity and social justice more clearly than other specialties in psychology as well as promoting the inclusion of environmental context and culture to more fully understand human behavior (Vasquez & Heppner, 2016). I did not initially have a clear idea about what a counseling psychologist was or what career opportunities were available when I first considered applying to a counseling psychology doctoral program. I am a first-generation college student. I obtained my undergraduate degree while living at home and attending my hometown university, Southwest Texas State University, which was then a Teacher's College (now Texas State University). I majored in English and political science and obtained secondary teaching certification. I taught in a middle school for two years in New Braunfels, Texas, while I worked on a master's degree in school counseling. Toward the end of the master's program, one of my professors, Dr. Colleen Conoley, for whom I had worked as a work-study student throughout my undergraduate program, encouraged me to apply to the counseling psychology program at the University of Texas at Austin, 30 miles north of my hometown. She tried to describe what a counseling psychologist was and assured me that it would be a good fit. She was right. The opportunities for employment as a counseling psychologist have been abundant, and I thoroughly enjoy all the work I do, even when there is a bit of drudgery (such as sitting and writing).

I was told at the time that this was a four-year program. Because I did not have a psychology background, I had to take three "vestibule" courses, so I took summer classes every year of my program to catch up and finish the program on time. At the end of my first year in graduate school, I received an American Psychological Association (APA) Minority Fellowship grant that provided partial financial support for my last three years of graduate school, which helped considerably. The directors of the APA Minority Fellowship program, Drs. Dalmas Taylor and then James Jones, also served as mentors and facilitated my entry into the profession by encouraging me to attend national conventions and participate in leadership activities.

I believe that my mother predisposed me to trust others who held similar values, and to be open to mentoring. Because no one in my family had obtained a college degree, I initially had no confidence in my academic skills. Some of my University of Texas at Austin faculty were very supportive, and although I had no faculty of color in my counseling psychology program, people like Lucia Gilbert, June Gallessich, Ira Iscoe, Gary Hansen and Earl Koile were supportive of research on women of color.

I graduated from the APA-accredited scientist-practitioner Counseling Psychology Program at the University of Texas at Austin in 1978. Although there were no minority faculty, most of the faculty there were helpful and supportive, and my peers in the graduate program were largely supportive, although there were at times hurtful experiences and microaggressions. Exposure to national conferences allowed for me and one of my peers, Anna Gonzalez (now Sorenson), to be exposed to wonderful mentors "from afar," including Drs. Marta Bernal and Amado Padilla.

I consider myself fortunate to have had the opportunity to explore the career paths and opportunities of a counseling psychologist. I found that the doctoral degree in counseling psychology opened doors to a varied, diverse, outstanding, and highly rewarding career. I began my career as a university counseling center psychologist at Colorado State University (CSU), where I also held an assistant professorship in the Psychology Department. I taught graduate courses in the doctoral program in counseling psychology and also supervised doctoral practicum and intern students. In addition, I provided individual, group, and relationship psychotherapy to university students. I consulted with faculty and staff, served as advisor for student organizations, and conducted an ethnic minority needs assessment for Dr. Jim Banning, the vice president of student affairs,. I also provided numerous workshops on topics such as stress management, test-taking skills, communication skills, date rape, and death and dying. I had wonderful mentoring from the then Director of the Counseling Center, Dr. Donna McKinley and from the Head of the Psychology Department, Dr. Richard Suinn.

After four years at CSU, during which time I became Training Director of the APA-accredited training program, I took a similar position at the University of Texas at Austin, where I did virtually the same kind of work for an additional nine years; the Director at the time, Dr. David Drum, was also a kind and supportive mentor; I met colleagues and peers who have become lifelong friends (Vasquez, 2017a, 2017b)!

My husband, Jim H. Miller, moved with me from Austin to Ft. Collins, Colorado. He took a large cut in salary to support the prioritization of my career. After four years, we moved back to Texas as we considered it was "his turn" to prioritize his career. We have alternated in prioritizing each other's goals, reflective of a very long-term and mutually supportive relationship. Jim was a school principal, and he eventually took early retirement and obtained a second master's degree, this time in Social Work. I feel very grateful and appreciative to have such a supportive spouse. As I indicated before, he has been one of my best consultants in dealing with a variety of challenges and dilemmas over the years!

Professional History and Scholarship

When I first acquired my doctorate, I was insecure about my ability to publish enough to serve as a tenured faculty member. I had been socialized by faculty members to view a Research I University tenured position as the ultimate career goal. Instead, I spent the first 13 years of my career primarily as a senior psychologist and internship training director at two university counseling centers. I also served as an assistant professor in the Counseling Psychology doctoral program at Colorado State University and taught courses in the Counseling Psychology doctoral program at the University of Texas at Austin. Despite no requirement to publish, my curiosity and engagement in scholarship has resulted in my authorship or co-authorship of over 50 book chapters, over 35 journal articles, five editions of an ethics book (Pope & Vasquez, 2016), an ethics code commentary and case book (Campbell, Vasquez, Behnke, & Kinscherff, 2010), and a practice resource book (Pope & Vasquez, 2005). Most of my publications are related to multicultural psychology, professional ethics, social justice, and approximately a third are related to women's issues and concerns. It seems to have been important, especially for graduate students and early-career professionals, that those of us who are more senior psychologists of color contributed to the literature to empower women and racial/ethnic minorities and to promote social justice. I have served on several journal editorial boards. Perhaps I was also proving to myself that I could have accomplished a tenure-track position!

I entered independent practice in 1991, intending to do so temporarily until I could apply for university administrative positions. In the late 1980s, when I was ready to apply for one such position, the directorship of a counseling center, my father died, and I did not feel that I could leave the state of Texas for the jobs that were available elsewhere. However, I fell in love with the individual and group practice of psychotherapy. I found that I could engage in independent practice, earn more money than I had in a counseling center agency (that was at least true at the time), and still engage in professional activities and leadership service. In addition to providing individual, group, and relationship psychotherapy, I have at times provided assessments for individuals entering various careers (e.g. police work, religious service). I have served as an expert witness in civil court on such issues as sexual harassment, workplace discrimination, sexual assault, and therapist violations (e.g. therapist-client sexual violations). I have provided consultation for various businesses, agencies, and nonprofit organizations regarding ethical issues, personnel issues, and conflict resolution, and I have provided skills training as well. I have been invited to serve as an instructor at various universities but have not had time to prioritize that activity. Instead, I have given talks to various classes each semester and have served as visiting professor for brief periods. I provide workshops and keynote presentations to various organizations and universities, particularly in the areas of multicultural psychology, professional ethics, self-care, a variety of women's issues and concerns, and leadership. I continue to provide psychological services in independent practice to this day, although I have cut back my practice to spend more time with my spouse and deal with my mother's health crises. It helps to have office-mates who are vibrant, professional, ethical, and good friends!

Key Leadership Activities

I was influenced by my mother's leadership activities; I am the firstborn of two firstborn parents, which implies that I have incorporated a sense of authority. I realize that I learned to take responsibility at an early age (Vasquez, 2001). Thus, taking the risk to take on leadership activities has felt natural from a young age. However, it frequently did feel risky and frightening. I found that one learns as one goes, and we can generally "rise to the occasion." I have served as president of APA Divisions 35 (Society of Psychology of Women) and 17 (Society of Counseling Psychology) as well as on various APA boards, committees and task forces. I served as president of the Texas Psychological Association in 2006.

My experience in initiating major new projects include cofounding The National Multicultural Conference and Summit in 1999 (now held every two years); APA Division 45, Society for the Psychological Study of Culture, Ethnicity and Race, for which I served as the first Council Representative; and APA Division 56, Trauma Psychology, for which I served as the first Treasurer. I served three terms on the Council of Representatives, APA's decision-making body. I also served a term on the APA Board of Directors (2007–2009). In 2011, I served as president of the American Psychological Association. The most recent leadership experience was as Co-Chair of the APA Ethics Commission, which was a Blue Ribbon Panel tasked with developing recommendations to improve the APA ethics processes, both of the APA Ethics Office and Committee and the Association in general. This was in response to the independent review conducted by Hoffman et al. (2015). I will describe some of the highlights of some of those leadership experiences.

National Multicultural Conference and Summit

One of my most gratifying experiences to date was the cofounding of the National Multicultural Conference and Summit (NMCS). The design, planning, and implementation of the NMCS counted as my primary presidential project when I served as president of APA Division 35, Society for the Psychology of Women. The division usually had an annual conference, in conjunction with its midwinter meeting, and at the APA Division Leadership Conference, we were encouraged to collaborate with other division presidents for meaningful projects. Therefore, in 1999, I helped to cohost the 1st Annual Multicultural Conference and Summit, with Rosie Phillips Bingham (president of Division 17), Lisa M. Porche-Burke, (past president of Division 45), and Derald Wing Sue (president of Division 45). One goal of the conference was to present state-of-the-art issues in topics that reflected the mission of our respective divisions: ethnic minority psychology, gender, and sexual orientation. We also wanted to facilitate difficult dialogues on those issues, forge multicultural alliances for political action and advocacy, and develop strategies for multicultural organizational change. Richard

M. Suinn was the 1999 president of the APA, the first Asian American to serve as APA president, and worked with us to have a successful event.

One of the most powerful sessions that I organized and chaired at the summit was "Honoring and hearing from senior women of color." The title of the panel discussion was "Surviving racism and sexism: Lessons we have learned." The panelists included representatives from each major racial/ethnic group and included Martha Bernal, Carolyn Payton, Reiko True, and Carolyn Attneave (represented posthumously by Teresa LaFromboise). The audience cherished the powerful and poignant stories; none of us had heard such an esteemed and powerful group of women talk openly about sexual harassment, racial/ethnic discrimination, and their coping strategies in response to those experiences. The biggest regret is that the panel was not videotaped. We were so glad to have honored these elder pioneers, and to this day, one of the most popular events at the conferences is the honoring of selected "elder" contributors at each NMCS.

We hoped, but did not assume that the Summit would be repeated, and it has indeed been held every two years. APA Division 44, Society for the Psychological Study of Lesbian, Gay, Bisexual and Transgender Issues, has joined as one of the hosts ever since the second conference was held. Various other divisions and organizations also help sponsor the NMCS. The 10th NMCS was held in 2017 in Portland, Oregon. The summit allows for a gathering of some of the most renowned researchers, educators, practitioners, and leaders representing issues of diversity, including gender, race and ethnicity, sexual orientation, and other aspects of identity.

Service as President of the APA

The most wonderful, exciting, and humbling period in my life was my service as president of the American Psychological Association. Because I did not have the "name recognition" that is often required to be elected by the APA membership, I traveled widely to provide presentations to state psychological associations and university and community workshops as well as keynote addresses to a variety of conferences and events. I provided 45 presentations in 25 states from late 2008 through 2009. I was thrilled and surprised when I was elected. I was able to do so because various colleagues of color and other allies encouraged their state psychological associations, universities or other organizations, such as the National Latina/o Psychological Association, to invite me to provide presentations. I will always be grateful for the overwhelming support.

I was the first woman of color, first Latina, and only the 13th woman elected president of the APA in its then 120-year history (Pickren & Rutherford, 2017). It was through the support of a wide range of members of my communities and allies that I campaigned and was elected. In addition to facilitating numerous Board of Directors meetings and two sessions of the Council of Representatives, I was able to engage in a variety of activities as president of the APA.

During my presidential year, I represented the APA at the Interamerican Society of Psychology (SIP) XXXIII Congress in Medellin, Colombia. The Interamerican Congress represents numerous Latin American countries and is attended by thousands of psychologists from those countries, and I was especially honored as the first "Latina" president of the American Psychological Association. I also represented the APA at the 12th European Congress of Psychology in Istanbul, Turkey; the Caribbean Conference of Psychology in Nassau; and during my past president's year, the XXX International Congress of Psychology (ICP) in Cape Town, South Africa.

Along with APA staff Rhea Farberman, my spouse, Jim Miller, and I attended the Voice Awards at Paramount Studios, Los Angeles, California, that the APA sponsors with the Substance Abuse and Mental Health Services Administration (SAMHSA) and the Center for Mental Health Services. The Voice Awards program honors consumer/peer leaders and television and film professionals who educate the public about behavioral health. It was a very inspiring event.

APA attorney Shirley Higuchi and her family were involved in ensuring that the APA helped sponsor the dedication and grand opening of the Heart Mountain Interpretive Center near Colby, Wyoming, about 60 miles from Yellowstone National Park. It was on the site where U.S. citizens of Japanese ancestry were imprisoned during World War II. This event featured speakers including journalist Tom Brokaw, Senator Daniel K. Inouye (D-Hawaii), former Senator Alan Simpson (R-Wyoming), and former Transportation Secretary Norman Y. Mineta. I also had an opportunity to speak, and I noted that more research on Japanese Americans' resilience during that time could inform work on modern-day discrimination against many, including Muslim Americans (Clay, 2011). The entire experience was very moving, poignant, and powerful! I was so proud of the APA's involvement with these events.

My special presidential initiatives included appointment of task forces to examine psychologists' perspectives on grand challenges in society, including immigration, discrimination, and educational disparities, and three very hard-working task forces produced the reports, all available on the APA website (American Psychological Association, Presidential Task Force on Educational Disparities, 2012; American Psychological Association, Presidential Task Force on Preventing Discrimination and Promoting Diversity, 2012; American Psychological Association, Presidential Task Force on Educational Disparities, 2012). The APA Presidential Task Force on Immigration, for example, developed an evidence-based report addressing the psychological factors related to immigration. The report provides an understanding of the psychological process of immigration and emphasizes the unique attributes and contributions of immigrant populations. Immigrants contribute significantly to the ever-expanding diversity of the population of the United States, and many challenges have resulted from inadequate federal immigration policy as well as anti-immigration legislation in several states. The report describes, in broad strokes, the diverse population of immigrants and then addresses the psychological experience of immigration, focusing on factors that impede and facilitate adjustment. Our hope is that widespread negative views of immigrants and their children will be informed and challenged by the increasing data available, rather than being driven by ideological impulses, and that this data will reduce the "disconnect" between research and policy (American Psychological Association, Presidential Task Force on Educational Disparities, 2012). Members of the task force and others have provided Congressional testimony on immigration using the report, including on the psychological distress experienced by disrupting families through deportation.

Discrimination is one of the grand challenges of society. I wanted the task force to identify and promote interventions to counteract and prevent the destructive processes of bias, prejudice, stereotyping, and discrimination on victims *and* perpetrators. The task force also identified the benefits of promoting inclusion, respect, acceptance, and appreciation of diversity. The term *diversity* encompassed individuals from racial, ethnic, (dis)ability, gender, class, age, and sexual identity groups who have been marginalized in some way. A theme in the report was that when the potential, capacity, and talent of all members of society are optimally developed, all of society benefits.

Educational disparities pervasively follow a pattern in which African American, American Indian, Latin American, and Southeast Asian groups underperform academically relative to Whites and other Asian groups. Task force members found that disparities: (1) mirror ethnic and racial disparities in socioeconomic status as well as health outcomes and healthcare; (2) are evident early in childhood and persist through the K–12 education; and (3) are reflected in test scores assessing academic achievement, such as reading and mathematics, percentages of repeating one or more grades, dropout and graduation rates, proportions of students involved in programs for those who are gifted or talented, and enrollment in higher education, as well as in behavioral markers of adjustment, including rates of being disciplined, suspended, and expelled from schools. The task force included recommendations that focus on psychological research, public policy goals, and the translation of psychological scholarship into educational practices.

As president, I was able to include social justice as one of the themes of the APA convention held in Washington DC in 2011. My presidential talk focused on the importance of social justice in psychology (Vasquez, 2012).

Dealing with Discrimination

I have written elsewhere about the experience of oppression, on individual and systemic bases, and the deleterious effects of those experiences (Vasquez & Daniel, 2011; Vasquez & Vasquez, 2016). I believe that it is impossible to take the risk of leading in a predominantly White male profession and/or organization without experiencing sexism, racism, classism, homophobia, and other forms of oppressions, microaggressions, and related offenses. The willingness to observe, take note, and decide whether and how to address those experiences is a lifelong process.

Learning how to seek support and care for oneself is a vital developmental task for all who must operate in and earn a living in a world in which society constructs gender, race, and other identity variables and where privilege is distributed unfairly. Mentoring (from and for others) and support from peers has been crucial in my ability to "survive" hurtful and humiliating experiences. I still smile as I remember a situation in which I was interrupted several times by a White male during a board meeting. A woman of color staff member came up to me during a break and said, "Dr. Vasquez, would you like us to beat that man up for you?!" The humor and significant expression of care in that simple statement will stay with me forever.

As I complete this narrative, *Time* magazine has named "The Silence Breakers" as the most influential "person" in 2017. The designation is a result of the social movement Me Too, designed to raise awareness of sexual harassment and sexual assault. It is being described as one of the fastest-moving social change movements in decades, initiated by courageous women and some men who came forward to tell their stories. It has been discouraging to see the sexual harassment and assault conducted by those from all walks of life, unrelated to race, political persuasion, etc., but it is an inspiring period of potential significant change. I am hoping that psychologists are able to incorporate this energy to promote and advocate for systemic changes in the values, attitudes, and behaviors associated with the worst of how society constructs gender, race, and other aspects of inappropriate privilege. Women can be supported and empowered to protect themselves if the changes are made at a systemic level, including in working-class environments.

Conclusion

It is clear to me that those who have influenced me have held values related to social justice in general and to the empowerment of women, especially women of color. I have been fortunate to experience the thrill of making a positive difference, both from a social justice perspective while serving in a governance position and when a student or colleague states how important an article I wrote has been for them.

I continue to learn from mentors, cohorts and colleagues, students and clients. My career has been rich, stimulating, and rewarding at many levels. I am so appreciative to my spouse, family, and friends for the support I have had throughout. I feel very fortunate to have been highly productive and to have made a contribution in my psychotherapy and consulting work, my scholarship, and my leadership activities. I am now in a stage of life where I am learning much about the caregiver role and am moving to spending time to be as present as possible with my life partner as his illness progresses.

I appreciate the patience of the editors to have my *testimonio* included in this publication. Given my mother's deteriorating health, I did not touch it for several months. Since I started this writing, my mother experienced a more significant brain stem stroke; we very reluctantly decided to remove the respirator she had for five days in October 2017. As my siblings and I sat with her the day she died, my sister Rachel said, "You know, she has probably already set up an appointment with God to discuss and negotiate how to make heaven better." She died on November 1, 2017, All Saints Day and the day that the Houston Astros won the World Series. My brother Gilbert expressed his belief that it was fitting: "Mom always liked good company for her significant events." We were gratified to have an outpouring of love and support from family, friends, and the community in which she had lived almost all her life. Our mother gave much to her family and community, and I believe she felt loved and respected as well. I feel tremendous appreciation to have had such a special mother. What an amazing influence! I dedicate this *testimonio* to my mother, Ofelia Trinidad Vasquez.

References

American Psychological Association, Presidential Task Force on Educational Disparities. (2012). *Ethnic and Racial Disparities in Education: Psychology's Contributions to Understanding and Reducing Disparities*. Washington, DC: American Psychological Association. Retrieved from www.apa.org/ed/resources/racial-disparities.aspx

American Psychological Association, Presidential Task Force on Immigration. (2012). *Crossroads: The Psychology of Immigration in the New Century*. Washington, DC: American Psychological Association. Retrieved from www.apa.org/topics/immigration/report.aspx

American Psychological Association, Presidential Task Force on Preventing Discrimination and Promoting Diversity. (2012). *Dual Pathways to a Better America: Preventing Discrimination and Promoting Diversity*. Washington, DC: American Psychological Association. Retrieved from www.apa.org/pubs/info/reports/promoting-diversity.aspx

Campbell, L., Vasquez, M. J. T., Behnke, S. & Kinscherff, R. (2010). *APA Ethics Code Commentary and Case Illustrations*. Washington, DC: American Psychological Association.

Clay, R. A. (2011, September). Muslims in America, post 9/11. *Monitor on Psychology*, 42(8), 72.

Hoffman, D. H., Carter, D. J., Lopez, C. R. V., Benzmiller, H. L., Guo, A. X., Latifi, S. Y. & Craig, D. C. (2015). *Report to the Special Committee of the Board of Directors of the American Psychological Association: Independent Review Relating to APA Ethics Guidelines, National Security Interrogations, and Torture*, July 2, revised September 4. Chicago, IL: Sidley Austin LLP.

Pickren, W. & Rutherford, A. (Eds.). (2017). *125 Years of the American Psychological Association*. Washington, DC: American Psychological Association.

Pope, K. & Vasquez, M. J. T. (2005). *How to Survive and Thrive as a Therapist: Information, Ideas and Resources for Psychologists in Practice*. Washington, DC: American Psychological Association.

Pope, K. & Vasquez, M. J. T. (2016). *Ethics in Psychotherapy & Counseling: A Practical Guide* (5th ed.). New York: Wiley.

Vasquez, M. J. T. (2001). Reflections on unearned advantages, unearned disadvantages, and empowering experiences. In J. G. Ponterotto, J. M. Casas, L. A. Suzuki, C. M.

Alexander (Eds.), *Handbook of Multicultural Counseling* (2nd ed.) (pp. 64–77). Thousand Oaks, CA: Sage.

Vasquez, M. J. T. (2012). Psychology and social justice: Why we do what we do. *American Psychologist*, 67(5), 337–346.

Vasquez, M. J. T. (2017a). A Latina's voice: Contributions to psychology. In M. Kopala & M. Keitel (Eds.), *Handbook of Counseling Women* (2nd ed.) (pp. 8–13). Thousand Oaks, CA: Sage.

Vasquez, M. J. T. (2017b). My professional journey. In F. P. Bemak & B. Conyne (Eds.), *Professional Journeys of Notable Psychology and Counseling Professionals: Stories of Courage, Innovation and Risk*. Thousand Oaks, CA: Sage.

Vasquez, M. J. T. & Daniel, J. H. (2011). Women of color as mentors. In C. A. Rayburn, F. L. Denmark, M. E. Reuder & A. M. Austria (Eds.), *A Handbook for Women Mentors: Transcending Barriers of Stereotype, Race, and Ethnicity* (pp. 173–187). New York: Praeger Press.

Vasquez, M. J. T. & Heppner, P. P. (2016). Counseling psychologists. In R. J. Sternberg (Ed.), *Career Paths in Psychology* (2nd ed.) (pp. 180–210). Washington, DC: American Psychological Association.

Vasquez, M. J. T. & Vasquez, E. (2016). Psychotherapy with women: Theory and practice of feminist therapy. In A. J. Consoli, L. E. Beutler & B. Bongar (Eds.), *Comprehensive Textbook of Psychotherapy: Theory and Practice* (2nd ed.) (pp. 299–314). New York: Oxford University Press.

PART VI
Conclusion

CONTRIBUTIONS TO A LATINA FEMINIST PSYCHOLOGY

Carmen Inoa Vazquez and Lillian Comas-Díaz

Yo misma fui mi ruta. (I was my own path).

Julia de Burgos

Our *testimonios* illustrate our journeys to thriving in the cultural borderlands. We struggled writing our *testimonios* and, thus, experienced intense inner tensions while revealing ourselves in these narratives. We are aware that therapist's self-disclosure can generate strong reactions of disapproval within some theoretical orientations. Nonetheless, we propose that when appropriate, therapist's self-disclosure and other cultural therapeutic adaptations can benefit Latina clients/patients. As such, we made a courageous decision to write in a candid manner, with the belief that our *testimonios* will be useful to Latinx providers and others who work with Latinx regardless of their ethnic identification. This decision is relevant because the number of Latinx individuals living in the United States has been reported to be 56.6 million, or 17.6 percent of the nation's total population (U.S. Census Bureau, 2016); and this continues to increase.

Our main goal for this testimonial project was to operationalize the centrality of the intersection of gender, ethnicity, (im)migration, sexual orientation, and class in the psychological understanding of Latinas. In particular, we discussed the oppressive structures that affect our clients/patients, students, and ourselves. To share our work, we opened the doors of our psychotherapy/consulting offices, classrooms, and research spaces. We kept our clients' and/or students' confidentiality and presented complex context-based viewpoints that contrast with the traditional psychological theories. Some of these gendered cultural adaptations include the application of *testimonio* therapy, *comadre* therapy, borderlands theory/method, *la facultad, conocimiento*, and theory in the flesh. When appropriate, we provide a supportive stance to facilitate discussions of spirituality/religion, *espiritismo* (spiritism), and sociopolitical issues – such as gendered racism – during psychotherapy, training, and/or consultation. All of these modalities are useful interventions that meet a Latina in her multiple intersecting contexts. Therefore, we strongly encourage you to read each of our personal narratives to find how we contribute to the growth of a Latina Feminist Psychology.

Contributions to the Growth of a Latina Feminist Psychology

The establishment of a Latina Feminist Psychology began over three decades ago in order to understand the structural variables that disempower Latinas in the United States (Russo & Vaz, 2001). Categories such as gender, ethnicity, race, class, and sexual orientation and their intersection were identified as barriers to attaining power. Hurtado and Cervantes (2009) added physical (dis)ability to these barriers. We propose language as another variable since speaking English with an accent frequently limits Latinas' attainment of social power. Moreover, we include ageism to the list of barriers for Latinas, particularly when we recognize that intersectionality does not go away when a woman has reached a certain age.

Oliva added to the understanding of Latina Feminist Psychology when she stated that, "Despite individual and theoretical variations, feminist therapists share a basic consensus that 'feminist therapy [... is a ...] transformation of the way in which therapy is understood and practiced'" (chapter 10, pp. 186–187). Each participant within this anthology has contributed to the way Latina Feminist Psychology is conceived and practiced. What is unique in this volume is that we formed a group of twelve women who share *diversity mindfulness* (Russo & Vaz, 2001), a focused analysis of gender, as a fundamental component in defining a Latina. Our aim is to add guideposts in the advancement of Latina Feminist Psychology. We go beyond the concept of diversity mindfulness to concentrate on Latinas' intersectionality of multiple oppressions. What has been amazing in the compilation of our experiences as Latina Psychologists is the resemblance we all share. In spite of differences in age, place of birth, skin color, sexual orientation, professional training, spirituality/religion, and social class, our experiences are very similar.

As Latina Psychologists, we deviate from cultural and theoretical mandates. This practice has required a great deal of self-awareness and pondering. Culturally speaking, Latinx expectation of us is about "*no sacar los trapos al sol*" (maintaining appearances and not sharing our inner secrets in public). When this cultural tenet is violated, the result is a feeling of discomfort. We have been mindful to follow the ethics of our profession, including setting boundaries with clients/patients and applying evidence-based modalities. Yet we agree with Celia's posture in chapter 1, where she said that sharing our experiences helps to show our work and determination to not blindly accept and apply findings or clinical interventions based on the mainstream Euro-American cultural models that have been advanced in the literature as universal truth, unwittingly marginalizing other cultural values, family forms, or societal experiences.

Applying a Latina Feminist Psychology

We apply a Latina Feminist Psychology by focusing on decolonization, healing, liberation, and social justice action. To foster decolonization, we use critical consciousness (Freire, 1973) to promote awareness of oppression and improvement of survival strategies. For these purposes, we apply a methodology of the oppressed (Sandoval, 2000) to nurture a series of strategies in the development of a coalitional consciousness. Moreover, we combat cultural imperialism, neocolonialism, gendered racism, and xenophobia, among other systemic oppressions. Following a decolonial orientation, we address soul wounds that support a colonial mentality applying self-reflection to challenge internalized colonization.

As conscious psychologists, we believe that healing is a collective effort, one that includes family, community, and environment. Moreover, we help clients to process soul wounds, challenge their colonial mentality, and promote collective liberation. Additionally, we empower Latinas to access their inner healer (Comas-Díaz, 2012). Specifically, we understand that when we heal ourselves, we contribute to healing the world (Comas-Díaz, 2010). As we apply this perspective, we aim to build a socially just society. Within this context, we promote a U.S. third world feminist oppositional consciousness (Sandoval, 1991), to emphasize geopolitical and transnational issues affecting Latinas. Ultimately, we believe that when Latinas recover their ancestral wisdom they nurture the emergence of a new consciousness – one that fosters thriving.

Latina Feminist Psychology Guideposts

We believe that our *testimonios* are so powerful that we cite the authors' voices in the following sections to illustrate relevant Latina Feminist Psychology guideposts. The twelve chapters exemplify in a vivid manner the challenging experiences we have endured, but they also mirror the reality experienced by many other Latinas. We identify significant topics as helpful guideposts in psychotherapy, in training, and in research. Let us walk you through each of these guideposts.

Testimonio *Therapy*

In the Introduction we discussed *testimonio* as a therapy that offers clients/patients an opportunity to find a voice, to understand their reality, and to cope with oppression and trauma. As Carrie elucidated in chapter 8 (p. 146),

> *testimonio* is a powerful tool to give voice to the individual experience situated within a communal and historical experience. Engaging in a process of developing one's *testimonio* requires adding a lens of critical consciousness that contextualizes the narrative in sociopolitical and historical contexts, recognizing that authenticity and vulnerability are critical.

Helping Latinas to narrate their *testimonios*, following the questions presented in the Introduction, has shown the impact of this therapy. Although very strong emotions can emerge during *testimonio* therapy, this method leads to self-reflection, critical consciousness, empowerment, and healing.

Culture and Gender

Even though the relevance of culture has received attention in psychology, we believe that culture does not represent the whole picture of a woman. As an illustration, Celia discussed the importance of acknowledging our multiple identities in order to appreciate both the cultural borderlands that we share and those that separate us (chapter 1, p. 29):

> the universals that unite us, the particulars (or idiosyncratic and unique features) that distinguish us, the culture-specific aspects (such as predictable religious rituals) and each person's ecological niche; i.e. the cultural and sociopolitical contexts of insertion and exclusion that create bridges of human connectedness or separation from each other.

Hortensia's red bicycle story, narrated in chapter 5, is a powerful illustration of the relationship between Latina gender and cultural socialization. Carmen had a similar experience where she did not even get a bicycle because, as a girl, she was not allowed to go far away and violate the tenets of her feminism (freedom and will); she still managed to ride in spite of all prohibitions. Time after time clients/patients will describe similar stories during treatment. For example, Susana (not real name), a woman in therapy, related that as a little girl she was given a beautiful bike, which was her pride and joy. She took such good care of this bike, added bells and flags and cleaned it daily. She became quite good at riding, but as she said, "the moment I developed breasts and a shape that could attract men, the bike was taken away." She was told, without much explanation, "this is for your own good." Although males may have a related experience, the prevalence of similar stories of girls and bikes in the Latinx culture is incredibly abundant. The symbolism of this component of Latinx culture may require working through in psychotherapy in order to connect insights that could translate into passivity and/or aggression and other debilitating behaviors.

Gender Specificity

There are other gender-specific cultural values that continue to exert significant pressure among Latinas. Marianismo, a cultural concept that encourages female passivity, self-sacrifice, and the repression of anger, is one example. In chapter 11 (p. 198), Patricia shared the following:

> Now, I would be less than honest if I did not also call out how roles, rules, and responsibilities also silenced Latina girls and women, gave us messages about being subservient and powerless, and placed undue burdens on us based on gender identity. *The Maria Paradox* … illuminated the ten rules of marianismo communicated both subliminally and overtly to most Latinas. Admittedly, I learned about putting others' needs first and not asking for help. I heard my mother say we did not discuss personal matters out of the house and that she had to be the consummate homemaker – making drapes and slip covers, baking three days a week, and following routines that modeled an ideal household.

Family responsibility and being a single parent is often cited as a gender-specific experience. You can read the chapters written by Carmen, Celia, Ester, Hortensia, and Margarita for applicable details. There, you will find how they shared their earlier experiences working and attending school and/or supporting family members while also moving along with their own aspirations.

Colorism and Being Biracial

Colorism is deeply ingrained in the colonized mentality. This experience frequently emerges during psychotherapy. As an illustration, a Latina client was quite alarmed when Carmen was getting "too dark" from playing tennis in the sun. According to the client, Carmen is considered white culturally. This was an opportunity where self-disclosure was helpful to the patient's narrative, allowing exploration into her low self-perception and the emergence of relevant dynamics, including the notion that if her therapist was "white," rather than black, then she was "the best therapist, and superior."

In chapter 11 (p. 199), Patricia stated:

> Fortunately, we now have literature by Latinas/os on the topic of colorism and how we must own what this represents to our sense of shared historical identities … . I am surprised when family from Mexico, or colleagues in the U.S. do not see me as a "person of color." The fact that this is verbalized by the latter always provides an opportunity to impart a brief history lesson about *mestizaje* and my mestiza identity.

Carrie, in chapter 8 (p. 147), described her experience of being biracial:

> Although I personally connect with aspects of the psychological literature about Chicanas and Latinas, my experiences of being biracial are not fully represented in Latino Psychology. I have blended many cultural values from both sides of my family; that is, a White mother and a Mexican American father. An added dimension to my identity is as a fourth-generation U.S.

> citizen. This identity is often compared to first-generation immigrants and characterized as more acculturated and less physically and mentally healthy than previous generations. … While research about Latino immigration provides important information about group trends and effects of acculturative stress …, little is known about the third and fourth generations of Latinos; thus, their rich experiences are overlooked.

Moreover, Carrie shares memories of a painful racial microaggression while in first grade when she was told by the other children that she could not play the role of a princess because she had brown hair and eyes. Carrie added: "These experiences were pieces in the puzzle of my identity development. I equated difference with confusion and exclusion" (p. 230).

Lillian eloquently stated her father's painful consequences of being mixed race (chapter 3, pp. 60–61):

> Being mulatto and poor in Puerto Rico was very difficult for my father. Due to his color, he was rejected by family, bullied during his military service, and subjected to many racial indignities. I still remember an incident during a beautiful sunny afternoon when my father, my brother David, and I were enjoying a walk in town. Holding our hands, Papi was flanked by his two children. All of a sudden, a man on the street shouted, "That girl looks like your daughter, but that blond boy is not your son!" Papi squeezed my hand hard, tensed his face, and said nothing. I stared at my father's face. I can still feel his pain today.

Many Latinx clients describe this type of aggression in psychotherapy.

The Effect of Language

In chapter 5 (p. 97), Hortensia gave a powerful description of the impact of language:

> Physical violence was one way to defend myself, but it did not prove useful. The indisputable way forward was to learn English. Papi spoke a little English; Mami did not. Papi taught us some basic words and phrases – "apple," "hello," "how are you?" "thank you" – but I knew I needed fluency to make it through this change. Having command of English meant what the *bicicleta* had meant: transportation and personal independence.

Later in the chapter (p. 101), she said:

> During many, many late nights studying in my UCLA cubicle, I eventually decided that knowledge was the best weapon to combat ignorance and bring forth change. An informed voice armed with facts might diminish social

> injustice, police brutality, racial and sexual discrimination, and societal suffering. You actually think that way when you're in college. I became convinced that there was a way to the heart through the head.

In chapter 10, as a linguistic empowerment strategy, Oliva highlighted the positive aspects of being multilingual: "The experience of living my life in the context of different languages has been significant in the development of the maps of my memory – an experience that is shared by many immigrants" (p. 188).

Being the Other

Carmen narrated, "In September, on the first day of school at James Monroe HS in the Bronx, the 'foreigners' were placed in a Tower of Babel where none of us spoke the same language" (chapter 2, p. 40). Also in relation to being the other, Patricia articulated (chapter 11, p. 197) the following:

> Growing up with my unique Mexican American identity in Lorain, Ohio, I was readily cognizant of my assumed "difference" from others, who were of European American and Mexican and Puerto Rican heritage. My early ethnic identity images were based on comparison of myself with others, primarily in terms of ethnicity, socioeconomic status, nationality, and color. I grew up working class but did not appreciate this fact until I studied sociology as an undergraduate. Just about everyone in South Lorain had immigrant heritage or was African American.

Coping with Grief

For Carmen (chapter 2, p. 50), grief extended to many areas, including the loss of a husband, a therapist, and parents as well as the Bilingual Treatment Program and clinic (BTP). "The BTP experience allowed me to understand the grieving process in the Latino culture and prompted the writing of my book *Grief Therapy with Latinos: Integrating Culture for Clinicians* together with my former supervisee and colleague Dinelia Rosa."

In chapter 1 (p. 27), Celia described her grief when losing her husband:

> A few years after moving to California, my husband died, at a time when we had two young teenagers and a new second-grader. His untimely death made it patently clear that one person can embody and signify a country and a culture for another person. Although I had reflected before on family transitions during migration, becoming a widow at a relatively young age brought another dimension. To the ambiguous losses of migration, the non-ambiguous loss of the premature death of my sole immigration life companion caused me to reflect on the intersection of migration with unexpected and untimely losses … .

In chapter 7, Pilar moved us through a heart-breaking story of losing her brother during her adolescence and clearly portrayed the significance of mayor losses and unresolved grief. Although stories of grief are often polyvocal – that is, each participant is affected differently by the loss – for most Latinx, the death of a significant family member is a loss for everyone; therefore, the suffering and pain are commonly shared. Additionally, grief in general often produces a reversion to emotionally ingrained cultural values (Eisenbruch, 1984; Vazquez & Rosa, 2011). But, grief renders individuals more vulnerable and in need of obtaining support from their cultural group.

Lillian provided an example of a cultural grounding for coping with grief (chapter 3, p. 65):

> Soon after my mother's death, I embarked a scheduled trip. While in India, a thousand miles away, my oldest niece *announced* her birth to me in a dream. This experience led me to process my mother's death and her first granddaughter's birth in my personal story – "In Search of the Goddess" … . Another painful loss made me re-examine my life-work balance. Elba, my *hermana del alma* and spiritual companion, succumbed to cancer. Once more, I resorted to cultural creativity to process grief. I celebrated Elba's life in a story. The publication of "A *Coquí* Serenade" … opened up new vistas for me.

Ester's contributions to the grief literature (chapter 9, p. 164) remind us to provide

> understandings of family experiences after a loved one's death. Grounded in our own lived experiences with bereavement while also listening closely to our clients/patients, we challenged dominant Freudian theories requiring "decathexis," or letting go of internalized/imagined relationships with the deceased, especially for children experiencing a parent's death – a deeply destructive belief contradicted by emerging evidence.

Melba gave us her *testimonio* (chapter 12) while undergoing the loss of her mother and her husband's debilitating illness at the same time. Her losses and deep grief did not stop her from contributing to this anthology, because this has been Melba's path as a Latina Psychologist. Her empowering journey serves as a remarkable role model of leadership, a strong Latina identity, a prolific writer, and someone always ready to "serve."

Family Conflicts

In Margarita's words (chapter 6, p. 113),

> Family conflict was an early dance that I had to master. My aunt and uncle went to family court to restrain my mother from taking me to live with her

> and her new husband in Scarsdale, New York. The entire family was involved in the decision of what should be done with Maggie. Under such circumstances, you confront what are family alliances, loyalty, familism, affiliative values, all head on. This positioned me in challenging circumstances where family members did not talk to each other or where I faced anger for not making the "right choice" and choosing "my family."

Family conflicts and other relevant struggles lead to Margarita's contributions to work with marginalized populations: "Some of the most important work we conducted during 1981–1988 dealt with marginalized populations (e.g. sex workers, the poor, women who used drugs) and the social and health conditions of the oppressed" (p. 115).

Understanding in the Flesh

An understanding in the flesh of the issues affecting Latinx has contributed to furthering research findings, as illustrated by Margarita in chapter 6 (p. 118):

> Conducting the study of the Mental Health Needs of the Puerto Rican Poor reinforced my admiration for the resiliency of poor people under conditions of extreme duress. Living check to check with almost no institutional supports left the family as one of the few sources of assistance. Families served the multiple roles of providing long-term care for the elderly, childcare services for the young, housing accommodations for extended family, and more. The intergenerational connection and cooperation was the buffer allowing people to move forward, even with slim to no resources. It also made apparent how many people saw their mental health problems as natural suffering with no cure.

From her understanding in the flesh, Ester shared her perspective on research (chapter 9, p. 163):

> Many of my students are intimidated or alienated by the term "research" until introduced to transdisciplinary and participatory action research ..., supported by cultural theorist Appadurai's vision of research as a human right: "Research is a specialized name for a generalized capacity, the capacity to make disciplined inquiries into those things we need to know, but do not know yet."

In chapter 4, Melanie narrated her understanding in the flesh, portraying an awareness, at first painful but then successfully adapted to apply to self and to those whose lives she touches in a daily basis. Melanie shared the following with us (p. 77):

> Over the years, teaching on diversity and multiculturalism, I have found myself grasping for a term that would capture the passive and pervasive ways in which individuals are shaped by their environments and that result in our unchecked implicit attitudes and biases. I call this *cultural programming*. I use this term as an instrument in teaching.

Melanie also echoed the impact of formidable role models of women in her life: "I remember Mami hosting her colleagues at our house for study sessions where everyone gathered, ate together, and collaborated toward a common goal. I listened to intellectual conversations that I could barely follow but which deeply shaped me" (p. 73). These role models also taught us about differences based on class, color of the skin, or sexuality preferences.

An understanding in the flesh is evident in Melba's contributions to the profession of psychology and, in particular, Latina Feminist Psychology; and just like all of us, one of her most important role models was her mother. This understanding in the flesh led Melba to fight oppression and discrimination, defend human rights, and advocate for women. In her own words (chapter 12, pp. 217–218):

> I was the first woman of color, first Latina, and only the 13th woman elected president of the APA in its then 120-year history … . It was through the support of a wide range of members of my communities and allies that I campaigned and was elected. In addition to facilitating numerous Board of Directors meetings and two sessions of the Council of Representatives, I was able to engage in a variety of activities as president of the APA.
>
> During my presidential year, I represented the APA at the Interamerican Society of Psychology (SIP) XXXIII Congress in Medellin, Columbia. … I also represented APA at the 12th European Congress of Psychology in Istanbul, Turkey; the Caribbean Conference of Psychology in Nassau; and during my past president's year, the XXX International Congress of Psychology (ICP) in Cape Town, South Africa.

Losing One's Voice

All of us have experienced the "loss of our voices" in relation to our racialized gender, but also as a result of a new culture, language, illness, and sexuality. Losing one's voice is a salient concept addressed during therapy with Latinas, and this, when combined with other methods such as a *testimonio* and/or engaging in creativity such as *autohistoria* (assemblages), can be empowering.

Lillian's description of her birth plight with a cleft palate – losing her voice at a very tender age and learning to negotiate these difficulties – is an example of fortitude and faith. Lillian's narration is a portrait of circular migration, weight issues, poverty, the pain of having an alcoholic father, racial aggressions, social and economic differences – all stressors minimized by the valuable support of the family, nuclear and extended, and her spiritual/cultural values. Additionally, she provided a valuable description of cultural melancholia. There are other powerful examples in this anthology that evidence finding one's voice and the relevance of addressing these issues clinically or in the classroom.

Impact of Migration Overall

The (im)migrant experience applies to each one of us either as first generation (as related by Celia, Carmen, Lillian, Melanie, Margarita, Hortensia, Ester, Oliva, and Pilar) or as subsequent generations (as related by Carrie, Melba, and Patricia). Separation issues experienced by children who may be left behind with relatives or other caretakers can contribute to difficulties adapting to many aspects of life, including a normal process of grief.

In most cases, the responsibility for the immigrant family falls on children, often on daughters, either due to change in poverty status and/or other stressors. In chapter 9 (p. 161) Esther articulated the following:

> Like all children, attuned to my family's grief and vulnerabilities, I worked hard to refashion myself in loyalty to the new story of our lives, in which our temporary sojourn in Cuba led us to the United States, the true Promised Land.

As Celia narrated in chapter 1 (p. 30),

> I have always been deeply interested in including the emotional impact of migration at an interpersonal level. I focus on migration relational stresses, such as ambiguous losses and gains, separations and reunifications, couple polarizations, the trauma of coaxed or unprepared migrations and the transformation of all relationships between those who came and those who stayed over time. These migration relational stresses have fairly defined clinical presentations at various life cycle points and require targeted therapeutic practices that are seldom addressed in cultural competence courses.

The Latinx migration experience frequently carries poverty and fear of discrimination. As Celia noted (p. 20),

> I cannot deny that getting off the subway two stops before the Jewish neighborhood was one of the attempts I made to hide where I came from. So were the vague answers I gave when people inquired about my family. Only many years later was I able to recognize that I was trying to "pass" for non-Jewish and perhaps for being from a higher social class. I reflect often on how easy and yet how painful it is for a person from a socially stigmatized group to feel ashamed or fearful of being seen with those negative attributes.

Later in the chapter, Celia said that she "began to see families as part of the solution, much more than as having the blame for their children's problems" (p. 25).

Melanie's recounting of temporary poverty in chapter 4 is a recurrent theme among many Latinx: "Our economic limitations were real, but also temporary. The experience of temporary poverty and the accompanying resilience it can afford has been captured in other testimonies" (p. 74). Carmen's narration also points to this: "While at the Latin American Institute, I became aware that I was without question the 'poorest' girl in the entire school" (p. 42).

The impact of immigration for Oliva resonates with many stories brought to our psychological practice (chapter 10, p. 184):

> As I have written before, having immigrated to another country, no matter how long ago, means you are always from somewhere else. You are always betwixt and between, neither here nor there. Many important events of your life have occurred in another place. Who you are is influenced by absence; the absence of people and places that shaped those events. Distance from your original place necessitates understanding yourself from a different geographical and cultural setting than the one in which many of your memories were encoded. You have to organize your memories in a certain way to make them intelligible in your new context; you have to explain details that would otherwise have been taken for granted. Sometimes I feel as if I have to explain myself constantly in order to be understood by those who matter to me in this new life and place.

*The Older Adult – "***Brilla por su Ausencia,***" or Conspicuously Absent*

Although the Latinx population is a young one, we need to pay attention to the elderly Latinx population. The patina of time causes a great deal of anxiety on most people, exemplified in avoidance of unpleasant topics such as death or infirmity; but old age does not only bring infirmity. When understood appropriately, old age can be viewed as a compilation of knowledge and wisdom, the attainment of sageness; and elderly Latinas can be empowered through this awareness. Although old age is venerated and appreciated within the traditional Latinx culture, ageism exists at the same time, and this must be recognized as part of a continuum of the same oppression afforded to the categories of sexism and racism (Vazquez, 2010).

Ageism is a topic that should be widely represented in the classrooms of all graduate schools, in therapy rooms, and in research efforts. This consciousness is very much needed, particularly when the present "culture of youth" exemplified in magazines, movies, greeting cards, and cartoons mocks the way older people look and portrays white hair and wrinkles as undesirable features, particularly in women. The difficulty of addressing this topic was evident in our avoidance of the following questions: "*Have you experienced discrimination, prejudice, racism, sexism, heterosexism, xenophobia, trauma, ageism, and/or oppression? Do you have significant others who have experienced these types of discrimination? If so, do you feel comfortable sharing how these experiences shaped your life and work?*" (Introduction, pp. 10–11).

Older Latinas bring to therapy conflicts with the cultural expectation that full accomplishment as a woman is primarily through motherhood and, then, grandparenthood. Grandparenting is a stage that is described as "fabulous" by those experiencing it. But these are not the only satisfying endeavors for Latinas. As evidenced by our stories in this anthology, some of us are mothers, others are not, some of us are grandmothers, others are not, but satisfaction in life can be achieved through mentoring, leadership, and many avenues.

Based on the life lessons presented in our *testimonios*, we now share with you ways to thrive.

Ways to Thrive

Embrace Living in the Cultural Borderlands

We have addressed the concept of cultural borderlands throughout this anthology and specifically refer you to Pilar in chapter 7 (p. 139):

> In the borderlands, there are translations back and forth; there are continuities and discontinuities. I am connected with my Indigenous ancestors through a way of thinking that places me as a part of a living world, where the use of plants and the flow of the word have a spiritual dimension and are intertwined in the processes of being and learning.

Practice Cultural Humility

In addition to our commitment to cultural competence, we practice *cultural humility* (Tervalon & Murray-Garcia, 1998), a concept within multicultural psychology. Cultural humility entails an interpersonal stance that is related to other rather than self. It involves critical self-reflection, lifelong learning, and institutional accountability. Research has shown that cultural humility is positively associated with stronger working alliances and better therapeutic outcomes (Hook, Davis, Owen, Worthington, & Utsey, 2013). You can practice cultural humility even if you are not a psychologist. This is a concept applicable to all.

Identify Strong Women as Role Models

As Latina Psychologists, we understand the importance of having strong female role models in our lives. We are fortunate that strong and caring women have guided, supported, and nurtured us. Narratives of strong female role models need to be included in Latina treatment and education and used as a way to thrive.

Commit to Social Justice Action

The examples presented in this anthology can also be found among other women of color, but here we share how Latinas thrive by contributing to social change and opposing an unjust status quo. Our writings serve to give voice to the voiceless, especially to the Latinx community. We have a lifelong commitment to social justice action exemplified in our psychological practice, research, scholarship, and advocacy.

Engage in Mentoring

We mentor as we engage in teaching, psychotherapy, research, writing, and social justice action. Moreover, we continue to mentor students and younger psychologists, who will carry on the torch for the development and understanding of Latinx communities. As Melba stated in chapter 12 (p. 220): "Mentoring (from and for others) and support from peers has been crucial in my ability to 'survive' hurtful and humiliating experiences." Although mentoring is a responsibility for those who have achieved leadership positions, we consider that all Latinas can mentor through peer mentoring. We strongly endorse mentoring as a form of collective care.

Nurture Your Creativity

We believe that creative expression fosters healing and thriving. Indeed, Anzaldúa (1999) recommended the practice of *autohistoria* (assemblages), an artistic self-narrative, to counter Latinas' legacy of silenced voices. Allow yourself to engage in creativity. For instance, you can express yourself through crafts, music, dance, theater, filmmaking, spoken word, and many other artistic forms.

Engage in Inner Work

Engaging in inner work is essential to your wellbeing and for those you love. A way of reflecting on your life, inner work nurtures your ability to thrive. Fortunately, there are various forms of participating in inner work. For instance, you can express your creativity, compose your *testimonio*, and/or connect with your *hermana del alma* (sister/friend). Additionally, you can practice mind-body-spirit techniques such as meditation, yoga, mindfulness, prayer, tai chi, creative visualization, and active imagination in addition to expanded awareness practices. You can also work with a psychotherapist who is committed to cultural competence and exhibits cultural humility (Comas-Díaz, 2012).

Conclusion

We conclude this anthology with a recommendation to transform your-self. Pilar (chapter 7, p. 139) summarized this concept as

> the process by which mestiza consciousness, or consciousness about hybridity, occurs is a journey whereby we confront multiple ways of knowing, some of which may challenge or coexist with the ones we are familiar with. In this journey, we … experience a dismantling of the identities we acquired within a colonial mindset.

Finally, living in the cultural borderlands helped us to create our own path. The development of this *testimonial arpillera* gave birth to a collective mission. We hope that you join us in the mission of transforming Latinx *testimonios* of oppression into epics of thriving.

References

Anzaldúa, G. (1999). *Borderlands/La Frontera: The new mestiza* (2nd ed.). San Francisco, CA: Aunt Lute Books.

Comas-Díaz, L. (2010). Healing the self, healing the world: A feminist journey. *Women & Therapy*, 33, (3/4), 1–5. doi: 10.1080/02703149.2010.484679

Comas-Díaz, L. (2012). *Multicultural care: A clinician's guide to cultural competence*. Washington, DC: American Psychological Association.

Eisenbruch, M. (1984). Cross-cultural aspects of bereavement II: Ethnic and cultural variations in the development of bereavement practices. *Culture, Medicine and Psychiatry*, 8(4), 317–347.

Freire, P. (1973). *Education for critical consciousness*. New York: Seabury.

Hook, J. N., Davis, D. N., Owen, J., Worthington, E. L., & Utsey, S. O. (2013). Cultural humility: Measuring openness to culturally diverse clients. *Journal of Counseling Psychology*, 60(3), 353–366. doi: 10.1037/a0032595

Hurtado, A., & Cervantez, K. (2009). A view from within and from without: The development of Latina feminist psychology. In F. A. Villarruel, G. Carlo, J. M. Grau, M. Azmitia, N. J. Cabrera, & T. J. Chahin (Eds.), *Handbook of U.S. Latino psychology: Developmental and community perspectives* (pp. 171–190). Thousand Oaks, CA: Sage.

Russo, N. F., & Vaz, K. (2001). Addressing diversity in the decade of behavior: Focus on women of color. *Psychology of Women Quarterly*, 25(4), 280–294.

Sandoval, C. (1991, Spring). U.S. Third world women feminism: The theory and Method of oppositional consciousness in the postmodern world. *Genders*, 10, 1–24.

Sandoval, C. (2000). *Methodology of the oppressed*. Minneapolis, MN: University of Minnesota Press.

Tervalon, M., & Murray-Garcia, J. (1998). Cultural humility versus cultural competence: A critical distinction in defining physician training outcomes in multicultural education. *Journal of Health Care for the Poor and Underserved*, 9(2), 117–125.

U.S. Census Bureau. (2016). Facts for features: Hispanic heritage month 2016. Retrieved from: www.census.gov/newsroom/facts-for-features/2016/cb16-ff16.html

Vazquez, C. I. (2010). The competent treatment of the diverse older adult. In A. E. Cornish, B. A. Schreier, L. I. Nadkarni, L. H. Metzger, & E. R. Rodolfa (Eds.), *Handbook of multicultural counseling competencies* (pp. 23–34). New York: Wiley.

Vazquez, C. I., & Rosa, D. (2011). *Grief therapy with Latinos: Integrating culture for clinicians*. New York: Springer.

INDEX